The African Transformation of Western Medicine and the Dynamics of Global Cultural Exchange

The African Transformation of Western Medicine and the Dynamics of Global Cultural Exchange

DAVID BARONOV

TEMPLE UNIVERSITY PRESS
Philadelphia

Temple University Press
1601 North Broad Street
Philadelphia PA 19122
www.temple.edu/tempress

Paperback edition published 2010
Cloth edition published 2008
Printed in the United States of America

Text design by Erin New

∞ The paper used in this publication meets the requirements of the American National Standard for Information Sciences—Permanence of Paper for Printed Library Materials, ANSI Z39.48-1992

Library of Congress Cataloging-in-Publication Data

Baronov, David.
The African transformation of Western medicine and the dynamics of global cultural exchange / David Baronov.
p. ; cm.
Includes bibliographical references and index.
ISBN 978-1-59213-915-6 (cloth : alk. paper)
1. Traditional medicine—Africa. 2. Medicine—Africa—History—19th century. 3. Medicine—Africa—History—20th century. 4. Anthropology, Cultural—Africa. I. Title.
[DNLM: 1. History of Medicine—Africa. 2. History, 19th Century—Africa. 3. Anthropology, Cultural—Africa. 4. History, 20th Century—Africa. 5. Medicine, African Traditional—Africa. WZ 70 Ha1 B266a 2008]
GN645.B37 2008
398'.353096—dc22 2008024426

2 4 6 8 9 7 5 3 1

ISBN 978-1-59213-916-3 (paper : alk. paper)

Dedication

para André y Jimena . . . y su madre

Contents

Acknowledgments

To begin, I wish to offer my deep gratitude to the Reverend Dr. Stephen Mbugua Ngari and his research team of multilingual graduate students at Egerton University in Nakuru, Kenya. Their invaluable assistance and keen observations took me along many valuable and unanticipated avenues of investigation. I am equally grateful to those Kamba healers in the Kitui region of Eastern Kenya who kindly shared their time and expertise. Their patience and generosity will not soon be forgotten. This travel and research in Kenya was made possible by a generous Faculty Development Grant from St. John Fisher College.

Among the many who have prodded and provoked me throughout the process of developing the ideas that comprise this work, I extend a special appreciation to Robert Brimlow, Paul Fuller, Ruth L. Harris, Festus N'Garuka, Barbara Rockell, Daniel Schaffer, and John Till. In addition, Timothy Madigan and the members of the Bioethics Reading Group at the University of Rochester Medical Center provided helpful comments and guidance for earlier drafts of select chapters. I have also significantly benefited from the critical feedback of my anonymous reviewers as well as the important insights and assistance of Micah Kleit, the executive editor at Temple University Press.

In the current age of library budget cuts and a general shift from paper to electronic library materials, the truly unsung heroes of contemporary research remain the interlibrary staff whose relentless detective work makes much of this work possible. In this regard, I offer a special thanks to Diane Lucas and John Gefell.

Lastly, I wish to acknowledge the essential contribution of Mrs. Druian, without whom this book would never have been possible.

1
The Origins of African Biomedicine

The popular image of Western biomedicine in Africa is that of a benevolent European gift, whose purpose—the improved health of Africans—bespeaks a spirit of unqualified generosity and kindness.[1] While directly fortifying the African body, biomedicine has also been credited with indirectly "civilizing" the African mind and spirit—introducing modern scientific principles to supplant primitive superstition and witchcraft. It follows that biomedicine is itself portrayed as a foreign (and Western) entity whose universal principles, properly understood, may be applied to equal effect across all societies and peoples. Given the force of this standard narrative, the impressive task set for those chronicling biomedicine's great trek to Africa is to document the ensuing cultural and social transformations that have reshaped the African peoples. Indeed, snapshots of medical care from a cross-section of African villages in 1900 would offer a dramatic contrast with similar snapshots in the year 2000. Thus, it can hardly be denied that the impact of biomedicine on African societies over the past century has been significant, and this is a story that has been ably documented by several generations of talented scholars. Biomedicine's transformation of Africa, however, is merely a partial rendering of a much larger process. Commonly

[1] Unless otherwise indicated, references to "Africa" refer specifically to Sub-Saharan Africa.

lost or diminished in these depictions, for example, are the contributions of local African societies and cultures to the development of biomedicine in Africa. Even more glaring, however, has been the near total silence with regard to the profound African transformation of biomedicine itself as a global cultural form. This silence, it is argued, is no mere oversight. Indeed, Africa's ongoing reconstitution of biomedicine has been persistently obscured by Western representations of biomedicine's African journey.

The familiar narrative of biomedicine in Africa is rather straightforward, though told from a variety of perspectives and disciplines. Critics decry the role of biomedicine as a form of "cultural imperialism" with which Europe has bombarded Africa with Western values and beliefs, which initially competed with and eventually undermined African values and beliefs. Proponents champion biomedicine as a force for positive change that has allowed Africans to enter the scientific age and, thereby, to improve their health and general well-being. Whatever the viewpoint, the introduction of biomedicine is presented as something that Europe does to Africa. Africans may respond favorably or resist biomedicine but ultimately they are the ones transformed by this encounter. Europe and biomedicine somehow remain remarkably unscathed by the entire ordeal. The story of biomedicine in Africa has typically been told through one of three basic disciplines—medical history, medical anthropology, and African political economy. Each of these disciplines provides an essential aspect of the story that differs appreciably from the others. However, each shares an underlying set of premises—focused narrowly on how biomedicine has transformed Africa—that fails to ask, and is conceptually incapable of asking, how Africa has transformed biomedicine.[2] This limitation follows from the manner by which each discipline conceptually frames biomedicine in Africa as a scientific, cultural, or political process.

Medical historians, for example, have produced a large and growing body of exhaustive scholarship, which details the actual arrival and development of biomedicine in Africa.[3] From the early missionary campaigns and the efforts of colonial medical officers to control malaria and sleeping sickness through the development of modern urban hospital care, medical historians provide a comprehensive and invaluable account of biomedicine's dramatic impact, as a set of universal, scientific practices, on standard med-

---

[2] Those occasional exceptions to this pattern, such as medical historians documenting the Western adoption of certain African pharmacopeia or political economists describing a potential European pandemic of African origins due to patterns of global migration, retain the notion of biomedicine as a narrow subfield of Western science. This is, thus, an African "contribution" that does not in any way alter the original Western premises of biomedicine.

[3] See, for example, Beck (1970, 1981), M. Gelfand (1976), and Iliffe (2002).

ical care in Africa. For medical historians, however, like the laws of physics, the basic precepts of biomedicine are not especially subject to cultural interpretation. By contrast, medical anthropology is largely predicated on the notion of Western biomedicine as a culture-bound phenomenon.[4] Accordingly, from this perspective, when biomedicine travels to Africa the story primarily concerns how biomedicine, as a Western cultural form, transforms African society.[5] This follows, in large part, from a disciplinary imperative that organizes anthropological research around locally bound subjects. The tendency, therefore, is to generate descriptions of outside (global) influences reshaping local cultures. The reverse would require a radically revised unit of analysis. Lastly, the vast literature of African political economy provides a well rehearsed overview of the exploitative nature of Western powers in Africa and the cynical role of biomedicine in this regard.[6] From such depictions one generally learns a great deal regarding Western aggression and African resistance, however biomedicine itself remains a distinctly foreign entity whose adoption represents simple acquiescence to Western subjugation. Thus, we learn very little about biomedicine itself as a scientific or cultural form and certainly nothing about how Africans may have helped to reshape it.

The challenge of inverting this standard Western narrative and asking not how biomedicine has changed Africa but *how Africa has changed biomedicine* is not merely a matter of expanding or revising any one or all of these three fundamental perspectives. The problem, rather, is a function of how each discipline frames its basic analysis of biomedicine in Africa. That which is required, therefore, is a perspective that both recognizes and incorporates the insights and contributions of medical history, medical anthropology, and political economy, while strategically reconceptualizing the organizing analytical principles that define biomedicine in Africa as an object for investigation. Such an approach must provide a reflexive framework that allows biomedicine simultaneously to transform Africa as Africa transforms biomedicine. Ultimately, the challenge is to identify an approach that allows one to turn from asking what the West can learn about Africans by studying their acclimation to biomedicine and to ask what the West can learn about Western medicine by understanding the African contributions to the development of biomedicine.

[4] See, for example, Comaroff (1993), Hahn (1995), and Kleinman (1980).

[5] See, for example, Buckley (1985a), Chavunduka (1994), and Janzen (1978).

[6] See, for example, Aidoo (1982), Fanon (1967, 1965), D. Ferguson (1979), and Turshen (1984).

World-Systems Analysis and Global Cultural Forms

To tell the story of biomedicine in Africa adequately, therefore, requires an analytical framework that is uniquely adept. It must allow one simultaneously to explore biomedicine as a culture-bound, historically contingent social form while also analyzing biomedicine as an instrument of Western expansion. At the same time, the analysis must be faithful to the fickle serendipity of the historical record, as opposed to allowing grand narratives to blindly shape the life story of biomedicine in Africa.[7] One of the more fruitful approaches in this regard, perhaps surprisingly, is that of world-systems analysis. To be sure, a frequent criticism of world-systems analysis concerns a pronounced tendency to construct large-scale, bird's eye analyses, which eschew local cultures. However, as discussed below, a basic failure to extend world-systems analysis beyond its initial, limited domain of investigation—economic and political structures and processes of the world economy at a global level—has resulted more from a lack of imagination than from deficiencies of the basic framework of analysis. In defense of this proposition, it is necessary to outline briefly the basic elements of world-systems analysis that make it ideal for an analysis of biomedicine in Africa as a global cultural development. Of particular interest in this regard are the early methodological debates among proponents of world-systems analysis whose insights have too often been neglected in later research.

First emerging in the 1970s, world-systems analysis provides a historical-analytical framework for interpreting long-term, large-scale social change. This framework borrows from a range of traditions across the historical social sciences, though it has been most influenced by the French Annales School and the work of Fernand Braudel, in particular, and by Marx.[8] A fundamental principle of world-systems analysis is that each historical era is distinguishable from other eras by virtue of the unique world-system that

[7] Comaroff and Comaroff (1993) frame this dilemma of global determinism versus local autonomy quite poignantly in the context of colonial and postcolonial Africa. "How do we write a historical anthropology of world systems that is not merely *the* History of *the* World System? Can we take sufficient account of the worldwide facts of colonial and postcolonial coercion, violence and exploitation, yet not slight the role of parochial signs and values, local meanings and historical sensibilities? How do we read European imperialism and its aftermath without reducing it to crude equations of power, domination and alienation? (emphasis in original, p. xiii). See also Appadurai (1995) in this regard.

[8] Marx's analysis of the accumulation of capital is an indispensable feature of world-systems analysis, explaining the expansion of the capitalist world-system (Hopkins, 1982a; Hopkins and Wallerstein, 1982). Additionally, members of the Annales school readily acknowledge their own debt to Marx. "The genius of Marx, the secret of his enduring power, lies in his having been the first to construct true social models, starting out from the long-term" (Braudel, 1972:39).

gives rise to it.[9] A world-system represents a coherent and integrated organizational structure that operates across a single spatial-temporal unit, with a basic governing logic (such as capital accumulation) that defines relationships between territorial units (such as nation-states) and shapes social interaction and societal and cultural development. In the current era, the globe is dominated by the capitalist world-system, a historical world-system with its origins in the mid-16th century. As a historical world-system, the current capitalist world-system is assumed to be time-bound with a beginning and an eventual end. "The capitalist world-economy has a 'natural history' in a way that no state structure does. It came into existence under specific historical circumstances; it manifests specific long-term secular trends; it will most likely one day have a demise" (Hopkins, Wallerstein, et al., 1982:55).

World-systems analysis originated in the context of the modernization debates of the 1950s and 1960s. As such, global political and economic structures and processes (for example, the global division of labor or the interstate system) have been the primary subjects for research, with a notable neglect of consideration for cultural forms. At the same time, as two of the primary proponents of world-systems analysis have argued, the cultural sphere is by no means only of secondary interest. It is in fact, a "third fundamental aspect" alongside and of equal rank with the domain of political and economic structures and processes.

> There is a third fundamental aspect of the modern world-system, in addition to the specifically "economic" aspect and the specifically "political" aspect. That is the broadly "cultural" aspect which needs to be mentioned even though little is systematically known about it as an integral aspect of world-historical development. Just as the world-system contains, as it were, a multiplicity of interrelated states, so too does it contain a multiplicity of interrelated cultural communities—language communities, religious communities, ethnic communities, races, status groups, class communities, scientific communities and so forth. (Hopkins, Wallerstein, et al., 1982:43)

Distinguishing themselves from other critiques of modernization (for example, Marxists, dependency theorists), Wallerstein and others argue that world-systems analysis proceeds from three conceptual premises—a single global unit of analysis, a multiplicity of social times, and a unidisciplinary perspective (Wallerstein, 2006, 1999). For those primarily concerned with

[9] The territories over which past world-systems have ruled never actually encompassed the entire globe. In this regard, the term "world-system" is a bit of a misnomer, as the first truly global world-system has been the capitalist world-system of the past century.

local- or national-level developments, it is this notion of a single global unit of analysis that evokes the strongest protest. Within world-systems analysis, the nation-state is not considered a sufficient unit of analysis for the purpose of understanding national or local developments. At the same time, a framework that offers only a global-level perspective is also inadequate. Rather, social and cultural developments at the local, national, or global level follow from the dynamic interaction of local, national, and global forces. Indeed, within this tri-level confluence, factors at the local level are generally understood to be the *most palpable and immediate* with respect to shaping people's lives and social organization. "A world-economy is defined as that kind of worldsystem in which the political and cultural 'structures' are multiple and the system-wide political and cultural structures are far less tangible and immediately constraining than more 'local' ones" (Hopkins and Wallerstein, 1987:764). Across the capitalist world-system, social space and social interaction are organized within a well-integrated zone of structures and processes, including cultural structures and processes, which reify systemic rules. One of the essential tasks of world-systems analysis has been to delineate the nature of these structures and processes in the context of the long-term, large-scale development of the capitalist world-system as it has grown over the past five centuries as a single spatial-temporal zone that cuts across political and cultural units at the local, national, and global levels.[10]

Two central concepts of world-systems analysis that follow from the notion of a single global unit of analysis, and with direct implications for biomedicine in Africa, are the core-periphery relationship and the process of incorporation. One of the basic social structures defining the capitalist world-system is an axial division of labor that links "core" and "peripheral" production processes in the pursuit of endless accumulation within a single expanding world-system. As a consequence, the core-periphery relationship is a fundamental organizing principle of the capitalist world-system.

> There is one expanding economy. This conventionally appears to us in the form of various "national" economies related through "international" trade. This one world-scale economy, which is progressively more global in scope, has a single or axial division and integration of labor processes ("division of labor"), which is both organized and paralleled by a single set of accumulation-processes, between its always more advanced, historically enlarging and geographically shifting core and its always less advanced, disproportionally enlarging, and geographically shifting periphery. (Hopkins, 1982a:11)

---

[10] See, for example, Abu-Lughod (1989), Arrighi (1994), Chase-Dunn (1989), Tomich (1990), and Wallerstein (1974, 1980, 1989).

While there is a rough correspondence between core activities and wealthy nations and peripheral activities and poor nations, conceptually the notion of "core" nation or "peripheral" nation is mistaken. Rather, depictions of the core or periphery pertain to descriptions not of specific nation-states but of a type of relationship between zones occupied by nation-states. The concepts of core and periphery within world-systems analysis, therefore, reflect an effort to depict conditions in various parts of the capitalist world-system (such as wealth and poverty) not as descriptive categories but as expressions of dynamic, system-wide relationships and processes. Biomedicine in Africa is a manifestation of this relationship. The core-periphery construct is thus fundamentally a relational concept and great mishap results when this basic principle of analysis is neglected.

> [U]nfortunately, the end-terms "core" and "periphery" all too often become themselves respective foci of attention, categories in their own right, as it were. And the relation which the joined terms designate slips into the background. When that happens the processes continually reproducing the relation, and hence the relational categories, also drop from sight, and we are left with only the categories, which, as a result, are now mere classificatory terms, neither grounded theoretically nor productive analytically. (Hopkins, 1982b:151)

World-systems analysis maintains that the basis for Western dominance is linked to its strategic position within an exploitive capitalist world-system, driven by the requirements of endless accumulation.[11] As a consequence, a central feature of the capitalist world-system over its five hundred-year history has been its periodic territorial expansion and the incorporation[12] of peoples and societies previously outside its system-wide, axial division of labor.[13] This represents the peripheralization of such peoples and societies, as they become increasingly ensnared in the structures and processes of production and consumption within the capitalist world-system. While whole societies are incorporated, this does not suggest that all persons and processes become direct participants within peripheral production. Rather, certain key

---

[11] See Amin (1974), Gunder Frank (1978), and Wallerstein (1974).

[12] For an extended treatment of the concept of incorporation as a historical process see the 1987 special issue of *Review—Fernand Braudel Center for the Study of Economies, Historical Systems and Civilizations* (Vol. X, Nos. 5/6, Summer/Fall, 1987).

[13] World-systems analysis draws a technical distinction here between the capitalist world-system and the world-economy. The expansion of the capitalist world-system, via the incorporation of new territories, is in fact precipitated by a cyclical period of contraction across the world-economy (Hopkins and Wallerstein, 1982; 1987).

export-oriented industries (such as mining or agriculture) are organized to meet the needs of core production, while others' activities are re-fashioned to support these expanding industries. Political and cultural institutions and practices are thereby transformed, as the newly peripheralized territory both resists and succumbs to core pressures. While guns and warships are the major tools of initial conquest in this period of incorporation, a broad phalanx of less lethal instruments secure subjugation (that is, missionaries, doctors, and teachers). Among these less lethal instruments in Africa, the introduction of Western biomedicine was an essential element. Both an ideological ramrod and a tangible social benefit, Western biomedicine effectively contributed more generally to the conditions for Western influence.

The second premise of world-systems analysis concerns the role of time (or temporal frames) as an organizing principle for social analysis. At the heart of world-systems analysis is a concerted effort to grapple with the challenge of including a multiplicity of social times as a feature of social development (Wallerstein, 1993). The underlying theoretical notion of a multiplicity of social times originated with the French Annales School and Braudel.[14] "Whether we are dealing with the past or present, a clear awareness of the plurality of social time is indispensable to a common methodology of the social sciences" (Braudel, 1972:13). The "plurality of social time" emerged by way of a critique of traditional historiographic work, which tends to emphasize one of two temporal extremes. On the one hand, there are those historical accounts that revolve around specific moments or events of great importance, such as a revolution or war. Such history offers fantastic descriptions of dramatic battles or colorful personalities but generally lacks a broader context or perspective for analyzing the events in question. At the other extreme, there are those nomothetic social scientists who treat their findings as timeless and universal—hence, subject to no temporal boundaries. Accordingly, Braudel depicts the nomothetic social sciences as the province of unexamined, ahistorical distortion.

> [T]he researcher into the world of today arrives at the finer components of structures only if he too "reconstructs," i.e., puts forward hypotheses and explanations, rejects reality in the crude form presented to him, cuts it up and goes beyond it—processes all entailing reconstruction, which lets us escape from the given pattern and re-arrange it. I doubt whether the sociological record of the present is any "truer" than the historical picture of the past; and the further it tries to place itself from the "reconstruction," the less "true" it is. (Braudel, 1972:23)

---

[14] See Braudel's (1972) seminal essay regarding social time and the historical social sciences.

Braudel sought to analyze history with the aid of two temporal measures found between these two extremes. The first he referred to as structural time, or the *longue durée*. The *longue durée* captures the life history of a particular historical world-system, such as the capitalist world-system. Structural time can, therefore, cover vast stretches of time—five hundred years plus—and over this period a great many structures and processes internal to a world-system are themselves subject to distinct temporal durations vis-à-vis the history of the system as a whole. An example would be the era of mercantile capitalist trade or of the Atlantic slave trade economy. The second temporal measure concerns midrange cycles, or the "conjuncture." These are medium-length, repeating periods (twenty- to fifty-year episodes) that mark the cyclical patterns of development of a particular world-system. For example, within the capitalist world-system this temporal measure may refer to routine business cycles or to those regular periods of expansion or contraction of the world-economy. New areas, such as Africa, are generally incorporated into the capitalist world-system during periods of cyclical contraction. The challenge is to frame specific and multiple structures and processes within a combination of overlapping, temporal frames to analyze simultaneously short-term or middle-range developments while chronicling the life narrative of a historical world-system—the *longue durée*—without reducing the former to the latter nor neglecting the latter for the former.

> [G]etting a grasp of what the world is about means defining a hierarchy of forces, currents and individual movements, and refashioning the pattern of their totality. At each moment in the search, distinctions will have to be made between long-term movements and sudden growths, the latter being related to their immediate sources, the former to the long-term span. . . . The long-term, the "conjuncture" and the event fit together easily because they can all be measured on the same scale. (Braudel, 1972:21, 36)

Importantly, while the present analysis of biomedicine in Africa borrows Braudel's notion of social times largely intact, there is one significant modification. The term "middle-range episode" replaces "conjuncture" to better capture those noncyclical developments (colonial rule, mercantilism) that persist for many decades and that possess qualities (including racial ideologies) that endure beyond their decline. The export of biomedicine to Africa trespasses any number of overlapping social times that correspond with various historical structures and processes that give shape to the capitalist world-system. The colonial era, African incorporation, the narrative of Western scientific discovery, and the age of European imperialism are, for example, each periods of momentous import by themselves. However as integrated structures and processes within the development of the capitalist world-system—an angle of vision made stark by a world-systems analysis of the processes associated with the introduction of biomedicine into Africa—these developments both account for biomedicine in Africa and are themselves shaped by biomedicine in Africa. Hence, the narrative of biomedicine in Africa, comprising a distinct social time, must be located within the longer train of historical development, in part to place it in broader perspective and, in part, to tell the story of the capitalist world-system more completely. With respect to economic or political structures and processes (such as Korean industrialization or the Soviet Union's rise and fall) this may seem self-evident. It is argued here, however, that conceptually within world-systems analysis the inclusion of cultural developments, such as biomedicine in Africa, provide no less insight regarding the capitalist world-system and are no less essential for its complete depiction.

The third premise of world-systems analysis concerns the notion of unidisciplinary research. It is argued that world-systems analysis requires a unified notion of the historical social sciences to analyze properly "total social systems over the *longue durée*."[15] Unidisciplinary research differs conceptually from the conventional interdisciplinary course of investigation. Interdisciplinary work implies a type of cooperation between individuals from separate and distinct scholarly spheres all of whom retain privileged expertise in their unique fields. Such orchestrated cooperation, in fact, reinforces division. Unidisciplinary work rejects the traditional apartheid structure of academia and advocates creating nonsectarian disciplines, which borrow from a range of fields, free of professionalized turf battles. Such work obviously clashes with the established academic norms of separation. In the present study, for example, among the disparate and overlapping professional fields are those of medical anthropology, medical sociology, medical history, African studies, political economy, and colonial/postcolonial studies—to name the most obvious. Lamentably, the reception for unidisciplinary research from disciplinary specialists often fluctuates between tepid indifference and outright hostility.

Finally, world-systems analysis raises unique methodological challenges for analyzing a historical world-system whose development results from the dialectical interaction of local, national, and global structures and processes over long stretches of time.[16] The development of biomedicine in Africa as a feature of the capitalist world-system presents a case in point. Biomedicine in African did not develop as a spontaneous and isolated cultural form. Nor was

---

[15] See Hopkins (1982b), Wallerstein (2001), and Wallerstein et al. (1996).

[16] See Bach (1982), Hopkins (1982a, 1982b), McMichael (1990), and Tomich (1994, 1997).

it the case that even the most detailed knowledge of the capitalist world-system would have allowed one to anticipate the unique patterns of biomedicine's local manifestations across Africa. World-systems analysis asks us to capture faithfully, somehow, the manifold history of biomedicine in Africa while simultaneously placing these developments within the flow of historical structures and processes that constitute the capitalist world-system across a single global unit of analysis, comprising a multiplicity of social times. Such work suggests a number of methodological challenges of considerable complexity.

By way of entry into such matters, a brief comment regarding the use of language is in order. At times, the terminology of world-systems analysis may appear to lack a degree of precision—especially from the perspective of analytical philosophy. Indeed, the use of language often lies closer to the metaphoric allusions of Nietzsche than to the strict correspondence rules of the Vienna Circle. As explored below, from the perspective of world-systems analysis, the difficulty of language follows, primarily, from the issue of concept-formation and from an investigative procedure that emphasizes the relationships between social phenomena rather than a given phenomenon's discrete properties. In general, this seeming lack of linguistic rigor is tempered by the rich details of the historical narratives that comprise much of the literature of world-systems analysis. At other times, however, such as when introducing a novel conceptual construction, this looseness of language presents certain difficulties. Here, for example, the task will be to consider "historical-cultural formations" (such as biomedicine in Africa) in a fashion that is parallel to analyses of the economic and political structures and processes that comprise the capitalist world-system.[17]

To begin, therefore, it is necessary to establish the proper conceptual language and corresponding methodological procedures for an investigation of a historical world-system—and specifically the capitalist world-system. Methodological considerations within world-systems analysis can be seen, in fact, as interventions in an ancient debate concerning parts/whole constructions applied to historical social analysis and laden with a terminology heavily influenced by Marx. In the language of such debates, a historical world-system represents a concrete whole, which is comprised of combinations of interrelated structures and processes. In isolation, each structure or process is an abstraction

[17] As understood in the present analysis, the term "structure" suggests orderly and regular patterns of social organization that direct and govern social interaction. The term "process" refers to a collection of linked social phenomena with expanding and contracting entanglements that develop across space and time. The economic and political entities that comprise the capitalist world-system, such as the division of labor or the interstate system, represent both structures and processes simultaneously. This is no less true for historical-cultural formations (e.g., biomedicine). Thus, the term "historical-cultural formation" refers to an entity comprised of structures and processes that are constituent elements of the capitalist world-system.

and cannot be meaningfully analyzed as such. It is only in relation to the concrete whole (the capitalist world-system) that these abstract elements are defined and made substantive. Analysis of the concrete whole, therefore, requires consideration of its structures and processes and the relations between them. Indeed, it is the relationships between structures and processes that constitute the capitalist world-system. Importantly, because these structures and processes are analyzed across a single spatial-temporal unit, they are "singular" structures and processes. This signals an important break from conventional, analytical-comparative methods which generally do not incorporate the contingency of historical time as an element of inquiry itself. "Long held strategies of concept formation and comparative analysis are challenged by the insistence upon singular processes as the starting point for inquiry. Perhaps the clearest impact is on the necessity to pursue the construction of structures in their time-place coordinates and in relation to the construction of structures elsewhere" (Bach, 1982:167).

The analysis of any historical development, such as biomedicine in Africa, emerges from an analysis of that development as a singular (and abstract) structure or process—the common starting point for inquiry in world-systems analysis. If biomedicine in Africa is conceptualized as a "singular process," then what distinguishes it is not its external properties but its relationships to other structures and processes that comprise the capitalist world-system (for example, colonialism in Africa). At the same time, world-systems analysis rejects reductionist notions whereby structures and processes are mechanically determined by their position within the capitalist world-system. Thus, one does not identify a singular structure or process and try to fit it into a pre-existing world-system (or concrete whole). Rather, in dialectical fashion, structures and processes determine (constitute the conditions for) a world-system. The capitalist world-system and its constituent elements are mutually conditioning.

> For the world-system perspective, then, the whole consists of singular processes which *form* and *reform* the relations that express patterns or structures. Parts are "pieces" of a process, not independent of the remainder of the process but located within a specific time-place coordinate. To "sum" the parts means to bring them together successively as each produces the particular time- and place-bound relations and traits. (emphasis in original, Bach, 1982:166)

As follows from this basic formulation, world-systems analysis rejects the conventional analytical-comparative methodology, which assumes a world of discrete "cases" (such as nations, ethnic/religious groups) that vary according to select properties. Such comparisons pay too little heed to the relationships between cases. Instead, world-systems analysis emphasizes the investigation of historical developments as elements within a set of interrelated structures and processes that, through their combination, form a single concrete whole.[18] The analysis takes the form of a continual juxtaposition between historically connected structures and processes rather than direct comparisons. Procedurally, this entails an initial movement from more immediate abstract elements to the concrete whole (the capitalist world-system).[19]

> The part-whole directive . . . says to keep moving out by successive determinations, bringing in successive parts—themselves abstract processes—in continuing juxtaposition and in this way form the whole which you need for interpreting and explaining the historical changes or conditions under examination. . . . [I]n the fullness of the whole so formed, one "interprets" observational statements; or, alternatively, one "measures" selected and partial "outcomes" of the complex processes. (Hopkins, 1982b:147)

Thus, in relation to the capitalist world-system (a concrete whole), various historical-cultural formations—such as biomedicine in Africa—represent singular, abstract structures and processes. Further, the term "historical-cultural" denotes a cultural formation that is dynamic, ever-developing, and thus subject to change. Methodologically, one would be in error to treat these historical-cultural formations as discrete phenomena comprised of unique properties, such as the scientific method or germ theory, in an effort to draw comparisons with other historical-cultural formations (for example, African pluralistic medicine). Historical-cultural formations found among societies across the capitalist world-system represent constituent elements of the capitalist world-system itself. Outside this relationship to the whole they are distorted abstractions. Thus, a historical-cultural formation's relation to the whole (its role as a constituent element)—as well as its relation to other historical-cultural formations—simultaneously defines that historical-cultural formation and further develops the capitalist world-system as a concrete whole. This would suggest that it is necessary to construct biomedicine in Africa, as a historical-cultural formation (1) in relation to the self-expanding capitalist world-system and (2) in relation to the ongoing structures and

[18] McMichael (1990) provides an example of this from the perspective of world-systems analysis through his use of the concept of "incorporated comparisons."

[19] This formulation, of course, mirrors that described briefly by Marx in his passage from *Grundrisse* on "Method of Political Economy." Additionally, though developed in a different context, this emphasis on abstract parts in relation to a concrete whole is clearly influenced by the analyses of Kosik (1976), Lefebvre (1968), and Lukacs (1971).

processes of Western expansion in Africa. Similarly, one must not view biomedicine in Africa, Western expansion, or the capitalist world-system as complete or fully constituted absent these relationships. In this respect, consideration of historical-cultural formations is similar to that of economic and political structures and processes.

With respect to biomedicine in Africa, world-systems analysis, therefore, presents a basic dilemma. On the one hand, world-systems analysis offers a decidedly compelling account of long-term, large-scale social development with respect to the political and economic structures and processes that comprise the capitalist world-system. On the other hand, world-systems analysis makes little, if any, effort to incorporate historical-cultural formations as integral (and indispensable) features of these long-term, large-scale developments. Two options emerge. One can simply abandon world-systems analysis and thereby sacrifice the robust potential of its basic framework. Or, working within this framework, one can attempt to broaden its conceptually sound though incomplete precepts to schematically include historical-cultural formations as essential features of the capitalist world-system. Opting for the latter, it is our intent to extend world-systems analysis in a fashion that treats biomedicine as a core-based, singular historical-cultural formation whose introduction to Africa has been integral to the expansion of the capitalist world-system and to the further development of biomedicine itself. As such, this framework will allow one to analyze how biomedicine has transformed Africa as well as how Africa has transformed biomedicine.

The Empirical, Conceptual, and Interpretive Realms of Historical-Cultural Formations

One of the most basic distinctions between historical-cultural formations and other elements of the capitalist world-system concerns their ontological status. As discussed above, economic and political structures and processes are abstract expressions of the capitalist world-system whose analysis is, in part, an empirical question and, in part, a conceptual question. Consider, for example, the division of labor. Its relation to the capitalist world-system and its simultaneous reflection of local social conditions is both a matter of empirical investigation and the result of conceptual analysis. For a variety of programmatic reasons, world-systems analysis has largely limited its research to economic and political structures and processes for which the empirical-conceptual methodological strategies described above largely suffice (Hopkins, Wallerstein, et al., 1982). Biomedicine is a historical-cultural formation whose structures and processes, from one angle of vision, are also abstract expressions of the capitalist world-system. More immediately, however, biomedicine is an expression of collective social meaning. The study of historical-cultural formations differs for this reason from most of the work of world-systems analysis and suggests the need for additional analytical strategies—beyond the empirical and conceptual—that permit interpretive methodological procedures.

As expressions of collective social meaning, the analysis of historical-cultural formations as constituent elements of the capitalist world-system introduces an ontological line of inquiry. Within world-systems analysis, the ontology of the division of labor (that which can be known about it) is essentially limited to the empirical-conceptual realm. As a historical-cultural formation, the ontology of biomedicine necessarily extends beyond the empirical-conceptual realm and includes the social worlds of interpretive communities.[20] Indeed, as it develops, not only do biomedicine's empirical forms and conceptual roles within the capitalist world-system change, so too do its social meanings. Biomedicine, therefore, is comprised of multiple ontological spheres across empirical, conceptual, and interpretive realms. But what types of phenomena, forms, and categories constitute biomedicine as a subject for investigation across these ontological spheres? From an empirical perspective, biomedicine consists of concrete facts (truths) and objects that are subject to observation and measurement. From a conceptual perspective, biomedicine represents a social relation, a form of social organization that is itself a historical abstraction (an expression of underlying social power relations). From an interpretive perspective, biomedicine is a symbolic-cultural expression that serves as a social representation whose meanings reify collective values and beliefs.

Each sphere signals a unique set of ontological phenomena. Each reveals a particular facet of biomedicine and thus all are necessary for its full understanding. Privileging one facet above another would distort one's view and replace biomedicine, as a product of the dynamic interaction (and creative tension) between multiple ontological spheres, with a flat, three-sided figure—a figure comprised of three discrete sides, versus a figure constituted by the ongoing articulation of its manifold forms. Integrating these three ontological spheres necessarily results in a conceptual representation that sustains internal contradictions as a premise of its being. Thus, understood as an ontological whole, biomedicine is the product of multiple ontological spheres. Representations of biomedicine neglecting any one of these spheres will be distorted and one sided. Representations incorporating all of these spheres will be contradictory and subject to constant revision. The task, therefore, is not to unite or reconcile these three spheres—biomedicine as an empirical object and biomedicine as a symbolic-cultural expression, for example, suggest

[20] The same could technically be said for economic and political structures and processes, such as the division of labor, and this remains a fertile area of investigation open to further inquiry.

alternative logics of inquiry. Rather, the task is to develop all of these spheres simultaneously as interdependent reflections of the multifaceted nature of biomedicine, as a historical-cultural formation comprised of multiple ontological spheres.

A further complication surfaces when one begins to analyze any one of these ontological spheres. Biomedicine remains in motion across both space and time vis-à-vis the capitalist world-system, and its analysis as an ontological form must reflect this. Consequently, it follows that each sphere is itself comprised of varying levels of abstraction depending upon one's spatial-temporal location across a single global unit of analysis with multiple social times. As noted, these levels of abstraction correspond with the *longue durée* at the level of the capitalist world-system, with middle-range episodes that encompass the development of the structures and processes that comprise the capitalist world-system, and with short-term events that punctuate and dramatize the life and times of middle-range episodes. For example, when analyzed across the capitalist world-system, biomedicine as a symbolic-cultural expression reflects interpretive meanings at the level of the concrete whole across the *longue durée*. However, when analyzed as a moment in Africa's incorporation, biomedicine is a symbolic-cultural expression of the structures and processes at the level of a middle-range episode. Lastly, when presented through the prism of a specific medical campaign to eradicate sleeping sickness, biomedicine takes on the appearance of a short-term event. Each of these sets of interpretive meanings is an equally integral aspect of biomedicine as a symbolic-cultural expression. Furthermore, that which is true for biomedicine as a symbolic-cultural expression holds equally for biomedicine as an empirical object or biomedicine as a social relation. Thus, each ontological sphere contains its own set of embedded levels of abstraction, corresponding to varying spatial-temporal locations across the capitalist world- system.

The extension of world-systems analysis to incorporate historical-cultural formations as integral features of the capitalist world-system, therefore, begins with an ontological dissection. The first step is to distinguish the multiple ontological spheres—empirical, conceptual, and interpretive—that comprise biomedicine and to sketch the relationships between them. The second and simultaneous step is to distinguish between the multiple levels of abstraction that comprise each ontological sphere and that correspond with varying spatial-temporal locations across the capitalist world-system. Importantly, just as the structures and processes that comprise the capitalist world-system stand in a relation of mutual conditioning to that world-system, the multiple levels of abstraction constituting each ontological sphere are also mutually conditioning. In other words, just as no single ontological sphere—empirical, conceptual, or interpretive—is primary, there is no single level of abstraction that *determines* the others. Alas, the search for a single governing logic at the "highest" level of the concrete whole (that is, *Geist*) resolves itself as pure illusion. Ultimately, the relationships between ontological spheres, as well as the relationships between each ontological sphere's levels of abstraction, determine the development of biomedicine as an ontological whole. The analysis of biomedicine in Africa as a feature of the capitalist world-system, therefore, begins with an ontological unpacking of biomedicine, itself a historical-cultural formation comprised of multiple, embedded ontologies.

Medical Systems, Western Expansion, and "Syncretic" Worldviews

As the expanding capitalist world-system incorporates and transforms more and more societies around the globe, deeply embedded sociocultural values, beliefs, and practices are reshaped in broad conformity with patterns of capital accumulation and the agenda of the Western powers. It is argued here that a medical system embodies a type of historical-cultural formation that is uniquely suited for the purpose of tracing these transformations of local sociocultural values, beliefs, and practices in the context of a society's incorporation into the expanding capitalist world-system. This approach locates such historical-cultural formations (and their inherent internal contradictions) at the nexus of a dynamic tension between the transformative pressures exerted by structures and processes at the level of the capitalist world-system and local forms of collective social expression (and resistance), which shape and define these historical-cultural formations. Furthermore, as symbolic-cultural expressions, a principle feature of historical-cultural formations is that they convey collective worldviews that are actualized through social praxis and interaction. In this sense, a worldview provides a representation of how societies interpret the meaning of its members' lived experiences, including of course, those foreign encounters precipitating dramatic social change. Importantly, historical-cultural formations are only one of the many sociocultural influences shaping collective worldviews. It merely happens that historical-cultural formations, such as biomedicine, provide an especially rich and detailed window into these.

By the late 19th century, biomedicine had begun its reign as the predominant form of healing in the core region of the capitalist world-system. Indeed, alongside the Bible and the gunship, it was the syringe that greatly hastened Europe's global ascendancy. As a practical matter, the Scramble for Africa would have met with far less success had it not been for the advent of "tropical medicine" (see Chapter 3), which granted the European soldier the requisite fortitude to survive conquest. Therefore, in concert with the 19th-century incorporation of Africa, the Western powers propagated a specific medical system, biomedicine, whose associated health beliefs and practices embodied a unique approach to medicine and healing. A potent agent of colonization, biomedicine provided the West with a powerful tool for "civilizing" Africans via the introduction of values and beliefs that challenged established African values and beliefs. The Europeans ultimately brought biomedicine to Africa as both a gift and a weapon.

The role of biomedicine as a strategic counterpoint to Africa's "primitive" and "brutish" cultural values and beliefs underscores the importance of biomedicine as a form of symbolic-cultural expression. Indeed, as a reflection of a society's health beliefs and practices, medical systems offer a particularly valuable perspective with respect to a society's collective worldviews. Health beliefs and practices reflect a fundamental understanding of how societies view an individual's and a community's place within the world and how societies interpret an individual's and a community's relation to the natural, supernatural, and social worlds. The worldview embraced by biomedicine limits health-related phenomena almost exclusively to the natural world. By contrast, the worldviews expressed by the pluralistic-medical systems, which predominated across Africa prior to biomedicine, generally associated health-related phenomena with a broad spectrum of overlapping forces that intersect the natural, supernatural, and social worlds. Consequently, the introduction of biomedical beliefs and practices can present significant challenges to a society's established worldviews. The result has been the emergence of a mix of syncretic health beliefs and practices across Africa that combine biomedical and pluralistic-medical elements. Over time, these evolving syncretic health beliefs and practices have the potential to reshape and reconstitute a society's worldviews radically with respect to how people understand and interpret their place within the natural, supernatural, and social worlds. At the same time, as is asserted here, through these same syncretic health beliefs and practices Africans have the potential to expand and reshape biomedicine itself as a "singular" historical-cultural formation.

This latter potential turns, in part, on how one conceptualizes African syncretic-medical systems in the context of the capitalist world-system. To begin with, the notion of an African pluralistic-medical system does not imply a medical system that is somehow frozen in time, embracing an ancient and primordial set of health beliefs and practices. Rather, African pluralistic-medical systems are dynamic, evolving medical systems that combine a wide variety of traditions, values, and cultural influences. In this sense, it can be argued that, even absent biomedicine, African pluralistic-medical systems are themselves syncretic insofar as they comprise a mix of medical systems. It is merely for clarity of presentation, therefore, that only medical systems that commingle aspects of biomedicine and aspects of African pluralistic medicine are referred to here as syncretic. African syncretic-medical systems are thus no less "African" than African pluralistic-medical systems. This, however, begs an obvious question. Why is it that when biomedicine travels to different regions of Europe or North America and the resulting medical systems represent a number of common health beliefs and practices as well as the influence of distinct local cultural traditions (see Chapter 2) it is labeled biomedicine, but when the same process occurs on the continent of Africa it is labeled African syncretic medicine? The distinction betrays a basic Western ignorance both of Africa and of biomedicine.

The ignorance of Africa concerns an alleged clash of conflicting worldviews that first originated with colonial rule. That which distinguishes biomedicine from African pluralistic medicine in the Western mind is the role of science. As detailed below, however, in actual practice there is little justification for labeling biomedicine "scientific" and African pluralistic medicine "unscientific." It is true that African pluralistic medicine often incorporates elements of the supernatural and social worlds (such as witchcraft and divination) that are very much at odds with the cultural beliefs and practices of Western biomedicine. However, it is also true that scores of pluralistic-medical practitioners rely on the same so-called scientific procedures associated with biomedicine, such as empirical observation and trial-and-error testing. Thus, in actual practice, African pluralistic medicine reflects a mindset that is no less grounded in science.

The ignorance of biomedicine concerns a mistaken notion of biomedicine as a medical system that is frozen in time, embracing an ancient and primordial set of beliefs and practices narrowly construed as a scientific enterprise. Medical knowledge and technology may change but the fundamental framework of biomedicine is considered eternal. In fact, as a singular historical-cultural formation, biomedicine is subject to continual transformation and renewal. As biomedicine infects different medical systems around the world, these medical systems are transformed. However, the resulting "syncretic" medical systems are merely the most recent and most up-to-date incarnations of biomedicine as a singular historical-cultural formation. These new incarnations of biomedicine, in turn, hasten the formation of new collective worldviews (grounded in praxis) that are both in harmony with and in opposition to the prevailing structures and processes that comprise the capitalist world-system. It is for these reasons that tracing the development of syncretic-medical systems in peripheralized regions of Africa after the introduction of biomedicine provides insight into how historical-cultural formations are transformed and, in turn, how these formations then transform the capitalist world-system.

Biomedicine in Africa: An African Appropriation

To unravel the genesis of African biomedicine, one must grapple with three distinct aspects of biomedicine before and after its Africa sojourn. There is first the matter of biomedicine itself. Like other historical-cultural formations, biomedicine represents an ontological whole that is comprised of multiple, mutually interdependent ontological spheres. The interrelated nature of these spheres indicates that biomedicine, far from embodying a fixed and universal set of scientific truths, is in fact a dynamic medical system, which is subject to ongoing change and development. Biomedicine framed as an ontological whole, therefore, is a basic prerequisite for the 20th-century emergence of African biomedicine. The journey of biomedicine to Africa is a second consideration. This journey served as an extension of European conquest and colonial rule over the African continent. More generally, however, it also signaled a moment in the incorporation of Africa into the capitalist world-system. After reaching the African shore, biomedicine emerged quite clearly as a singular historical-cultural formation. As such, biomedicine invariably pulled Africa more and more tightly into the orbit of those economic, political, and historical-cultural structures and processes that comprise the capitalist world-system. The basic features of African pluralistic-medical systems represent a third aspect of biomedicine in Africa. Upon arrival, biomedicine encountered a heterogeneous patchwork of African pluralistic-medical systems across the continent. The rich diversity of these pluralistic-medical systems notwithstanding, a fair number of common elements could be distinguished. Many of these elements, such as holistic interpretations of illness and pragmatic attitudes toward other medical systems, have facilitated the adoption of certain aspects of biomedicine without sacrificing the cardinal values and beliefs of African pluralistic medicine. The result has been African biomedicine, a unique African contribution to the development of biomedicine as a singular historical-cultural formation and constituent element of the capitalist world-system.

Biomedicine as an Ontological Whole

Before biomedicine could serve as a tool of colonization in Africa, it first had to establish its domination over Europe. Detailing the manner by which biomedicine came to monopolize health and medicine in the West from the 18th century through the early 20th century begins with an ontological interrogation of biomedicine itself—its empirical, conceptual, and interpretive spheres. The multiple ontological spheres that comprise biomedicine each frame biomedicine as a distinct subject of investigation. From an empirical perspective, biomedicine takes on the appearance of a scientific enterprise and is defined as a derivative category of Western science more generally. As a scientific enterprise, biomedicine represents a combination of specialized knowledge, complex technology, and scientific rigor and is subject to the critical scrutiny of like-trained peer scientists. From an interpretive perspective, biomedicine represents a symbolic-cultural expression whose avowed adherence to the principles of scientific objectivity conceals an ideological agenda. As a symbolic-cultural expression, biomedicine propagates a set of values and beliefs that reify a narrow and distorted (mis)understanding of health and medicine that attributes illness to "natural" conditions and, thereby, absolves the toxic social environment. From a conceptual perspective, biomedicine represents an expression of social power that reflects structures of class-based divisions in capitalist society. As an expression of social power, biomedicine is a type of social relation that links the parallel processes of the commodification of medicine and the concentration of power among biomedical practitioners with the historical structures and processes of capital accumulation that comprise the capitalist world-system.

The image of biomedicine as a scientific enterprise is today ubiquitous. Most commonly, the life story of biomedicine is placed within the narrative of modern Western science, dating from the 16th century and roughly paralleling the duration of the capitalist world-system. Indeed, while many of its applications would need to await the industrial-technological advancements of the 19th century, biomedicine's fundamental ethos and approach to health as a matter of applied scientific principles originated with the dawn of modern science and the heroic "objectivity" of Bacon, Locke, Galileo and Newton. Science equaled truth and medical science equaled the true understanding of health and illness. Over the centuries, biomedicine's development has at times been slow and at other times more rapid. Ultimately, however, it has been a linear and cumulative process, building at each new stage upon the lessons of the past. Ancient superstitions, such as humoral theories of disease, were put to the test and vanquished. As an ontological sphere, therefore, biomedicine as a scientific enterprise details a rich world of complex medical-scientific paraphernalia organized by the logic and rigor of a scientific-technical expertise. This would be a most welcome gift for Africa, no doubt.

Further analysis of biomedicine as a scientific enterprise reveals that this ontological sphere combines multiple integrated levels of abstraction pertaining to three spatial-temporal locations across the capitalist world-system. At the level of the capitalist world-system and corresponding with the *longue durée*, biomedicine exemplifies the proud narrative of scientific progress. In this sense, its development parallels advances in the forces of production, to borrow from Marx, and is integral to the accumulation of capital. At the level of the core region of the capitalist world-economy and corresponding with a middle-range episode, biomedicine is linked to distinct biomedical-scientific eras of discovery. The era of pathological anatomy in the early 19th century, for example, provided a better understanding of mortality patterns during a period of rapid industrialization linked to deteriorating urban centers. At the level of a local development within the capitalist world-system and corresponding with short-term events, biomedicine parades triumphantly in the guise of a pioneering, new advance. The establishment of the Paris School at the turn of the 19th century, for example, proved an innovative organizational structure for enhancing medical treatment and research. This organizational structure was later generalized to create the modern research hospital. Each of these features of biomedicine as a scientific enterprise—the narrative of scientific progress, advances in pathological anatomy, and the Paris School—is shaped by, and in turn helps to shape, the other two. The organization of the Paris School, for example, as a laboratory that gathered large samples of patients, directly aided scientific progress and provided the basic data for pathological anatomy. Likewise, the spirit of scientific progress inspired the Paris School, and the field of pathological anatomy validated their efforts.

A second ontological sphere, biomedicine as a symbolic-cultural expression, stands in opposition to the first ontological sphere. On the one hand, it rejects the empirical-objectivist premises of biomedicine as a scientific enterprise. Where the latter sees scientific categories built on careful observation and analysis, the second ontological sphere sees crude ideological constructions that reflect vested social interests. Consequently, whereas biomedicine as a scientific enterprise prefers methods of inquiry that follow the sound, positivist principles of experimental science, the methods of inquiry informing biomedicine as a symbolic-cultural expression involve interpretive procedures designed to understand biomedicine as a constructed world of meaningful items. The standard portrayal of biomedicine as a detached and objective science, for example, conceals how stoic indifference turns social problems into technical problems via ideological subterfuge. "The new scientific medicine tended to place the focus of research on the individual and especially the sub-individual (cell or organ). This not only helped to mask the reaction of the external environment to disease but also tended to focus curative and preventive research on the individual rather than the collectivity. This had the effect of making the individual responsible for his or her own health, and, in effect, of taking this responsibility away from society" (Berliner, 1975:577). That which distinguishes the second ontological sphere, therefore, is the shift from formal techniques promoting empirical explanations to a critique of biomedicine (and of science) that results in a process of inquiry grounded in interpretive understanding.

Like the previous ontological sphere, biomedicine as a symbolic-cultural expression is comprised of three integrated levels of abstraction. At the level of the capitalist world-system and corresponding with the *longue durée*, biomedicine exudes the ideology of scientific-technical knowledge and the accompanying cult of objectivity. This is in conformity with the scientific-cultural norms and values of core-based societies from the 16th century forward. At the level of select regions across the capitalist world-system and corresponding with a middle-range episode, biomedicine is linked to periods of deepening social consensus based on technology-driven invention and advancement. The mid-19th century, for example, saw a spate of technological breakthroughs permitting more precise observations of the human body (such as the ophthalmoscope and otoscope in the 1850s, the sphygmograph in 1860, and the electrometer in 1872). Such devices were critical for the cultural popularization of biomedicine both by linking it to the imagery of scientific progress and by offering people tangible evidence of its scientific content. At the level of a local development within the capitalist world-system and corresponding with short-term events, biomedicine celebrates the periodic, science-affirming medical breakthrough. Louis Pasteur and Robert Koch's simultaneous discoveries of *anthrax bacillus* as the cause of anthrax in animals in 1876 is a case in point. The scientific rationale behind this discovery, the germ theory of disease, resulted in a popular understanding of biomedicine, which focused narrowly on physical phenomena as the cause of illness. Each of these levels of abstractions interacts with and shapes the others. The discovery of *anthrax bacillus* (and its attendant social meanings), for example, followed from a collective social abeyance to a deified scientific- technical knowledge and the general public's reception for Koch and Pasteur's findings was prepared, in part, by the mid-19th century period of celebrated medical inventions. In turn, the ideological grip of scientific-technical knowledge was furthered by this discovery and the cultural impact of these medical inventions was realized.

A third ontological sphere, biomedicine as an expression of social power, reveals a further essential aspect of biomedicine. The links between biomedicine, as a social relation, and structures of power within capitalist society take several forms. On the one hand, the ongoing commodification of medical care beginning in the mid-19th century has today generated a large, U.S. biomedical-industrial complex, a sprawling conglomerate of private physician groups, government agencies, state and private universities, corporate foundations, research and teaching hospitals, biotech firms, transnational pharmaceutical corporations, and the insurance industry (Clarke et al., 2003).[21] Indeed, in practice in the West, biomedicine is largely predicated on the

[21] By the 1950s, most of Europe had removed patient care from the marketplace and provided national healthcare. Nonetheless, much of the basic infrastructure of biomedicine—e.g., the biotechnology and pharmaceutical industries—remains in private hands.

marketplace as the primary site of care and as a distribution center for its products. The premise of medical care as an item of exchange is not unique to biomedicine. However, the combination of biomedicine's commodity form and advanced capitalist society have created unique conditions for intensifying this process, especially in the United States. Thus, one of the major tasks of biomedicine in the West has been the methodical elimination of its competition and the resulting concentration of power. The concerted efforts of biomedical proponents (a combination of elite biomedical practitioners and leading industrialists) to establish exclusive controls over the education and licensing of medical practitioners has created a medical system thoroughly monopolized by an ever-expanding biomedical-industrial complex. This third ontological sphere, therefore, concerns biomedicine's imbricated social relations and details both its rampant commodification and its calculated self-positioning vis-à-vis the realms of social power.

Biomedicine's third ontological sphere is again comprised of three integrated levels of abstraction. At the level of the capitalist world-system and corresponding with the *longue durée*, biomedicine provides direct ties to the accumulation of capital via the commodification of medical care. Given biomedicine's development into a multibranch, medical-industrial complex, medical care today is as much a source of investor profit as it is a source of healing. No depiction of biomedicine, therefore, is complete without due attention to its bottom line. At the level of territorial governance (national or state/provincial levels) across the capitalist world-economy and corresponding with middle-range episodes, the systematic elimination of biomedicine's competition proved essential to its dominance. In the United States in the early 20th century, a variety of nonbiomedical practitioners (for example, homeopaths, eclectics, Thomsonians) provided medical care in competition with biomedical practitioners. Equally troubling, the actual population of self-proclaimed biomedical practitioners was growing unchecked and largely unregulated. Over the course of several decades, working primarily at the level of individual states, biomedical proponents were able both to marginalize nonbiomedical practitioners (barring them, for instance, from hospital practices) and simultaneously to winnow down the number of "legitimate" biomedical practitioners by controlling medical education and licensing. At the level of a local development within the capitalist world-system and corresponding with short-term events, biomedicine's rise was punctuated by the publication of the Flexner Report in 1910, sponsored by the Carnegie Foundation. The report served as a scathing indictment of the state of U.S. medical education and sounded a clarion call for radical reform, which, just coincidentally, placed biomedical proponents at the helm of creating the new criteria for U.S. medical schools. Again, each of these levels of abstraction interacts with and shapes the others. The Flexner Report, for example, directly contributed to the further commodification of medical care and the marginalization of nonbiomedical practitioners. At the same time, in advancing the establishment of an industrial-medical complex linked to patterns of capital accumulation, the Flexner Report was manipulated as a strategic tool by representatives of biomedical interests seeking to eliminate their competition.

Biomedicine, therefore, framed as a historical-cultural formation and a constituent element of the capitalist world-system, is comprised of three ontological spheres. As an ontological whole, biomedicine is simultaneously a scientific enterprise, a symbolic-cultural expression, and an expression of social power. Each sphere is distinct from yet inseparable from the other two. At the same time, each ontological sphere is itself comprised of varying levels of abstraction depending upon one's spatial-temporal location within the capitalist world-system. It is the dynamic interactions between these levels that defines each sphere. Capturing biomedicine as an ontological whole results from efforts to chart the ongoing interactions both between individual spheres and between the varying levels of abstraction that comprise each sphere. The story of biomedicine in Africa must, therefore, proceed with an understanding that it is these three spheres in unison that made the journey. To lay too great an emphasis on any one ontological sphere to the neglect of the others would be to distort biomedicine's development as a singular historical-cultural formation and to obscure Africa's unique contributions to this process.

Biomedicine's Africa Journey

As biomedicine approached the African shore, the complexity of its arrival and greeting remained hidden beneath layers of ideological rationalizations. The three ontological spheres of biomedicine were equally present. However, the visible face of biomedicine revealed only those select aspects of each sphere as suited the conqueror's purpose. From an African perspective, this may have been confusing but it could not have been especially surprising given a relationship built from its inception on deceit and exploitation. It would appear, however, that Europe's calculated distortion of biomedicine in Africa was not only missed by Western scholars, but that, given the contemporary academic division of labor, which mirrors these distortions, its ideological premises have helped shape the actual representation of biomedicine in Africa. The primary academic fields responsible for the West's portrayal of biomedicine in Africa (such as medical history, medical anthropology) remain specialized disciplines with links to different aspects of Western conquest. This both reifies the original Western distortions and generates a scholarship that is ontologically incomplete. For purposes of professional self-identity each discipline retains its own autonomous intellectual sphere—protected by a time-honored system of apartheid, which separates journals, professional associations, and academic departments. Consequently, any description of biomedicine as an ontological whole, that is, one that is blind to these faux disciplinary boundaries, is fraught with peril. Efforts to capture the complexity of forcing biomedicine, as an ontological whole, upon non-Western subjects are thus especially difficult. Reinterpreting the introduction of biomedicine into Africa from a unidisciplinary perspective, which depicts this historical-cultural formation as an integral feature of Africa's incorporation into the expanding capitalist world-system, is a first step in re-framing the prevailing, distorted image of biomedicine's arrival from an African perspective. This begins by locating biomedicine in Africa within a unique episode in the life history of the capitalist world system.

The circumstances of biomedicine's arrival in Africa provide the bases for its analysis. The period of the late 19th and early 20th century, the so-called age of imperialism, signals a dramatic period of territorial expansion for the capitalist world-system. This period encompassed a series of expansionist territorial campaigns by Western powers, including the Scramble for Africa, the Open Door Policy, the Spanish-American War, and assorted land grabs from the remains of a dying Ottoman Empire. These were the caravan of events that prepared the path for biomedicine's African arrival. As such, the origins of biomedicine in Africa are found on three spatial-temporal levels across a single global unit of analysis. At the level of the capitalist world-system and the *longue durée*, biomedicine in Africa marked a transformation of collective worldviews in concert with participation in the global division of labor and processes of capital accumulation. At the level of newly incorporated African territories and a middle-range episode, biomedicine was a vital weapon against illness during conquest (for example, "tropical medicine") as well as a putative ideological rationale for domination. At the level of the village and the short-term event, biomedicine provided colonial authorities with pragmatic solutions to a variety of dire health crises. It is precisely because biomedicine's arrival in Africa took place across a single unit of analysis comprised of multiple social times that it must be treated as a singular historical-cultural formation whose development had implications at all three levels such that biomedicine transformed Africans as Africans transformed biomedicine.

The need for a unidisciplinary approach to capture these overlapping processes follows, in part, from a consideration of how each of the three ontological spheres of biomedicine contributed to social transformation in Africa during the period of colonial rule and how these spheres shaped the structure of the literature on biomedicine in Africa as a reification of each of these spheres. Biomedicine as a scientific enterprise is the province of medical historians and their depictions of biomedicine in Africa. Biomedicine as a symbolic-cultural expression falls within the domain of medical anthropology, and biomedicine as an expression of social power has been the purview of works in political economy. The contributions of each are essential. The contributions of none are sufficient. Nonetheless, even the most rudimentary review of the scholarship pertaining to biomedicine in Africa reveals three distinct camps, largely content to converse with and cite one another. It is not that the accounts provided by any one camp remain narrowly provincial. It is just that when medical historians or any of the others do venture beyond their preferred ontological sphere they rarely reflect on how perspectives from another ontological vantage point might reshape the interpretations of biomedicine in Africa from the perspective of their primary ontological orientation.

Much of the work of medical historians in Africa has been rich, detailed, and often brilliant in scope. The story of biomedicine in Africa from this perspective begins with the advent of "tropical medicine" and the establishment of makeshift African medical clinics across the nascent colonial landscape. Because Western scientific medicine was understood as the one "true" form of medicine, it was not so much a question of *replacing* African medical systems with superior medical systems. Rather, it was a question of explaining to the ignorant African masses that the enlightened European was bringing them a radical, foreign concept referred to simply as medicine. The primitive "medical" practices of the Africans that were observed and documented by the European were in no sense to be thought of as even in the same conceptual category as biomedicine. Consequently, medical historians have written stunning and often highly critical accounts of the development of biomedical systems under the auspices of colonial authorities alongside efforts to curb African pluralistic medicine by belittling and demonizing popular beliefs and practices.[22] The analysis of this ontological sphere of biomedicine in Africa, therefore, is well represented by medical historians and joins the longer narrative of Western efforts to promote scientific progress and the ideals of the enlightenment—hence the emphasis on how biomedicine changed Africa and not vice versa.

Medical anthropology joins the story of biomedicine in Africa, emphasizing a second angle of vision, and biomedicine as a symbolic-cultural expression is brought into view. The scholarly output of medical anthropology with respect to biomedicine in Africa easily matches that of the other two camps combined, and the contributions of medical anthropology in this regard have been far-sweeping and tremendously influential. For this reason, many aspects of their account have dominated the Western understanding of biomedicine in Africa. Foremost in this respect is the localized analysis of the cultural transformation of popular medical beliefs and practices. Medical

[22] See, for example, Aidoo (1982), Beck (1970, 1981), C. Good (1991), Hopwood (1980), and Lasker (1977).

anthropology offers spectacular accounts of the Africans' encounters with biomedicine—tales of skillful adaptations alongside ardent resistance—and how these encounters have transformed African life and society at times for the better and, at times, for the worse.[23] Given the great attention paid to local, community-level, ethnographic detail, the profound nature of biomedicine's transformation of African cultures has been especially well documented. In part, due to the powerful imagery of these compelling and often moving accounts of social disruption, the focus on biomedicine's impact on Africa has largely muted the story of Africans' impact on biomedicine. Indeed, in light of the volume of materials produced by medical anthropology, this ontological sphere has tended to cast the longest shadow across the Western imagination with respect to biomedicine in Africa.

In comparison with the first two ontological spheres, biomedicine as an expression of social power has received only modest attention. Those writing from the perspective of political economy tend to present biomedicine in Africa as secondary to the analysis of Western imperialism or of capitalism in African. As such, biomedicine frequently appears more as a bit player in a larger geopolitical drama, than as the central character. Consequently, analyses of biomedicine (and medical care in general) serve the purpose either of revealing the great depths of social poverty across Africa or of providing a proxy for the maldistribution of social resources. Given the breadth of approaches informing international political economy, those describing biomedicine in Africa from this perspective represent a wide variety of views.[24] Depictions of biomedicine's third ontological sphere generally provide glimpses of biomedicine in Africa as an extension of colonial rule and a multipronged point of contact between the African and European. There is a tendency within this literature, however, to frame African health and medicine as a direct function of social inequality and Western exploitation. It follows that it is primarily the lack of sufficient biomedical resources and not any attendant patterns of cultural disruptions that are viewed as the major catastrophe for Africa. The contemporary AIDS epidemic is a case in point. The underlying rationale of this perspective, therefore, shares certain ideological beliefs with the medical historians' camp regarding the virtues of scientific progress as a one-way transaction from the West to Africa and offers few insights regarding Africa's impact on biomedicine.

A common feature of Western depictions of biomedicine's introduction to Africa, addressed in varying fashion by all three camps, are the "African medical campaigns"—those heroic Western efforts to combat long-standing

[23] See, for example, Comaroff (1993), Evans-Pritchard (1937), Janzen (1978), Ranger (1988), and Vaughan (1994).

[24] See, for example, D. Ferguson (1979), Lyons (1988a), Marks (1996), and Turshen (1984).

African plagues such as malaria, yaws, or sleeping sickness. The African medical campaign presents biomedicine as an ideological metaphor for the benevolent, developmental colonial intentions of the West. Indeed, African medical campaigns are strategically situated at the center of explicit efforts to advance medical science, improve the general health of Europe's colonial subjects, and reshape African worldviews. Efforts to treat yaws in East Africa are a case in point. The 1920s yaws eradication campaign was unique among African medical campaigns both for the attention given to a disease that tended only to impact Africans and for the campaign's rapid medical successes. Over the course of a decade, a vast assembly of medical missions and satellite government dispensaries was able to reach well over seven hundred thousand persons in Kenya alone (Dawson, 1987a:425). The scale of the campaign's success, along with the novel use of syringes, offered opportunities for the popularization of biomedicine. As a means of cultural conversion, however, the yaws campaign ultimately proved less than overwhelming.[25] Nonetheless, the campaign advanced a vital ideological interest of the British by positioning them as champions of science-based medicine and as kind and compassionate overlords who strove mightily to improve the health of their African subjects. This ideological interest, in fact, explains why such tales of valiant medical campaigns, from Dr. Livingston forward, occupy so central a role in standard Western narratives of biomedicine in Africa.

The complexities of depicting biomedicine's introduction to Africa, therefore, reflect the need, on the one hand, to capture biomedicine as an ontological whole and, on the other hand, to detail its journey to Africa on three spatial-temporal levels across a single global unit of analysis. To do all this, however, still leaves us with a story that is fundamentally flawed. From an African perspective, after all, the story of biomedicine in Africa concerns how Africans borrowed select elements from a provincial European medical system, which allowed them, thereby, to deepen and further develop their own African medical systems. For Africa, it was not a matter of the universalization of biomedicine at the expense of African medicine. It was a matter of "particularizing" biomedicine to permit its appropriation by Africans. Detailing this perspective allows one better to appreciate how Africa transformed biomedicine.

Africa's Appropriation of European Medicine

Contemporary African syncretic-medical systems are the products of ongoing historical-cultural exchanges between Western biomedicine and African

---

[25] See Clyde (1980), Dawson (1987a), and Ranger (1981).

pluralistic medicine, as shaped by the development of the historical structures and processes that comprise the capitalist world-system. The distinct collective worldviews reflected by these African syncretic-medical systems reinforce the prominence of local influences over global influences in shaping medical systems. These worldviews also represent Africa's reinterpretation and enduring transformation of biomedicine as a historical-cultural formation at the global level. With respect to collective worldviews, the actual African syncretic-medical systems that resulted from Africa's encounter with biomedicine reflect many more African elements derived from African pluralistic medicine and far fewer elements of Western biomedicine than may appear to be the case at first glance. This follows primarily from two basic circumstances. First, prior to biomedicine, African pluralistic-medical systems already featured many of the fundamental organizing principles of biomedicine. Second, given the far more narrow worldview reflected in Western biomedicine, it only stood to reason that biomedicine would be absorbed into African pluralistic medicine rather than vice versa. This is made most apparent via a brief inventory of the common elements that inform the collective worldviews of African pluralistic medicine, absent biomedicine's influence, and that are no less relevant for African syncretic medicine *after* biomedicine's influence.

One of the principle distinctions between biomedicine and African pluralistic medicine—and the basis for claims of an African/Western cultural dualism—are contrasting notions of disease etiology.[26] Whereas biomedicine restricts explanations of disease to the natural world of physical phenomena, African pluralistic medicine generally frames disease within the broader category of personal or collective misfortune and attributes causes in holistic fashion across the natural, supernatural, and social worlds. In other words, from an African perspective, biomedical etiology is largely compatible with the precepts of African pluralistic medicine. It follows that from an African perspective, notwithstanding a broader cosmological sensibility, most of the etiological precepts of biomedicine are already present in African pluralistic medicine. Indeed, as detailed by Evans-Pritchard and others (see Chapter 4), explanations of disease attributed to the natural world are frequently the first and only cause of illness treated by African pluralistic-medical practitioners who routinely adhere to the basic principles of empirical-rational investigation. However, because disease is inseparable from the larger category of misfortune, it is often the case that African pluralistic-medical practitioners combine the diagnosis of a natural cause with a supernatural or social explanation to identify the underlying malevolent forces that brought on the

[26] See, for example, Horton (1967), Mbiti (1970), and Mburu (1977).

natural cause. Consequently, the vast literature on witchcraft, magic, and sorcery in Africa has significantly distorted the West's understanding of African pluralistic medicine, emphasizing that which dramatically distinguishes it from biomedicine and minimizing that which complements biomedicine. From an African perspective, therefore, there is very little about the etiology of biomedicine—save for its oddly narrow perspective—that is foreign or incompatible with the more holistic approach of African pluralistic medicine.

A second feature of African pluralistic medicine with respect to its incorporation of biomedicine concerns its pragmatic attitude toward "foreign" medical systems. African pluralistic-medical systems are the result of an ongoing historical-cultural exchange of values, beliefs, and practices across peoples which freely mixes and combines elements from the medical system of one ethnic group with those of another. It is for this reason that the idyllic notion of discovering a pure and unadulterated African medical system is so untenable. Through the centuries, prior to biomedicine's arrival, the primary sources of such influence were neighboring African medical systems and, in certain regions such as East Africa, the regular contact with Arab traders. Over time, such exchanges have not resulted in a uniform or universal set of African pluralistic-medical systems, but a collection of medical systems that reflect at a general level certain common elements. Thus, not only were biomedicine's natural explanations of disease compatible with the belief system of African pluralistic medicine, in addition it was a long-established practice to borrow liberally from other medical systems. As a consequence, though the harsh colonial context of biomedicine's imposition significantly clouded its greeting, it would not have been inconsistent with African past practice to try to learn from and incorporate key aspects of biomedicine with their own medical systems.

An additional characteristic of African pluralistic medicine that caused it both to mesh and conflict with biomedicine concerned the conceptualization of medical care as both a valuable item of exchange and as a form of social obligation. While not a point of major emphasis in the vast library of Western ethnographies on African pluralistic medicine, this literature is nonetheless notably replete with examples of practitioners across African pluralistic-medical systems who provide services either on the condition of compensation (with fees ranging from modest to exorbitant) or in fulfillment of communal services linked to ancestral obligations. Prior to any contact with biomedicine, therefore, the commodity form of African pluralistic medicine was well established. The social attitudes and values reflected in the practice of individuals using their specialized healing knowledge either for personal gain or to fulfill communal obligations was, in fact, directly challenged by the outwardly munificent and selfless initial overtures of biomedicine. The earliest African contact with biomedicine, offered through missionaries and through colonial government dispensaries, ran very much counter to established African values and practices. In these cases, services were invariably free, suggesting biomedicine entailed little or no exchange value. (To this day, routine care through biomedical clinics is commonly less expensive than the care of African pluralistic-medical practitioners.) At the same time, given their foreign status, the provision of biomedicine could not be tied to any communal obligations of the European to the African. Operating well outside the norms of African pluralistic medicine, the European claimed to want nothing in return but the good health and possible goodwill of Africans. Alongside the more destructive and exploitive colonial practices, this offer no doubt must have seemed less than convincing.

The introduction of biomedicine thus precipitated a protracted process of historical-cultural transition from African pluralistic medicine to African syncretic medicine. In the context of colonial rule, this was certainly at times a violent and bloody affair. From the perspective of shifting worldviews, however, the transition was significantly less contentious. This was because, while colonial proponents of biomedicine may have rejected many features of African pluralistic medicine, Africans found many core features of biomedicine itself to be quite compatible with the health beliefs and practices of African pluralistic medicine. Indeed, those syncretic medical systems that have emerged across Africa are but among the latest incarnations of biomedicine, as a historical-cultural formation, to result from the combination of local medical beliefs and practices in peripheralized societies and the beliefs and practices of core-based biomedicine. That is why the notion of "African syncretic medicine" is, in fact, a misnomer. More accurately, it is simply African biomedicine.

Capturing local social change in the context of but not reduced to global forces, while simultaneously recognizing that the global system is itself subject to the influences of local peoples and societies, remains an analytical challenge of the first order. For the reasons discussed above, it is believed that an expanded treatment of world-systems analysis will accomplish this. The analysis of biomedicine in Africa that follows is an attempt to validate this claim as well as to re-position Africans at the center of their own history and athwart the gathering winds of world-historical transformation.

2

Dissecting Western Medicine

Biomedicine emerged in the mid-19th century, as a hybrid branch of the biological sciences, at a unique historical moment in the socio-cultural development of the capitalist world-system.[1] By the early decades of the 20th century, having demonstrated its value as an effective tool for the diagnosis, treatment, and prevention of disease, Western scientific medicine had become singularly identified with biomedicine. The techniques and symbols of biomedicine (such as vaccinations, laboratory testing, and high-tech gadgetry) captured the popular imagination of the West and its methods were associated with advanced, "scientific" medical care. At the same time, as an emerging profit-generating venture, biomedicine was the source of fierce battles among physicians and between physicians and corporate interests. A unique combination of scientific-material, symbolic-cultural, and social-institutional influences has thus shaped Western interpretations of biomedicine from its beginnings and through its ongoing formation. The image of biomedicine that has emerged is

[1] Use of the term "biomedicine" here connotes a set of underlying epistemological and ontological rationales that is unique to Western scientific medicine. "[T]he term biomedicine emphasizes the established institutional structure of the dominant profession of medicine in the West, and today worldwide, while also conjuring the primary of its epistemological and ontological commitments, which are what is most radically different about this form of medicine" (Kleinman, 1993:16). At the same time, "It is no longer only Western, in its site of practice or in its locus of knowledge production and technological innovation" (Kleinman, 1995:25).

multifold—biomedicine as a scientific enterprise, biomedicine as a symbolic-cultural expression, and biomedicine as an expression of social power. Each of these interpretations corresponds with a unique ontological sphere comprising a set of phenomena subject to distinct investigative techniques. Importantly, therefore, both the actual material forms thought to comprise biomedicine and the methods by which meaning is attached to these material forms vary across ontological spheres. Each sphere is not merely a separate world; it is a separate perception of reality.

The analysis of biomedicine thus begins with a dissection of its multilayered appearance which reveals, at one and the same time, several manifold and overlapping ontological spheres, each intersecting and interdependent with, and yet distinct from, the others. The relationships and mutual influences that constitute these spheres develop in a reflexive, rather then determinative or reductionist, fashion. Thus, where differences of interpretation emerge, they reflect basic tensions and contradictions within biomedicine itself as an ontological whole, and not merely the inherent ontological limits of a particular perspective. Furthermore, as a singular historical-cultural formation across the capitalist world-system, biomedicine contains ontological spheres that are comprised of varying levels of abstraction, which correspond with specific spatial-temporal locations across a single global unit of analysis with multiple social times. In other words, the manifest phenomena (material, ideological, cultural, and so forth) that comprise each ontological sphere must be located in a specific temporal dimension (the *longue durée*, middle-range episodes, or short-term events) and a corresponding spatial unit of analysis. Capturing biomedicine as an ontological whole, therefore, requires both the dissection of its multiple ontological spheres and the unraveling of each sphere's multiple social times and spatial locations.

Understood as a scientific enterprise, biomedicine's scientific-material content reifies those forms of technical-utilitarian knowledge associated with scientific reason and the 18th-century rise of the physical sciences. From this perspective, biomedicine's universal beliefs and practices are located within the progressive train of scientific history and modern biomedicine is celebrated as the summative achievement of four hundred years of Western Enlightenment thought. Thus beholden to an Enlightenment ethic of ceaseless, utilitarian progress and innovation, biomedicine embraces medical practices that follow the strict empirical norms of the experimental sciences. Human health or disease is defined as any variance from the normal statistical ranges for the species's regular physiological functioning, and the human body itself is laid before biomedicine as a soulless, multifunctional machine whose detailed internal structures require precise probing via a sophisticated complement of capital-intensive biotechnology. As such, biomedicine today is unmistakably identified with a range of scientific-material forms (from syringes to CAT scans) that mediate the relationship between physician and disease, between physician as active investigator and patient as passive object, and between the patient (a full person) and his or her body (a mass of biochemical functions and reactions). As a scientific enterprise, objectivity, standardization, and the peer-reviewed rigor of the scientific method provide biomedicine with the only conceivable investigative techniques for its phenomenal forms. Science as praxis is thus essential to any representation of biomedicine. It is one side of biomedicine as an ontological whole. While it would be mistaken to accept what is found within this sphere (its scientific-material forms) uncritically, it would be equally foolish to lose sight of biomedicine's material content. It is necessary, therefore, to hold this side of biomedicine in view while simultaneously bringing its other sides into the frame.

Understood as a symbolic-cultural expression, biomedicine represents a multifaceted social construct that reveals the material-ideological contours of Western capitalist societies from the mid-19th century forward. As such, the symbolic content of biomedicine rests precariously upon the universal claims made on its behalf as a product of objective, scientific reason—the one true form of medical understanding free of sociocultural contingency. Those who view biomedicine as a symbolic-cultural expression, therefore, attempt to isolate those unique, cultural vestiges that distinguish it from medical systems in other non-Western cultural settings.[2] Were biomedicine treated as just one ethnomedicine among others, then the veracity of its beliefs and practices would merely be relative to those of other cultures and contingent on, and therefore limited to, Western capitalist societies.[3] For this reason, from a symbolic-cultural perspective, biomedicine's phenomenal forms are intentionally framed (by the West) to demonstrate both their intrinsic value and their universal superiority over all others. The appropriate methods for investigating these forms, and thus revealing the perception of reality open to biomedicine as a symbolic-cultural expression, call for a battery of interpretive techniques of investigation. The self-ascribed beliefs and practices of biomedicine are subjected to cultural critique in an effort to expose their internalized social meanings and thereby to understand and represent biomedicine as a unique ethnomedicine. The distillation of its symbolic-cultural content, therefore, reveals a further side of biomedicine,

[2] For the purposes of analysis here, "non-Western" refers to those societies that are not today among the advanced capitalist nations and were not direct participants in the post-Enlightenment ferment of the 18th and 19th centuries.

[3] Feierman (1985), for example, argues that, "[African pluralistic medicine] and biomedicine are forms of ethnomedicine: They are embedded within a system of social relations, and give concrete form to assumptions about reality drawn from the wider culture, which in turn influences the wider culture" (p. 110).

exposing elements not visible to the positivist gaze.[4] Biomedicine as a symbolic-cultural expression, therefore, peers beneath the veil of scientific dogma, and the ideological images that emerge are no less a part of biomedicine than is penicillin or the mammogram.

Understood as an expression of social power, biomedicine represents a complex of social institutions (manifest forms of contentious social power relations), which reflects its origins among competing social forces in the late 19th century. Biomedicine was born in an era of large-scale social and political upheaval across the Western world. The rise of industrial capitalism unleashed unprecedented forms of concentrated economic power and staggering social dislocation.[5] In effect, both biomedicine and industrial capitalism were products of an Enlightenment heritage that spawned the intellectual lineage of Galileo, Bichat and Claude Bernard alongside that of Smith, Bentham and Mill. For this reason, biomedicine as a complex of social institutions has proven remarkably compatible with the interests of corporate power. Its values, practices, and organizing principles reflect the utilitarian, profit-motivated, and commodifying ethos of capitalist production. As such, biomedicine's ubiquitous social-institutional forms—such as centralized hospitals, medical universities, biotech firms, physicians' professional associations—are generally mistaken for natural features of a medical system itself rather than points of tension that reveal contentious social power relations. Biomedicine as an expression of social power thus exposes a third side of biomedicine. Just as the scientific-material content and symbolic-cultural elements of biomedicine require unique methodological strategies, so too does biomedicine as an expression of social power. In this case, exposing the underlying dynamics of social power entails analyzing biomedicine as a social institution whose development coincided with a unique period in the history of the capitalist world-system.

Thus, the apparent contradictions between biomedicine as an objective science and biomedicine as a value-laden cultural form are further complicated by the story of biomedicine as the product of a struggle for the vested interests of competing social factions. Ultimately, there is no one true image or representation of biomedicine as an ontological whole and it is only by unraveling the multiple, embedded ontologies that comprise biomedicine that

---

[4] As Rhodes observes, "The issue is not simply the description of biomedicine but the discovery of strategies that will make visible its nature as a cultural system" (1996:167).

[5] Hobsbawn captures the two-fold transformation of industrial capitalism in this era. "On the one hand there was the concentration of capital, the growth in scale which led men to distinguish between 'business' and 'big business,' the retreat of the free competitive market, and all the other developments which, around 1900, led observers to grope for general labels to describe what plainly seemed to be a new phase of economic development. On the other hand, there was the systematic attempt to rationalize production and the conduct of business enterprise by applying 'scientific methods' not only to technology but to organization and calculation" (1989:52–53).

an understanding of biomedicine can begin. In other words, the manifold forms and multiple sides of biomedicine must not be envisaged as different truths about biomedicine. Rather, these are evolving constituent elements, whose dialectical combination and ongoing reconstitution make the conceptualization of biomedicine possible. The analysis that follows attempts to make plain the contours of each of these spheres that comprise biomedicine as an ontological whole.

Biomedicine as a Scientific Enterprise

Biomedicine is informed by a coherent and totalizing worldview that organizes and universalizes its values, beliefs, and practices. The analysis of biomedicine as a scientific enterprise thus presents a certain paradox. On the one hand, it is true that the representatives of biomedicine (physicians, medical researchers, lab technicians, and so forth) largely conceive of it as an objective, value-neutral science that is essentially independent of cultural and social influences.[6] On the other hand, few if any, historians of biomedicine adopt this simple caricature. Rather, several generations of medical historians have provided rich descriptions of the social and political factors shaping the development of biomedicine.[7] Nonetheless, inclusive as such accounts of biomedicine may be, the history of biomedicine as a scientific enterprise remains faithful to an underlying narrative that conceives of it as an objective science whose progressive development—notwithstanding occasional external influences—has unfolded with linear precision as a series of scientific discoveries and breakthroughs. The purpose here is to trace the outline of this narrative.

Contemporary biomedicine slowly crystallized as a scientific enterprise over the 18th and 19th centuries. It was in this period that the scientific method (empirical, experimental research) solidified its prominence as an epistemological orientation within the physical sciences.[8] In this manner, the birth of biomedicine introduced a radical new way of thinking (and worldview) among practitioners as well as a growing body of knowledge. The major medical developments across these centuries are as much associated with efforts to supplant anachronistic modes of thought (for example, humoral pathology) as with actual advances in knowledge (such as bacteriology). It is, therefore, difficult to understand biomedicine, as a scientific enterprise,

---

[6] See Bynum (1994), Engel (1977), Gillett (2004), and Wright and Treacher (1982).

[7] McNeill (1976), Miller (1957), and Porter (1997), for example, are typical of the medical historians' more nuanced approach.

[8] For a discussion of the influence of 18th-century positivist, mechanistic developments within the physical sciences on medicine see Engel (1977), Gadamer (1996), Magner (1992), Osherson and Amarasingham (1981), and Shryock (1969).

absent the social and ideological transformations wrought by Bacon, Locke, Newton, and the Age of Reason. The empirical sciences provided biomedicine with a set of tools for investigation as well as a new, self-assured identity. "[M]edicine's burst of development came with the displacement of the criterion of truth from tradition and rationality to 'look and see'" (Gordon, 1988:33).

This triumphant era of science signaled two major reforms. First, there was a seismic shift in attitudes. A basic belief in progress and the ability to control nature replaced long-standing traditions that relied more fatalistically upon God's will.[9] The doctrine of the new age of science called for calculated, proactive intervention for specific and predictable ends. A utilitarian, instrumentalist ethic prevailed. Second, there were important epistemological developments associated with empiricism and rationalism. Observation, measurement, and experimentation, modeled after the investigative techniques of Galileo and Newton, became the customary methods for assuring truth and objectivity. Any deviation from these strict empirical procedures was thought to risk allowing individual subjectivity to influence the results. Stephen Hale's measurement of blood pressure (1733) and Albrecht von Haller's 18th-century experimental physiology exemplified the new influences of empiricism and rationalism.[10] "[T]he basic principle of science of the day, as enunciated by Galileo, Newton and Descartes, was analytical, meaning that entities to be investigated be resolved into isolable causal chains or units, from which it was assumed that the whole could be understood, both materially and conceptually, by reconstituting the parts" (Engel, 1977:131).[11]

---

[9] "Religion and medicine were closely associated in Europe until relatively recent times. In the medieval period, it was the religious orders that maintained the hospitals and infirmaries and this association has continued in some institutions to the present day. Religious interpretations were placed upon illness and relief from suffering was sought in the healing rites of the church. The central theme in the theistic response to man's vulnerability to disease and suffering is resignation to the will of God" (Powles, 1973:17).

[10] Reflecting the era's relatively loose disciplinary boundaries, there were, likewise, considerable contributions by those trained in medicine to the fields of physics, chemistry, and biology—including, Helmhotz and Du Bois-Reymond in physics, Davy, Wöhler, and Berzelius in chemistry, and Johannes Müller, Huxley, and Haeckel in biology (Shryock, 1969:120).

[11] Comaroff's experience in Southern Africa is instructive with respect to the inherent limitations of Western science and the basic differences between Western science and some non-Western cosmologies that follow from these limitations. "In parts of Southern Africa, indigenous peoples are aware of the connection between the louse and typhus fever, and will often avail themselves of Western treatment if they develop appropriate symptoms. However, they frequently also seek divination and indigenous therapy. Here, the fact that Western treatment may relieve symptoms is often evident; but it does not solve the fundamental experiential problem of 'who sent the louse?'" (Comaroff, 1978:251).

Consequently, from this perspective, biomedicine represents the culmination of a long history of (Western)[12] advancements in medical knowledge from Galen's humoral pathology through Thomas Sydenham's doctrine of specificity to the current genome mapping, which were made possible by dramatic shifts in how medical science was conducted and understood. This history is marked by major moments of advance (for example, bacteriology) and long periods of stagnation. Greek tradition weighed heavily on Western medicine from the time of Galen's death around A.D. 200 through the 18th century (Nutton, 1983). The humoral theories advanced by Galen attributed illness to imbalances between the essential body fluids (blood, bile, and such). Treatment focused on efforts to restore corporeal harmony as a general state of the body. Consequently, the investigation of distinct causal agents outside the body was not a concern. "[A]s long as one general state of the body was assumed to underlie all illness, there was no great interest in causal factors (etiology) . . . What had originally caused the bilious, the dropsical, or the feverish state of the system was not so important as was the question of how one dealt with such a condition once it had appeared" (Shryock, 1953:224).

Humoral pathology continued to inform and frame medical thinking in the West until the mid-18th century when a handful of Sydenham's followers, building on the 16th-century insights of Paracelsus, sought to overturn its influence by proposing that, in fact, there were a great many types of diseases and that each had a unique and specific cause.[13] Sydenham's ideas have been attributed, in part, to the fact that he primarily concerned himself with clinical care (and, therefore, the empirical description of symptoms) rather than with the investigation of the specific causes of disease (Hahn, 1984; Shryock, 1969). This made him especially cognizant of the variety of disease types he was confronting.[14] These empirical observations, along with the skepticism of Paracelsus, William Harvey and others, prompted Sydenham to push medicine to abandon humoral pathology.

---

[12] The literature treating biomedicine as a scientific enterprise focuses overwhelmingly on the history of Western medicine, with the assumption that non-Western medicine is increasingly influenced by Western medical practices over time. For a discussion of this exclusive focus on Western traditions see Temkin (1977a).

[13] In a parallel fashion, Engelhardt and Tristam trace the contrast between ontological and physiological theories of illness (1975). See also Fábrega (1997) and Temkin (1977d) in this regard.

[14] The analytical and cultural distinctions between the terms "disease" and "illness" have been widely discussed. See L. Eisenberg (1977), Engelhardt and Tristam (1975), Gadamer (1996), and Hahn (1984). In general, disease refers to observed abnormalities in the function and/or structure of body organs and systems. Illness refers to how people subjectively experience abnormal health conditions (both as individuals and as members of larger groups). It is often said that patients suffer illness, while physicians treat disease.

The primary task of scientific medicine thus shifted to mapping the variety of distinct diseases and their causes. After Sydenham helped found nosology (the science of classifying diseases), Charles Linné, François Boissier de Sauvages, William Cullen, and others went on to create the grand nosological systems of the 18th and 19th centuries based on symptom clusters that classified diseases into orders, families, genera, and species. This was one of the first concrete steps to integrate the precision of science as an organizing principle of biomedicine. Engel (1977) details how this basic approach to disease has remained a cornerstone of biomedicine throughout the 20th century. "[T]axonomy progresses from symptoms, to clusters of symptoms, to syndromes and finally to diseases with specific pathogenesis and pathology. This sequence accurately describes the successful application of the scientific method to the elucidation and the classification into discrete entities of disease in its generic sense" (p. 131).

Advances in the study of human anatomy, beginning in the 16th century with the publication of Andreas Vesalius's *De Humani Corporis Fabrica* (1543), along with Harvey's description of the circulation of the blood, complemented these developments in nosology and culminated in G. B. Morgagni's highly influential *On the Seats and Causes of Diseases* (1761) which correlated disease patterns with findings from morbid anatomy. Just as nosology allowed physicians to link certain symptoms with specific diseases, pathological anatomy allowed researchers to link certain postmortem anatomical findings with specific diseases. All of these developments helped to advance the evolution of experimental pathology, and medicine was finally able to jettison its ancient humoral notions of disease when all such efforts culminated with the establishment of the Paris School—a hospital-based medical school dedicated to the development of the medical sciences—at the start of the 19th century.[15]

The highly influential Paris School played an instrumental role in reframing medicine as a scientific enterprise. It was here that biomedical researchers for the first time on a large-scale could simultaneously pursue clinical care and medical research as integrated activities.[16] One of the major

[15] Ironically, prior to the establishment of the Paris School, though Parisian scientific inquiry was much the envy of the world, it was in the one area of medicine that the French lagged. "The Paris of 1770–1800 became—so far as any one town could be—the world's scientific capital. In no city could there be found more brilliant and intensive research in mathematics, physics, chemistry and biology . . . All the sciences were advancing, one should add, except medicine" (Shryock, 1969:151–152).

[16] Importantly, it was the French Revolution (and the subsequent reorganization of social institutions) that gave the Paris School access to essential resources and material. "Building on its success in institutionalizing major reforms like the unification of medicine and surgery and the integration of the hospital clinic, the so-called Paris school became the world centre for medicine during the first half of the nineteenth century. Pathological anatomy, another innovation with

innovations of the Paris School was its use of the hospital system to generate a large sample of clinical cases to observe and from which to draw broader generalizations (T. Gelfand, 1993; Rosen, 1974b). Typical of this approach was the work of Pierre Louis, a clinician who sought to apply his "numerical method" (a form of statistical reasoning) to clinical understanding. Louis was highly critical of his physician colleagues for their sloppy, haphazard approach to diagnosis and therapeutics. "Physicians, he observed, witnessed a few fatal cases where no blood-letting was employed, and thereupon jumped to the conclusion that this process would have saved them. Other practitioners, noted a few cases where death *followed* a resort to blood-letting, and denounced the practice as the whole cause of death. In neither instance did they employ any check or test of their sweeping conclusions. '*Quels faits*!' exclaimed Louis, '*quelle logic*! [sic]' " (emphasis in original, Shryock, 1969:160). By the 1840s, large-scale clinical observations, combined with statistical reasoning, was firmly established as a norm of medical practice across much of the West.[17]

As biomedicine attempted to develop as a basic science, its greatest obstacle concerned a lack of instruments to make precise observations in the manner of physics and chemistry. Pathological anatomy, for example, was initially of limited value to clinicians insofar as it required the observation of conditions within the body. The introduction of Auenbrugger's percussion technique (1761) and Laënnec's stethoscope (1819) allowed clinicians to make greater use of these findings. Prior to this, the physician had to rely on a patient's description of symptoms (Figlio, 1976; Osherson and Amarasingham, 1981). By the mid-19th century, the diagnosis of disease remained largely an art and only partially a science. This began to change in the second half of the 19th century with a flurry of inventive activity, highlighted by Hermann von Helmhotz's ophthalmoscope, otoscope, and laryngoscope to examine the eye, ear, and throat in the 1850s; Etienne-Jules Marey's sphygmograph to measure pulse rates in 1860; Samuel von Basch's sphygmomanometer to monitor blood pressure in 1876; Augustus D. Waller's use of the electrometer (an 1872 invention) to record the electrical currents generated by the heart in 1887; and Wilhelm Röntgen's discovery of X-rays in 1895.

The technological inventions of this era allowed physicians further to develop medicine as a quantitative, empirical science and to view their work

---

eighteenth-century antecedents, particularly within surgery, and heavily dependent on the large numbers of cadavers furnished by the state charity hospitals, emerged as the basis for a new science of disease" (T. Gelfand, 1993:1132).

[17]"J. F. Double observed in 1842 that all critics now admitted the great value of statistics in therapeutic studies, despite the disadvantages involved" (Shryock, 1969:167).

as contributing to scientific progress more generally.[18] The new bio-tech gadgetry instilled physicians with a sense of detached objectivity and greater certainty—on par, at last, with their peers in physics and chemistry—with respect to the precise measurement of physiological phenomena.[19] Biomedicine could finally rely upon a common set of diagnostic instruments that would minimize the subjectivity of the physician (and of the patient) and the human body could be studied as a complex organism with integrated, functional systems, whose discrete parts were subject to direct observation and measurement.[20]

> The conversion of physiological signals generated by respiration, circulation and heat production into graphs and numbers allowed physicians to obtain clear and accurate records; to preserve these signals so that changes in pattern could be studied over time; to free these signals from the limitations of private analysis—necessary when they were individually monitored by the natural senses—and open them to group inquiry; to make them objective and to invest them with unambiguous meanings that were evident to all physicians. (Reiser, 1978:121)

The delayed popularization of the thermometer (and temperature monitoring) illustrates the evolution of physician attitudes toward technology in light of biomedicine's scientific advances. The thermometer had been available to physicians for several centuries, however by the mid-19th century, its clinical use remained the exception. This changed dramatically in 1868 when

[18] See Osherson and Amarasingham (1981), Reiser (1978), Turshen (1977a), and Wightman (1971).

[19] Advances in the techniques of diagnosis notwithstanding, physician judgment continued to play a key role. A 1930 study found that, though presented with similar cases, physician judgments could vary widely (Reiser, 1978). A group of 300 school children were examined by 20 physicians to determine if any required a tonsillectomy. Roughly one-half were recommended for the procedure. The other half was then examined by a second set of physicians. Again, one-half were recommended for surgery. The remaining half was then examined by a third set of physicians and again tonsillectomy was recommended for one-half of this group. By the 1950s, it was recommended that further studies of observer disagreement among physicians be discontinued as it was harming professional morale.

[20] As explored below, these new technologies marked a significant shift in doctor-patient relationships. Previously, the doctor had relied on the patient's subjective account of symptoms. Increasingly, physicians came to view disease as a localized disorder in the body that was accessed via objective readings of specialized instruments. "The localization of illness changed the status of the patient's body; no longer was it primarily the seat of subjective impressions interpreted by the patient to the doctor, but rather it became the site of specific disease entities to be detected and evaluated by the doctor independently of the patient" (Osherson and Amarasingham, 1981:224). See Hahn (1982), as well, for a discussion of the evolving medical notion of the patient.

Carl Wunderlich published *On the Temperature in Diseases.* Wunderlich's massive study of temperature fluctuation and clinical care involved nearly twenty-five thousand patients and millions of individual temperature readings. Particularly impressive for physicians was Wunderlich's demonstration of the thermometer as an objective, unbiased measure of temperature. "Wunderlich's treatise elevated thermometry to a highly regarded diagnostic technique in the 1870s. Many physicians declared that thermometer readings were beyond control of the patient's will, or of extraneous circumstances, and thus were unerringly accurate" (Reiser, 1978:118).[21]

All of these technological developments, alongside significant progress in the field of experimental pathology, led to a period of extraordinary advances in medical knowledge with respect to the causes and prevention of disease. Most dramatic in this regard were the breakthroughs witnessed in the area of bacteriology (and insect-born diseases). Between 1800 and 1850, the disciples of Sydenham and Linné had moved beyond general symptoms and were able to classify a great many diseases that are recognized today, such as diphtheria, gastric ulcer, multiple sclerosis, typhoid fever, and malaria. Indeed, by the mid-19th century, the medical sciences were avidly pursuing specific causal agents for these newly identified diseases, culminating in Robert Koch's discovery of *tubercle bacillus* in 1882 and Louis Pasteur's rabies vaccine in 1885. Medical science, in the form of bacteriology, now focused on specific pathogenic microorganisms.

Disease came to be seen as a reaction of particular parts of the body (organs, tissues, cells) to certain stimuli. Though it only addressed infectious diseases, the influence of bacteriology on the general notion of disease was

---

[21] At the same time, the role of technology to establish "normal" levels of biological function raised more fundamental issues. King (1954) describes the circular logic that predominates within biomedicine, for example, when establishing the "normal ranges" of specific physiological traits.

> I recall a very precise young physician who asked me what our laboratory considered the normal hemoglobin level of the blood (with the particular technique we used). When I answered, 'Twelve to sixteen grams, more or less,' he was very puzzled. Most laboratories, he pointed out, called 15 grams normal, or perhaps 14.5. He wanted to know how, if my norm was so broad and vague, he could possibly tell whether a patient suffered from anemia, or how much anemia. I agreed that he had quite a problem on his hands, and that it is a very difficult thing to tell. So difficult, in fact, that trying to be too precise is actually misleading, inaccurate, stultifying to thought and philosophically very unsound.
>
> He wanted to know why I didn't take one hundred or so normal individuals, determine their hemoglobin by our method, and use the resulting figure as the normal value for our method. This, I agreed, was a splendid idea. But how were we to pick out the normals? The obvious answer, just take one or two hundred healthy people, free of the disease . . . But that is exactly the difficulty. We think health as freedom from disease [sic], and disease as an aberration from health. This is traveling in circles, getting us nowhere. (p. 195)

profound and far-reaching.[22] "It was not only the substance of bacteriology, but its role as a vehicle for the infusion of the ideology of science into medicine, which made it pivotal in the history of scientific medicine" (Maulitz, 1979:92). Diseases, it was believed, had specific and definite causes. The study of invading microbes and the manner of their transmission became the primary focus, as applications of the germ theory of disease increasingly organized medical research. For biomedicine, the body as a whole (the person) was no longer a primary point of reference.

The basic idea behind the germ theory of disease was not new. Scores of dogs and cats had been routinely destroyed as a prophylactic measure during plagues throughout the Middle Ages. Marcus Plenciz had proposed a germ theory of disease in 1762, based on the earlier work of Antony von Leeuwenhoek and others. However, developments in experimental pathology following the establishment of the Paris School gave germ theory a firmer foundation. So long as one disease was indistinguishable from another (for instance, diphtheria from malaria) it was not possible to identify distinct pathogenic organisms. Earlier speculation about living microorganisms as a source of disease contagion was also better understood after the development of the achromatic microscope in the 1830s and its later refinements. However, as the search for pathogenic organisms grew among 19th-century medical researchers, it remained for a definitive causal link to be established between a specific microorganism and a specific disease.

In 1840, faithful to the basic principles of the scientific method, Jacob Henle outlined the criteria for asserting a causal relationship. First, a parasite must be consistently associated with a specific disease and *not* with others. Second, a parasite must be isolated and it must be demonstrated that it is capable of causing the disease. It was not until 1876 that Robert Koch, a student of Henle, was able to identify a definitive, causal link between *anthrax bacillus* and disease in animals based on this criteria. (Pasteur reached the same results independently at roughly the same time.) Following Koch and Pasteur's breakthroughs, laboratories and special medical institutes were established across Germany and France and a period of rapid discoveries ensued.[23] In 1882, Koch identified *tubercle bacillus* as the cause of tuberculosis. This was followed by the discoveries of *comma bacillus* (cholera's origin) and *diphtheria bacillus* in 1883, and then *typhoid bacillus* and *tetanus bacillus* in 1884. The causes behind the bubonic plague and syphilis were identified in 1894 and 1905, respectively. Using similar scientific principles, the roles of certain insects and worms were

---

[22] See Brandt and Gardner (2000), Dubos (1959), Maulitz (1979), and Temkin (1977b).

[23] The first U.S. laboratories were established in 1892 at the University of Pennsylvania.

discovered for other diseases such as malaria (1898), yellow fever (1901), and sleeping sickness (1905). Finally, for the first time, medical science was able to demonstrate definitively the ability to prevent some of the dread diseases that had haunted the West for centuries. Biomedicine was firmly established as the dominant form of medical explanation in the West.[24]

It was not long before the science of immunology made use of these breakthroughs in bacteriology. Earlier efforts to inoculate against smallpox had already demonstrated that inoculation with a weak virus could produce a mild case of a disease that afforded protection from a later, more severe case.[25] The identification of specific organisms that caused diseases now provided a rationale for developing further immunizations. These efforts were led by the same medical scientists who had engineered advances in bacteriology. Shryock recounts Pasteur's "happy accident" that contributed to his development of vaccines for anthrax and rabies.

> Having isolated the organisms he thought responsible for chicken cholera, he proceeded to prove this by injecting them into healthy fowls. The latter promptly died and the organisms were recovered from their bodies. This would ordinarily have been viewed as the end of the project; the cause of the disease had been found. It happened, however, that some virulent cultures were put aside for several days in the course of the experiments. Then the birds, into which these were later injected, failed to die as expected. More remarkable still, the same birds refused to die even when inoculated with fresh cultures ordinarily lethal for their kind. Pasteur, quick to sense the significance of the seeming accident, realized that the inoculation with stale, attenuated cultures had in some way provided protection against further infection. Perhaps the attenuated virus was able to arouse a protective mechanism in the bird, which in turn was powerful enough to ward off later attacks of a more serious character. The analogy with smallpox inoculation was now apparent. Perhaps every pathogenic virus could be attenuated as soon as it was discovered, and then be employed to provide protection against the very disease for which it was responsible. (Shryock, 1969:294–295)

[24] Of course, for all of the impressive developments by those advocating germ theory, it remained the case that many respected physicians of the era continued to maintain that germs alone were insufficient to cause disease. See Dubos (1959) and Shryock (1969). In a rather miraculous bit of medical chutzpah, Max von Pettenkofer, a Munich sanitarian, confidently drank an entire glass of water swimming with cholera bacilli—a feat that should have killed him—and survived with no ill effect.

[25] See, for example, McNeill (1976) and Miller (1957).

The story of biomedicine as a scientific enterprise appears to unfold in a conveniently linear fashion following discovery after discovery on through the era of bacteriology and immunology into the early 20th century. Indeed, biomedicine's hegemonic grip on the popular imagination is inseparable from its impressive breakthroughs in the areas of bacteriology and immunology. These breakthroughs, however, were preceded by (and intersected with) waves of social activism in the form of public health campaigns that confronted unsanitary working and living conditions.[26] For this reason, a full accounting of biomedicine as a scientific enterprise must also include the unique contributions of working-class agitation and the scientific discoveries that followed therefrom.

With 19th-century industrialization came expanding areas of concentrated poverty. Urban populations were increasingly forced to live and work in highly unsanitary and unhealthy conditions. Given this link between poverty and disease, those advocating sanitary improvements shared much in common with those pushing for more generalized social reform.[27] "The significance of the sanitary movement of the 1830s for the history of mankind resides in the fact that it was the first conscious and organized effort not for the treatment of disease but for the creation of a healthier, happier world. Its leaders approached the problems of health with much practical skill, but it must never be forgotten that a philosophical and humanitarian doctrine was the inspiration of their pragmatic genius" (Dubos, 1959:182–183). Given advances in germ theory that made clear connections between pathogens and disease, by the second half of the 19th century many officials sought to protect the larger public from contagious diseases lurking in the swelling slums through investments in preventive public health measures. Such campaigns were certainly not new, as evidenced by the earlier efforts to inoculate the public against smallpox and yellow fever.[28] Nonetheless, while the principle of contagion may have been understood, the precise means of transmission (for example, insect or contaminated water) was not always clear.

Prior to the advent of the public health movement and developments in bacteriology, it was common to approach health and disease within a broader framework that included social factors. Rosen's history of "medical police" in the West is a case in point. "Awareness of the social problems of health and

---

[26] "The English sanitarians who became prominent in this period, were not usually in direct association with such radical reformers as [Francis] Place, [Robert] Owen and the Chartists. But like the latter, the sanitarians were brought face to face with the basic problems of poverty. There was in consequence much latent socialism in the views of such leaders as [Edwin] Chadwick, [John] Simon and [Thomas] Southwood Smith" (Shryock, 1969:221).

[27] See Dubos (1959), Stark (1977), and Zola (1972).

[28] See McNeill (1976), Miller (1957), and Porter (1997).

disease is evident throughout the early 19th century and is often found expressed in terms of medical police. Thus Gordon Smith in his *Principles of Forensic Medicine*, published in 1821, defined medical police as 'the application of medical knowledge to the benefit of man in his social state'" (Rosen, 1974a:153). Public health efforts in the first half of the 19th century produced a number of influential studies that assessed the impact of unsanitary conditions on health and morbidity. Such studies mirrored the advances in nosology that preceded the discovery of links between specific parasitic microbes and diseases. In 1828, Louis René Villermé developed a series of studies examining the relationship between neighborhoods and disease in different parts of Paris. In 1842, a comprehensive survey of national health in England was organized by Edwin Chadwick and presented in the form of a report to the Poor Law Board. In 1848, following a typhus epidemic in Silesia, Rudolf Virchow[29] led an investigation into the living conditions associated with the disease's spread. In 1850, the Massachusetts Medical Society prepared a massive statewide public health survey. Such reports did not always lead to immediate action on the part of governments. However, by the end of the 19th century, most Western nations had established public policies regarding sanitary conditions and a network of public health boards to respond when necessary.[30]

These boards provided a practical means for rapidly testing (and applying) the medical advancements in bacteriology and immunology. Prior to the advent of bacteriology (and a fuller understanding of the nature of disease transmission), the impact of these public health surveys was significant but somewhat muted by an inability to devise definitive responses to outbreaks. Ultimately, it was the combination of a basic medical understanding of how cholera spread alongside a detailed description of unsanitary living conditions across urban slums that provided public health officials with the capacity to address serial epidemics. Indeed, even prior to the breakthroughs associated with bacteriology, major health epidemics such as smallpox, typhus and malaria were already well under control due to the reforms implemented by those working to improve basic sanitary conditions.[31] "The conquest of epidemic diseases was in large part the result of the campaign for

[29] Virchow was typical of the medical researchers of the era who linked public health concerns to wider political movements. He joined the first major working-class revolts in Berlin in 1848 and later became an ardent supporter of the Paris Commune (Waitzkin, 1978).

[30] In 1907, the Rome Conference established the International Office of Public Health in Paris, an antecedent to the creation of the World Health Organization in 1946.

[31] See Berliner (1975), Canary and Burton (1983), Dubos (1959), Mishler (1981), and Powles (1973).

pure food, pure water, and pure air based not on a scientific doctrine but on a philosophical faith" (Dubos, 1959:127).

By the 1930s, biomedicine and its self-confident worldview were firmly established in the West as the premiere form of medical care and the standard by which all other forms of medicine were to be measured. Biomedicine's exalted status followed from its rapid-fire discoveries over the previous half century as well as its ideological adherence to the principles of experimental science and utilitarian social progress. Biomedicine's value and utility had been tested and proven through spectacular medical advances that the public experienced firsthand, such as the eradication of age-old scourges within a single generation. Because this was also the age of science, with major advances in physics and chemistry, biomedicine's close ties to science brought even greater public adoration. The days of medical quackery and physician uncertainty were over and biomedicine prepared to march arm in arm alongside science to unlock further mysteries of health and disease.

The story of biomedicine as a scientific enterprise is certainly a powerfully inspiring one. The link between scientific principles and medical progress has been played out on a public stage. Nonetheless, as a description of biomedicine itself (as an ontological whole), this conventional story remains rather flat and one dimensional. Particularly suspect are the universal claims of biomedicine that its principles and methods can be applied across all populations and societies to equal effect. In addition, the notion of applying the attitudinal norms of the purportedly value-neutral physical sciences to the world of health and disease have been seen as increasingly problematic. Thus, biomedicine as a scientific enterprise revealed significant underlying tensions and unsettled concerns. Among the first to address biomedicine's extravagant (and socioculturally decontextualized) scientific claims and its supposed value-neutral objectivity and universality were those who depicted biomedicine not as a scientific enterprise but as a symbolic-cultural expression.

Biomedicine as a Symbolic-Cultural Expression

Of the three perspectives discussed here, biomedicine as a scientific enterprise clearly represents the most pervasive and predominant image of medicine across virtually all facets of Western societies. Indeed, those who present biomedicine as a symbolic-cultural expression or as a social institution do so, in large measure, in juxtaposition to this hegemonic interpretation. In effect, biomedicine as an ahistorical and acultural scientific enterprise is presented as just the way things are. Biomedicine as a symbolic-cultural expression begins, therefore, as an interrogation of the implicit and taken-for-granted conceptual precepts underlying biomedicine as a scientific enterprise. The essence of this analysis turns on the belief that the portrayal of biomedicine as a scientific enterprise has unwittingly adopted biomedicine's positivist ontology, not merely as a faithful description of biomedicine's self- understanding (its scientific framework for understanding the world), but as an actual description of biomedicine itself. It is one thing to illustrate how biomedicine as a scientific enterprise interprets the world based on a law-like, positivist methodology. It is quite another thing to characterize biomedicine—the product of a complex sociocultural history—as the *result* of the same law-like, positivist methodology.

Biomedicine as a symbolic-cultural expression, therefore, stands in opposition to positivist representations that purport to provide transparent depictions of biomedicine merely as it appears. The goal is to peel back the visible layers of scientific medicine's internalized identity. Biomedicine is treated as a social construct—a notion that is today commonplace. The intent here is not, therefore, merely to restate this well-worn critique but to incorporate this perspective as one dimension of biomedicine as an ontological whole—and thereby avoid substituting one, one-dimensional description for another. The differences between medicine as a scientific enterprise and biomedicine as a symbolic-cultural expression do not revolve around empirical facts, as such. Rather, the differences concern how one interprets those facts, as well as the criteria for positing such facts. By penetrating and exposing its symbolic-cultural forms, biomedicine as a symbolic-cultural expression seeks to de-mystify the social origins of the world of biomedicine that are obscured by its scientific pretensions—and its claims of universality. The goal is to expose the symbolic-cultural content of a biomedical worldview that uncritically reifies the norms and values of the physical sciences. This worldview, in effect, reduces the human body to a machine, while explicitly marginalizing the social, cultural, and institutional contexts of health and healing.

The Ideological Content of Biomedicine

As outlined above, one of the most fundamental attributes of biomedicine is its self-conscious identification with the physical sciences[32] and, in particular, the epistemological assumptions underlying the experimental model of science.[33] Hence, biomedicine provides a way of understanding health and

[32] This is notwithstanding the numerous studies detailing a significant gap between the ideal of scientific knowledge and pragmatic medical practices. See Gordon (1988) and Hahn (1983, 1995). Thomas Chalmers has estimated that "perhaps five percent of procedures currently [1993] in use in medical practice are supported by solid evidence such as randomized clinical trials" (quoted in Hahn, 1995:150).

[33] See Brady (2001), Comaroff (1982), Hahn (1984), and Loustaunau and Sobo (1997).

disease (for generating and assessing medical knowledge) based on the rules and procedures associated with the physical sciences. "[Biomedicine] assumes that the language of chemistry and physics will ultimately suffice to explain biological phenomena. From the reductionist viewpoint, the only conceptual tools available to characterize and experimental tools to study biological systems are physical in nature" (Engel, 1977:130). A fundamental distinction is drawn between findings based on observable, testable causal evidence and claims that rely on nonreplicable, metaphysical practices.

The consequences of this science-based, positivist orientation are multifold. To begin with, there is a strong tendency to treat biomedical categories as things rather than as social constructs. Empiricism limits the ontological world of health and healing to observable and measurable physical phenomena. The scope of biomedical practice cannot go beyond one's immediate sensory apprehension. Ultimately, the cause of any disease or illness must be traced to certain phenomena within the physical environment (or within a given organic entity). Any attribution of disease either to one's social environment or to mischievous spirits is well beyond the ken of empirical science and is thus considered primitive superstition. By contrast, for instance, many nonbiomedical health and healing systems identify a number of extraphysical factors in disease causation. "An alternative model defines illness as a disturbance in social relationships; questions of etiology are then framed with reference to social rather than biological processes" (Mishler, 1981:1).

For purposes of empirical investigation, biomedicine is largely limited to the human body as its physical matter. It follows from this that the "doctrine of specific etiology," which assumes that individual diseases are associated with specific biophysiological processes, represents a cardinal, organizing principle of biomedicine (Mishler, 1981). From Sydenham forward, biomedical practitioners have adopted the practice of moving in linear fashion from the initial recording of presenting symptoms, to symptom clusters, to syndromes, to diseases with specific pathogeneses and pathologies. Today, the basic measure for how "advanced" the biomedical community's knowledge of a disease is follows from how far along this path it has traveled. Biomedicine's universal aspirations lead it to claim that all such disease symptoms and categories apply equally and in the same manner across the human species. The world is thus comprised of hundreds of disparate societies and populations who confront a common set of generic diseases. These diseases—as naturally occurring objects in the world—exist prior to and independent of their discovery by biomedicine (Manning and Fábrega, 1973; Wright and Treacher, 1982). Thus, no disease is unique to a given society or culture, either in its symptoms or in its etiology.

However, from the perspective of biomedicine as a symbolic-cultural expression, the notion that these disease designations are somehow culture-free is very difficult to sustain. Indeed, culture-bound syndromes seem as much the rule as the exception (Hahn, 1985). As Janzen has observed, "[O]nly 55 percent of the entries in the World Health Organization's widely used 'International Classification of Diseases' (ICD) [8th edition, 1965] are 'scientifically diagnosable entities,' that is reducible to single, universal and duplicable, sign-symptom complexes. Remaining entries of the ICD are independently varying signs and symptoms classified somewhat arbitrarily according to body parts or problem focuses. In other words, cultural assumptions, rather than laboratory experiments, pervade much of the ICD" (1978:192).[34] The epitome of biomedicine's acultural pretensions is the *Diagnostic and Statistical Manual for Mental Disorders* (*DSM IV*), the modern incarnation of Sydenham's nosology for physical diseases, as applied to mental illness.[35] It neatly catalogues and classifies all known mental disorders for purposes of diagnosis and treatment. The goal is to remove any hint of ambiguity or subjective judgment from the diagnostic process. Each mental disorder has distinct features that are thought to be universal across all human populations. These features are ultimately determined by neurophysiological factors and, as such, the idyllic mental illness is one that remains unaffected by local custom or beliefs.[36] In light of actual biomedical practice, however, the notion of universal disease types suggests a more fundamental ontological confusion with respect to disease as a thing versus disease as a constructed social category. Biomedicine as a symbolic-cultural expression frames disease as a social construction (a reflection of ongoing social interactions with multiple, embedded meanings) and not as a material entity. "Diseases are not *things* in the same sense as rocks, or trees, or rivers. Diseases represent patterns or relationships, which are not material. The problem then

[34] King also captures the arbitrariness of such classifications. "There is only one reason why we should not regard fever as a disease entity and that is, such an entity is so broad and inclusive, so general and nondiscriminating, that it lacks utility" (1954:201). See also Prince and Tcheng-Laroche (1987) and Wig (1983).

[35] The American Psychiatric Association (APA) published the first edition (*DSM I*) in 1952, with a second edition (*DSM II*) in 1968, a third edition (*DSM III*) in 1980 and a revised third edition (*DSM III-R*) in 1987. *DSM IV* was published in 1994 and the APA is currently preparing a fifth edition to be published sometime after 2010.

[36] Grob (1994) recounts the battles that erupted within the American Psychiatric Association in 1946, when a group of brash upstarts formed the Group for the Advancement of Psychiatry (GAP), suggesting that greater heed be given to links between the social environment and psychological disorders. These efforts were mocked by senior colleagues who responded by forming GUP, the Group of Unknowns in Psychiatry. "Opponents of GAP were determined to keep psychiatry rooted within a more somatic and presumably medical tradition and were less inclined to elevate psychological and environmental phenomena to a position of paramount significance" (p. 199).

becomes, how real is a pattern, what is the ontological status of a relationship?" (emphasis in original, King, 1954:199).[37]

A further consequence of biomedicine's scientific legacy is its adherence to an ethic of value-neutrality and stoic objectivity with respect to medical knowledge. A central feature of biomedical training[38] is the cultivation of an attitude and disposition toward health and healing that is objective, dispassionate, rational, and professional.[39] "Physicians tend to view themselves as bioscientists. Their self-image as practitioners reflects a view of medicine as a discipline that has adopted not only the rationality of the scientific method but the concomitant values of the scientist, namely objectivity and neutrality" (Mishler, 1981:15). Indeed, the primary value distinguishing science from other endeavors is vigilant objectivity. The products of a medical laboratory are neither inherently good nor bad. They are indifferent facts. One test might indicate someone has diabetes or that another person is free of cancer. Medicine, as a science in the pursuit of pure knowledge, is counseled to refrain from any value judgments one way or the other. "[I]n medicine it is frequently assumed that illnesses 'happen' to people and that sickness has no special attraction to virtue or vice. It is merely mechanism, not good, bad or righteous behavior that counts. Instead of judging, medicine diagnoses, explains 'how,' and treats" (Gordon, 1988:28).

As a value-neutral science, biomedicine remains focused on disease at the expense of patient suffering or broader social issues. It is feared that the subjective aspects of patient suffering may unduly interfere with the physician's reasoned judgments. "The patient's and family's complaints are regarded as subjective self-reports. The physician's task, wherever possible, is to replace these biased observations with objective data: the only valid sign of pathological processes because they are based on verified or verifiable measurements" (Kleinman, 1993:18). Biomedicine promotes a detached, impersonal (technocratic) approach to medical care in which this cult of objectivity separates the physician from the patient as a full and sentient human being. It also helps to marginalize the roles of social, cultural, and political influences when setting biomedical research agendas. As a greater number of social issues continue to trespass upon the pristine laboratory (for example, stem cell research, cloning, RU486), this fiction, of course, becomes less and

---

[37] This is not to deny an actual biological reality. As Lock and others insist, "There is, of course, a biological reality, but the moment that efforts are made to explain, order, and manipulate that reality, then a process of contextualization takes place in which the dynamic relationship of biology with cultural values and the social order has to be considered" (1988:7).

[38] The classic U.S. studies of the medical students' world are *The Boys in White* (Becker et al., 1961) and *The Student Physician* (Merton et al., 1957).

[39] See B. Good (1994), Gordon (1988), Lock and Gordon (1988), and Stein (1990).

less tenable. It is increasingly evident that the decisions taken by dispassionate biomedical scientists significantly reflect the social norms and cultural values of the larger society. The notion of biomedicine as a science, therefore, can distort as much as it reveals.

The standard metaphor of a machine (in need of occasional fine-tuning and repair), remains today the most common biomedical image of the human body and stands as a lasting testament to biomedicine's 18th-century Enlightenment roots.[40] "In the 1700s a positivistic, mechanical science developed that was influenced by and in turn influenced the practice of medicine" (Osherson and Amarasingham 1981:222). In this scheme, the human body—a mechanical device comprising a complex, multifunctional system—is comprised of discrete parts and subsystems governed by intricately connected, cause-and-effect relationships.[41] Biomedicine as a symbolic-cultural expression is especially attentive to the consequences (distortions) that follow from the machine metaphor. Subject to particular scrutiny is the machine metaphor's embrace of the mind/body duality and how it structures the practice of medicine and rationalizes a technology-driven medical system.

The machine metaphor is firmly rooted in the Cartesian mind/body duality.[42] The Western notion of a soulless body and a bodyless soul provides biomedicine with a ready rationale for treating the body as a high-functioning, nonsacred, human vessel. Viewing the soul (one's essential, eternal humanness) as separate from and unrestricted by the limits of the body, allows biomedicine to diagnose and treat a person's body without compromising his or her spiritual essence.[43] "Biomedicine was founded on a Cartesian division of man into a soulless mortal machine capable of mechanistic explanation and manipulation, and a bodyless soul, immortal, immaterial, and properly subject to religious authority, but largely unnecessary to account for physical disease and healing" (Kirmayer, 1988:59). It follows that, for purposes of diagnosis and treatment, biomedicine maintains strict lines of distinction between the somatic (the body) and the mental (the mind). Material reality (disease) exists separate and apart from how we think about it (the mind)—one's psychological or emotional state. Disease is a physical reality of the body and, as such, biomedicine can only account for explanations of disease function that are based on narrow physiological criteria (Kleinman, 1981).

---

[40] Harvey's description of the circulation of blood, to take just one example, was celebrated as a direct application of Newton's mechanical physics (Wightman, 1971).

[41] See Engel (1977), B. Good (1994), Kleinman (1981), and Manning and Fábrega (1973).

[42] See Gordon (1988), Kirmayer (1988), and Kleinman (1993).

[43] "The Cartesian schema was a stroke of scholastic genius; it legitimated the study of the body as a mechanism by the science of physiology and preserved the soul as the domain of theology" (L. Eisenberg, 1977:10).

"Medicine exemplifies materialism. 'Real' illness corresponds to the degree to which physical traces show up in the body" (Gordon, 1988:24).

The machine metaphor reduces the role of the biomedical physician to that of a tinkering mechanic, attempting to patch up this or that malfunctioning (disease-ridden) body part. He or she is trained to quarantine disease within specific tissues or organs. This, effectively, isolates the diseased tissue or organ—as the site of diagnosis and treatment—from the rest of the body. The primary recipient of care is the diseased tissue; the whole body (or full person) is secondary. First, biomedicine isolates and separates the patient from his or her social world via the doctrine of specific etiology. Then, invoking the machine metaphor, biomedicine isolates and separates the disease from the patient. "A prominent feature of *Stedman's* [*Medical Dictionary*] definition of the domain of medicine is the designated subject of medical work: medicine prevents and cures, studies and treats, not persons, nor their bodies, but the diseases of the body" (Hahn, 1995:133).

This rationale of finite subdivision dictates the professional organization of biomedical practice. For biomedicine, the human body is comprised of discrete and interconnected physiological systems. Therefore, it is believed that medical knowledge and skill areas should mirror this functionalist system through specialization (and subspecialization) based on organ systems—for example, gastroenterology, ophthalmology, psychiatry (Stein, 1990). "The object of diagnosis and treatment and prognosis is fragmented into a single organ system. Expert judgment is further legitimated over that of the generalist" (Kleinman, 1995:38). At the same time, depending on the level of one's analysis, biomedical knowledge about the physical structures of the body are, likewise, compartmentalized into discrete categories—anatomy, physiology, biochemistry, microbiology, and pathology.[44] These formal subdivisions within biomedicine reinforce the separation of disease (as an organic form) from the patient (as a full person).

Lastly, there is a direct link between the machine metaphor and biomedicine's profound reliance on technology.[45] As detailed above, beginning in the mid-19th century, a series of inventions were designed to provide physicians with an increasing number of techniques for observing and measuring vari-

[44] This was further reflected in the medical school curricula by the late 19th-century. "Nineteenth-century medical reformers envisioned the physician as a bedside scientist. Medical practitioners must think and talk like scientists. They must be trained in anatomy, physiology, bacteriology, pathology, pharmacology, and the physical sciences. They must think of health and disease not holistically as general relationships between bodily systems or between the person and the environment, but in terms of the micro-concepts of physiology and anatomy, bacteriology and cell pathology. These sciences and their reductionist concepts were gradually recognized in the late 19th century as the foundations of medical education" (Brown, 1979:80–81).

[45] See B. Good (1994), B. Good and M-J. D. Good (1993), and Rosenberg (1979).

ous physiological functions. On the one hand, along with emerging statistical methods, these inventions allowed physicians to generate enormous volumes of normative data for large populations—such as Wunderlich's study of body temperatures and disease—for the purpose of gauging an individual patient's progress vis-à-vis group norms. "[A]ssertions about the normality of levels of biological functioning, or about the normal structure of an organ, must be based on the relationship between the observed instance and the distribution in a specified population of these structures and functions. Further, implicit to any specified norm is a set of presupposed standard conditions with regard to when, how and on whom measurements are taken" (Mishler, 1981:4). Once technology became available to reliably establish the human population's "normal" blood pressure, pulse, body temperature, and such, it became a routine function of the physician to monitor fluctuations in human physiology based on such measures as evidence of disease (or recovery). Today, biomedicine offers a battery of technological apparatuses (primarily diagnostic) for each disease and organ of the body. Given biomedicine's heavy dependence on this biotechnology to observe and treat the body, there is a strong bias in favor of cure-oriented treatments that are (reflexively) invasive and technology-driven.

> Dr. Kass, writing of her Harvard Medical School education, says, "As a medical student, I knew I was being trained to rely heavily on technology, to assume that the risk of action is almost always preferable to the risk of not acting . . . My class in medical school was absorbing the idea that more is better. No one ever talked about the negative aspects of intervention, and the one time a student asked about the appropriateness of fetal monitoring, the question was cut off with a remark that there was no time to discuss issues of 'appropriateness.' " (Payer, 1988:133)

The expanded role of technology further separates the physician from the patient (as a full person) and marginalizes the patient's subjective impressions (Leon Eisenberg, 1977; Powles, 1973). One consequence of this separation is greater physician indifference regarding how patients actually experience illness.[46] There is a general neglect of how disease impacts an individual's life and overall wellbeing. Eisenberg quotes a physician treating

[46] Kleinman (1993) bemoans the "dehumanizing" aspects of technology when applied to medicine. "This radically reductionistic and positivistic value orientation is ultimately dehumanizing. That which has been such a successful blueprint for a bio-chemically oriented technology in the treatment of acute pathology places biomedical practitioners into a number of extremely difficult situations when it comes to the care of patients with chronic illness" (1993:18).

acute myeloid leukemia who reflected on biomedicine's substitution of disease management for attention to a patient's basic quality of life. "'The present preoccupation with intensive therapy appears to blind physicians to the poor quality of life which their patients lead. The aim of treatment is too often to induce a hematological remission (an irrelevance to the patient) rather than to improve quality of life'" (1977:19). Whereas in the past, physicians had relied almost entirely on patient self-reports to document and assess disease, physicians were now able to turn to laboratory reports that provide "direct" physiological data, with less concern for the specifics of individual patient suffering.

> These inventions were part of a shift in the doctor-patient relationship from a patient-centered focus in which the doctor was dependent on the patient for information to a more technical focus in which concern centered on objective signs of illness and in which illness could be seen for the first time as being localized in the body. The localization of illness changed the status of the patient's body; no longer was it primarily the seat of subjective impressions interpreted by the patient to the doctor, but rather it became the site of specific disease entities to be detected and evaluated by the doctor independently of the patient. (Osherson and Amarasingham, 1981:224)

It follows that if disease is perceived as a deviation from the normal functioning of a human machine then the role of biomedicine will, in turn, be to provide episodic repairs. Biomedicine is episodic in the sense that a person's state of health is divided into "normal" periods when she or he is well and "abnormal" periods when she or he is not well (Engel, 1977). Mishler (1981) has noted the ironic parallel between the contemporary notion of disease as a variation from normal function and previously rejected ancient Greek humoral theories of imbalance and disharmony as the origin of disease. Whereas humoral theory asserted that any imbalance between certain essential bodily fluids might cause a disease, biomedicine appears to believe that the state of imbalance is itself the actual manifestation of the disease. What was cause is now effect. Biomedical care is thus provided during abnormal times and has little application during normal times. Consequently, people conceive of biomedical health care as an occasional, episodic concern rather than an ongoing, daily experience that is an extension of one's lifestyle.[47] This cure-oriented care emphasizes aggressive therapeutic intervention with the goal of moving a person from an abnormal state (disease) to a normal

---

[47] See Corin (1995), Helman (2000), and Rhodes (1996).

state (healthy). The biomedical physician remains at the ready for persons who, otherwise, go about their lives hoping to avoid the need for biomedicine. Therefore, beyond occasionally providing a cure for disease, biomedicine remains peripheral to one's immediate life. This contrasts sharply with a great many non-Western medical systems which view health and healing as integrated with (and inseparable from) one's everyday material, personal, emotional, and spiritual well-being.[48]

The Sociocultural Autonomy of Biomedicine

Given that disease is ultimately reducible to physiological abnormalities within a particular human organism, it follows that biomedicine has historically evolved as a medical system that largely ignores broader social, cultural, and institutional contexts.[49] The logic is clear. Insofar as social, cultural, or institutional factors play a role in the perpetuation of disease, this is secondary to the actual physiological mechanisms of disease transmission. Social relationships, for example, may contribute to stress that then triggers certain physiological responses, perhaps, in the form of disease. However, the proper role of biomedicine is to eradicate disease in a manner that is narrowly restricted to addressing the body's physiological response to such stress—not the stress itself.[50] Engel describes the ultimate consequence of eliminating social factors from disease in his critique of biomedicine and psychiatry (Engel, 1977). In essence, all human behaviors (and emotions) are reducible to a finite chain of biochemical reactions governed by neurophysiological properties. "The biomedical model not only requires that disease be dealt with as an entity independent of social behavior, it also demands that behavioral aberrations be explained on the basis of disordered somatic (biochemical or neurophysiological) processes" (Engel, 1977:130).

Inherent in biomedicine's underlying etiological rationale is a type of fortress mentality (with respect to disease and the body) that places social or interpersonal concerns well beyond the physician's proper sphere of interests. As noted, if the social inequities or psychological stresses of today's world

---

[48] See Corin (1995), M-J. D. Good (1995), Helman (2000), and Kleinman (1993).

[49] See Engel (1977), Kleinman (1993), and Wright and Treacher (1982).

[50] Kleinman attributes this, in part, to Western individualism and contrasts biomedicine, in this regard, with many African healing systems. "The attention of biomedicine is also focused on the body of the individual sick person because of Western society's powerful orientation to the individual experience. That illness infiltrates and deeply affects social relations is a difficult understanding to advance in biomedicine. Population- and community-based public health orientations run counter to the dominant biomedical orientation, which takes for its subject the isolated and isolatable organism. In contrast, African healing systems see illness as part of kinship networks and healing as a kinship community effort" (1993:22).

create conditions that give rise to disease, it is not the task of biomedicine to address these broader concerns. In fact, it is seen as a strength of biomedicine that its attention remains focused on organic disease, whose universal laws are indifferent to the ephemeral social conditions. In such uncertain times, the biomedical physician provides reassuring protection against the savage and ever-changing social and natural forces.

> [I]llness is explained predominantly as the result of the interaction of "pathogens" and "host," and also through processes of congenital deformity or natural degeneration, none of which imply the motivation of human interest or causal agency. These etiological models entail a specific image of man—and a tacit ideology. For they connote a view of disease as an asocial, amoral process, and a view of man as the decontextualized "host" to a set of unmediated natural processes, which call for technical intervention. Healing acts upon the symbolic domain of the body to emphasize the ontological primacy of physical existence, rendering cognition and emotions epiphenomenal, and excluding social relations as a separate order of reality . . . The healing process in our society emphasizes our alienation from ourselves as bio-physical beings, reinforcing our state of dependence on specialist knowledge in a ceaseless combat against natural threat. (Comaroff, 1982:59)

Biomedicine ignores not only the social, cultural and institutional contexts in which disease occurs among human populations, it also ignores the social, cultural, and institutional contexts in which biomedicine is practiced. In other words, it is assumed that biomedicine itself is the product of the value-free, apolitical pursuit of pure knowledge, as a scientific enterprise (Gordon, 1988; Powles, 1973). The presumption is that the sociocultural setting where biomedicine emerged was mere historical happenstance. Because the methods and truths uncovered by biomedicine are universal, had it first developed in India or Egypt, its basic features would be no different. Biomedicine, the one, true source of medical knowledge, is universal. All other healing practices are relative to each other and culturally specific (that is, limited in application) to a given society. Given biomedicine's idealized self-understanding, asking how social norms, cultural values, and political and economic interests have shaped the historical development of biomedicine, as a knowledge-generating activity, lies well beyond the scope of the biomedical sciences.

Biomedicine as a symbolic-cultural expression is made especially evident when considering the degree of pluralism within biomedicine itself. Were it the case that universal reason dictated biomedical practices, then one would expect a strong congruity between Western nations. If diseases are universal phenomena and each disease's diagnosis and treatment is determined by culture-free, experimental science, then it stands to reason that a common set of homogeneous, biomedical practices should predominate across the West. However, significant differences abound among Western nations with respect to biomedicine (Payer, 1988).

> Some of the most commonly prescribed drugs in France, drugs to dilate the cerebral blood vessels, are considered ineffective in England and America; an obligatory immunization against tuberculosis in France, BCG, is almost impossible to obtain in the United States. German doctors prescribe from six to seven times the amount of digitalislike drugs as their colleagues in France and England, but they prescribe fewer antibiotics, with some German doctors maintaining antibiotics shouldn't be used unless the patient is sick enough to be in the hospital. Doses of the same drug may vary drastically, with some nationalities getting ten to twenty times what other nationals get. French people have seven times the chance of getting drugs in suppository form as do Americans. (Payer, 1988:24)

The use of anesthesia during childbirth presents a further example of the nonuniversal aspects of biomedicine in the West (Hahn, 1995). Dutch physicians tend to use little anesthesia, with the belief that in the case of pain management, a woman's body knows best. In Sweden, there is an expectation of anesthesia, and the mother takes an active role in pain management decision making. In the United States, a woman must typically demonstrate significant pain before anesthesia is introduced. Loustaunau and Sobo (1997) and Payer (1988) detail more examples of differences in medical care that are difficult to account for without appealing to cultural differences. Unlike other Westerners, German physicians treat patients for low blood pressure and, in general, tend to use fewer antibiotics. French physicians place a greater emphasis on the therapeutic role of vitamins, diet, and exercise. U.S. physicians tend to be far more aggressive in treating disease. So stark are some of these differences that Payer claims that in some cases actual disease diagnoses can be a function of one's nationality. "The same clinical signs may even receive different diagnoses. Often, all one must do to acquire a disease is to enter a country where that disease is recognized—leaving the country will either cure the malady or turn it into something else" (Payer, 1988:25).[51] Such differences certainly reflect social and cultural rather then scientific differences.

---

[51] See also Feldman (1992) for U.S./French comparisons with respect to AIDS and Gaines (1992) for U.S./French comparisons with respect to psychiatric conditions.

Ohnuki-Tierney (1994) observes that, because "brain death" in Japan is the technical criterion for declaring an individual deceased and terminating life support, many advances in transplant technology have more limited utility. It is thus clearly the case that, as non-Western societies adopt biomedical models, there remains significant room for adaptation to cultural differences.

Biomedicine as a symbolic-cultural expression paints a social context that seeks to reveal the symbolic-cultural world (material, ideological) hidden within the heroic rhetoric of scientific medicine. Linking the meanings of such symbols to specific cultural settings qualifies the scope and power of biomedicine's universal discourse. Here then is a second side of biomedicine as an ontological whole that further illuminates our understanding of the first side. The first perspective of biomedicine as a scientific enterprise (grounded in positivist science) is not superseded by the second perspective of biomedicine as a symbolic-cultural expression (informed by hermeneutic and poststructural interpretations). Each merely brings out elements in biomedicine that are unavailable to the other perspective. Beyond its scientific-material content and its symbolic-cultural forms, however, biomedicine also constitutes a manifest form of social power relations. Examining the historical development of biomedicine as an expression of social power (a social institution) reveals this third side of biomedicine.

Biomedicine as an Expression of Social Power

To understand biomedicine as an expression of social power it is necessary to view it, above all, as a social institution that is subject to a range of social, economic, and political forces that have shaped its formation and continue to determine its further development. Biomedicine emerged in a specific place (Western Europe and North America), at a unique time (the latter 19th century), under particular social conditions (industrial capitalism and the consolidation of monopoly corporate power). Its development reflected titanic struggles between the representatives of powerful social classes who fought to guard competing interests. Ultimately, biomedicine's institutional forms are the result of a combination of victories, defeats, and compromises. These determined who could practice medicine, who profited from medicine, and who controlled the conditions under which medicine was practiced. For the purpose of considering biomedicine as an expression of social power, the period of its remarkable ascent in the United States provides a vivid illustration of the social ferment from which it grew.

Today, U.S. biomedicine represents a multibillion dollar industry organized around an enormous network of high-tech, capital-intensive medical research and clinical care enterprises forming a conglomerate of private physician groups, government agencies, state and private universities, corporate foundations, research and teaching hospitals, biotech firms, transnational pharmaceutical corporations, and the insurance industry.[52] In the mid-19th century, however, this rise of biomedicine to a position of exclusive control within the U.S. medical system was by no means a foregone conclusion. Biomedicine was still maturing as a scientific enterprise and its cultural forms had yet to penetrate very deeply into the social fabric. Biomedicine did not yet exist as a formal, institutionalized practice. Its social influence remained restricted to small circles of elite physicians trained in Europe.

Given the number of medical sects throughout the 19th century, to refer to someone as a "physician" at this time did not necessarily identify what type of medicine that person practiced, biomedical or otherwise. The largest and most influential of these sects, allopathic physicians, were the crude forebearers of modern biomedical physicians.[53] The allopaths' preferred means of therapy—aggressive sessions of bleeding, blistering, purging, and high-dosage medication—were often considered worse than the original ailment and their success rates were abysmally low.[54] As a consequence, among the general public, allopathic physicians were one of the most feared medical sects. The process by which allopathic physicians came to dominate medical care in the United States (in league with a powerful national lobby, a core group of elite medical schools, and major corporate sponsors) helps to explain, in part, the story of how biomedicine came to define and control U.S. medical care by the early 20th century. Each of these social actors, in turn, has its parallel when considering the development of biomedicine in Africa, as explored in Chapter 5.

The context for these developments was a unique period of U.S history—from the late 19th century through the first few decades of the 20th century—marked by the rise of concentrated corporate power.[55] This was a time when large corporations controlled by wealthy families (the Rockefellers, Carnegies, Vanderbilts, and the like), already yielding great influence over the larger economy, set out to refashion social and economic institutions to fit the new patterns of industrial capitalism. "Industrialization in 19th-century America

---

[52] Clarke, et al. (2003) refer to this as the "Biomedical TechnoService Complex, Inc."

[53] The term "allopathic" is not ideal. This label was developed by homeopathic physicians (homeopath meaning "same as disease") to denote those who treated disease with opposite remedies. Allopathic physicians—associated with the elite medical schools of the early 19th century, Harvard, Dartmouth, and the University of Pennsylvania—referred to their medicine as "regular" and that of all other sects as "irregular." For purposes of exposition, however, this language is far too prejudicial.

[54] See Baer (2001, 1989), Berliner (1985), and Porter (1997).

[55] See Burrow (1977), Chandler (1977), Hofstadter (1955), Josephson (1962), and Sklar (1988).

created many problems for those who owned and managed the corporations that came to dominate the economy . . . [T]hey had to reshape older social institutions or create new ones. Educational, religious, medical, and cultural institutions were some of the glue that held together the *ancien régime*" (Brown, 1979:13).[56] Like many social institutions, therefore, the evolution of biomedicine was in large part shaped by private corporate interests. These corporate interests were advanced via philanthropic foundations that funded the transition to capital-intensive, university-based programs of biomedical education and training. Whereas allopathic physicians sought to control who could practice medicine and thereby assure a monopoly for biomedical practitioners, corporations sought to control the conditions under which physicians practiced (and researched) medicine via medical school reforms.

The attraction of biomedicine for those at the helm of industrial capitalism was not difficult to fathom. The focus on a single pathogenic cause of disease appeared to absolve the excesses and inequities of capitalist society and to offer an antidote for diseases that spared any major social transformations.[57] Disease was presented as an engineering problem—reducible to a unifactorial model of disease. Much like in the industrial world, it was felt, medicine simply required the requisite technical knowledge and resources to progress.[58] Furthermore, insofar as industrial productivity was linked to fit and healthy workers, biomedical advances could serve as a boon to corporate profits.[59] Feierman (1985) presents a compelling case for this position from a South African sugar plantation.

> Dr. Lamont, employed by the Tongaat Group, owners of a large South African sugar plantation in Natal, reported on an acute form of cardiac failure among African field workers. According to Lamont's re-

[56] While distancing oneself from the functionalist analysis of Brown (1979) and others, it is possible nonetheless to join them in many of the conclusions they draw. "[M]embers of the corporate class, acting mainly through philanthropic foundations, articulated a strategy for developing a medical system to meet the needs of capitalist society" (Brown, 1979:4).

[57] See Baer et al. (2003), Berliner (1982), Navarro (1976), and Waitzkin (1978).

[58] The machine metaphor is especially apt, given the dominant image of capitalist production (and its engine) in the late 19th century on the part of those who came to subsidize the development of the biomedical industry. See Singer (1992) for an analysis of the political economy of biomedicine as a scientific enterprise.

[59] See Baer (1989) and Berliner (1982). Turshen (1977a) challenges this common assertion, arguing that, "In every recession, rather than spend money on medical services, capitalists find it more profitable to fire sick workers and replace them with healthy people picked from a labor pool that is swelled by widespread unemployment . . . In addition, this formulation deflates the victory of the working class by turning its health demand into a productivity gain for the capitalists" (p. 54).

> port the workers all live in compounds. They rise at 4:30 in the morning, eat a slice of bread, drink a cup of coffee and work in the sun until late in the afternoon, with only sour, watery maize porridge to eat until the evening meal. The plantation supplies large quantities of so-called "kaffir beer" on the weekend. Under these conditions, many workers experienced intractable heart failure, and were therefore sent back to the homeland from which they came. Dr. Lamont introduced a potassium-sparing diuretic, after which "not one case has needed to be repatriated. Furthermore, provided the patients continue on maintenance therapy, it has been found that they can be kept out of failure, doing heavy manual labor for lengthy periods of follow-up." Dr. Lamont appears to measure his own success as a physician in terms of the capacity of workers to keep working under inhuman conditions. The only possibility for making significant improvement in Tongaat workers' health is through improved conditions of work. (p. 115)[60]

Biomedicine was, therefore, both ideologically and materially consistent with the views and interests of corporate owners as well as those of the emerging, technocratically oriented professional class of managers, lawyers, and engineers (Braverman, 1974). "The medical profession discovered an ideology that was compatible with the worldview of, and politically and economically useful to, the capitalist class and the emerging managerial and professional stratum" (Brown, 1979:71).

A battle for control ensued between corporate foundations and the new class of biomedical practitioners. Biomedical practitioners organized to bolster their professional independence as well as their social and economic status. Their primary strategy was to create favorable licensing criteria for biomedical physicians. Corporate foundations maneuvered to weaken physician independence by influencing the content of medical education and dictating the conditions of medical practice. This took the form of reforming medical schools. At the same time, there was sufficient collusion to ward off nonbiomedical challengers. "The emerging alliance around the turn of the century between the American Medical Association, which consisted primarily of elite practitioners and medical researchers based in prestigious universities, and the industrial capitalist class ultimately permitted biomedicine to establish political, economic and ideological dominance over rival medical systems in the United States" (Baer et al., 2003: 329). Examining

[60] More recently, given the high rates of HIV/AIDS in South Africa combined with the prohibitive cost of Western drugs, three corporations—Anglo Gold, Anglo-American Corporation and De Beers—opted to provide their HIV positive workers with the necessary medications.`

these licensing campaigns and medical school reforms in the U.S. context thus reveals a third side of biomedicine, as an expression of social power.

The Origins of U.S. Biomedical Hegemony

At the start of 19th century, the social status and prestige of U.S. physicians varied tremendously. This was primarily a function of one's family background, the pedigree of one's medical school, appointments to prestigious medical colleges and hospitals (Harvard, Yale, University of Pennsylvania), and the social standing of one's patients. At the time, there were no broadly accepted criteria or qualifications for practicing medicine. Attending medical school itself was only an option. As a consequence, there were a great many persons from a great many medical sects who referred to themselves as physicians with wide-ranging preparation and skill (Jones, 2004).[61] Uniform licensing criteria was a major goal for those allopathic physicians seeking to distinguish themselves from the other medical sects. Indeed, with the advances in bacteriology and immunology, allopathic medicine (later referred to as biomedicine) was promoted as the only reliable and proven form of medicine. "Scientific medicine was held up as *the* nonsectarian medical theory and practice—the only one based on verifiable truths" (emphasis in original, Brown, 1979:78). As such, it was endorsed as the blueprint for licensing standards.

One of the major challenges for those who sought to impose tighter licensing restrictions for physicians was a basic lack of agreement concerning which techniques actually constituted the soundest medical practice. Other than the allopathic physicians, the most numerous sects were the Thomsonians, eclectics, and homeopaths. Developed by Samuel Thomson, the Thomsonians mixed radical politics with herbal medicine, while flatly denying the value of scientific medicine (Haller, 1997). This sect died out in the latter 19th century. The eclectics were botanic physicians who, as the name suggests, borrowed liberally from other sects. They accepted and taught conventional scientific medicine, however they opposed what they considered the excessive use of bleeding, drugging, and other aggressive medical interventions practiced by allopaths. Homeopathic medicine—introduced to the United States in the mid-1820s—was developed by Samuel Hahnemann, a German physician, in the early 19th century. Homeopathic physicians believed in the so-called law of similars (that which makes you ill makes you

[61] It was commonly argued that this lack of coherent standards was contributing to an "oversupply" of physicians in the United States. By 1900, the United States averaged one physician for every 568 persons. This compared with one physician for every 2,000 persons in Germany.

well) and maintained that the effectiveness of a drug could be increased by using smaller and smaller doses.

Allopathic physicians targeted homeopaths in 1855 through their newly formed (1847) American Medical Association (AMA).[62] The AMA adopted a code of ethics that denied membership for homeopaths and that forbade allopathic physicians from working with homeopaths in the course of their medical practice (effectively excluding homeopaths from most hospitals, medical schools, and public health programs). Nonetheless, eclectics and homeopaths thrived. By 1870, nonallopathic sects controlled fifteen of the nation's seventy-five medical schools and accounted for one-fifth of all physicians. Twenty years later, eclectics and homeopaths controlled twenty-five of 106 medical schools. In the 1880s, the AMA revised its strategy. Given the reality of the eclectics' and homeopaths' relative political power,[63] as well as the common need among all three groups to exercise greater control over who could practice medicine, the AMA opted to join with the others to pursue medical licensing on a state-by-state basis. By 1901, all states had some level of licensing. In twenty-five states (and Washington, DC) licensing requirements included a medical school diploma and an independent state medical examination. (Most state medical examination boards included representatives from all three sects.) In 1903, the AMA formally revised its code of ethics to permit member cooperation with the other sects, as had been the common practice for decades.

> The collaboration between regular physicians and sectarians [before 1903] clearly violated the AMA's code of ethics, but none of the doctors who served on joint licensing boards suffered excommunication. The code was simply ignored. By the turn of the century, prominent leaders in the AMA conceded the code was an anachronism and were anxious to put the issue of sectarianism behind them. So in 1903 the AMA adopted a revised code of ethics that said little about irregular practitioners. While noting that it was inconsistent with scientific principles for physicians to designate their practice as exclusive or sectarian, the new code elided any reference to the kind of medicine doctors actually

[62] The AMA's British counterpart, the Provincial Medical and Surgical Association, was formed in 1832, becoming the British Medical Association in 1856. The *Association Générale des Médecins de France* was formed in 1858. Germany did not form a national medical association in this period.

[63] The AMA remained relatively weak throughout this period in terms of overall numbers. In 1900, there were only 8,000 national members. The AMA suffered, in part, from an exclusive reputation. Its founding members had been elite medical educators or practitioners of high regard associated with reputable hospitals. Following its successful licensing campaign, however, by 1910, over one-half of all biomedical physicians were members, and by 1920 this grew to 60% (Starr, 1982:110).

> practiced. Within a few years, orthodox societies were seeking out members among sectarian physicians. (Starr, 1982:107)

Ultimately, the demise of the eclectics and of homeopathy was not attributable to AMA suppression alone. Rather, this followed from a combination of political and scientific factors. Over time both were assimilated by the allopaths, as the public grew more and more receptive of biomedicine's demonstrated scientific progress (as detailed above) and its diminished reliance on extreme practices such as bleedings and purges. "While regular medicine was producing important and demonstrable scientific advances, homeopathy generated no new discoveries. The contrast was not lost on many in the group. They edged further away from Hahnemann; the final dissolution came of itself" (Starr, 1982:108). The political maneuverings of the AMA, therefore, coincided with the era of bacteriological breakthroughs and other advances in scientific medicine that made an immediate impression on public attitudes. Importantly, the U.S. pattern was not commonly repeated in other Western societies. For example, homeopathic and other botanical traditions retained a strong influence within both German and Dutch medicine (Maretzki and Seidler, 1985; Schepers and Hermans, 1999). Molassiotis et al. (2005) found that at least 36% of cancer patients in Europe make use of alternative medicine. Furthermore, all of the above U.S. developments notwithstanding, one would be remiss in neglecting to mention the strong retention of a parallel (and thriving) U.S. market of nonbiomedical practitioners.[64]

Following its successes in the area of state physician licensing, the AMA turned to the other major source of surplus physicians flooding the field—unregulated medical schools.[65] For this purpose, however, it became clear that the AMA would need influential allies and it turned to corporate foundations for assistance. Doing so, however, inadvertently opened up a new battle, as physicians now found themselves struggling to retain their professional independence against corporate investors who sought to impose new restrictions on the medical field via reforms of medical education and training.

[64] See Davis and Darden (2003), D. Eisenberg et al. (2001), D. Eisenberg et al. (1998), and Elder et al. (1997), along with Baer's (2001) historical analysis of alternative medicine in the United States. Also attesting to the broad interest in nonbiomedical practices, in 1998, the two leading U.S. biomedical journals—*The Journal of the American Medical Association* and *The New England Journal of Medicine*—each dedicated an entire special issue to the topic.

[65] In 1850, there were 52 U.S. medical schools. This grew to 100 by 1880 and 160 by 1900. The number of students grew in tandem from 11,826 in 1880 to 25,171 in 1905 (Starr, 1982:112).

Prior to the 20th century, U.S. medical schools were considered woefully inferior to European medical schools.[66] Elite U.S. physicians typically traveled to Germany or France for their education. Between 1870 and 1914, fifteen thousand U.S. physicians studied medicine in Germany alone. In the 1890s, the AMA worked with the Association of American Medical Colleges (AAMC) to establish minimal standards for U.S. medical schools. Representing the top one-third of U.S. medical schools, the AAMC's activities were highly influential. The medical school at Johns Hopkins University—almost all of whose faculty had trained in Germany—became the model for reform efforts in which the overriding goal was to join science and research with clinical hospital practice as the foundation for a medical student's education.

> From the outset, Johns Hopkins embodied a conception of medical education as a field of graduate study, rooted in basic science and hospital medicine, that was eventually to govern all institutions in the country. Scientific research and clinical instruction now moved to center stage. The faculty, rather than being recruited from local practitioners, as had always been the pattern in America, were accomplished men of research, wooed from outside Baltimore. Students were also drawn from a distance and carefully chosen; they spent their first two years studying basic laboratory sciences and their last two on the wards, personally responsible for a few patients under the watchful eyes of the faculty. A hospital was built in connection with the school, and the two were conducted as a joint enterprise . . . Here were the glimmerings of the great university-dominated medical centers of the next century. (Starr, 1982:115–116)

With the progress of the AAMC, the AMA created the Council on Medical Education (CME) in 1904. Its purpose was to reshape state licensing standards for medical schools.[67] The Council drafted a set of guidelines for state licensing boards to adopt. The criteria required all physicians to complete a four-year

---

[66] Shryock (1953) attributes U.S. backwardness in the area of scientific medicine to the nation's utilitarian attitude toward scientific research. The surviving aristocracies in Europe remained open to funding research that was more in the tradition of knowledge for the sake of knowledge. "It even became a matter of pride with some (Europeans) that their research had no relation to 'mere utility' . . . Had the matter been left to (the U.S.), it is unlikely that modern medicine as we understand it would ever have evolved. At best, the process would have taken a much longer time" (p. 228).

[67] Two years earlier, the AMA had gone through a major strategic reorganization that significantly reinforced member conformity to AMA rules and guidelines. Branch societies were established on the local, state, and regional levels. Local medical societies were empowered to enforce AMA codes of conduct for physicians via the expulsion (or other sanction) of local members.

high school education, a four-year medical program, and to pass a state licensing exam. In 1906, based on these criteria, the Council inspected 160 medical schools and found eighty-two fully adequate, forty-six poor but redeemable, and thirty-two beyond help. The results, however, were never published for fear of the political fallout. Instead, the AMA worked with the Carnegie Foundation for the Advancement of Teaching to conduct a broader assessment. The Carnegie Foundation was considered an impartial outsider with fewer vested interests than the AMA.[68] Abraham Flexner, a professional educator who was well connected with university elites, was selected to conduct the study. Given his ties with the philanthropic Carnegie Foundation, medical schools welcomed Flexner. Ultimately, Flexner's critique was far more harsh than even that of the AMA.

> Though a layman, he was much more severe in his judgment of particular institutions than the AMA had been in any of its annual guides to American medical schools. The association was constrained by possible suspicion of its motives; Flexner felt no such compunctions. Repeatedly, with a deft use of detail and biting humor, he showed that the claims made by the weaker, mostly proprietary schools in their catalogues were patently false. Touted laboratories were nowhere to be found, or consisted of a few vagrant test tubes squirreled away in a cigar box; corpses reeked because of the failure to use disinfectant in the dissecting rooms. Libraries had no books; alleged faculty members were busily occupied in private practice. Purported requirements for admission were waived for anyone who would pay the fees. (Starr, 1982:119)

In the wake of Flexner's report it was evident that advances in medical education had not kept pace with advances in the biomedical sciences. It was recommended that all medical schools model themselves after Johns Hopkins and that the lower-ranked schools simply shut down. "Flexner saw his mission as translating the Hopkins medical school into a standard against which to judge all other medical education in the United States" (Brown, 1979:145). Shortly after the Flexner report, in 1912, the Federation of State Medical Boards was created. Though not a direct body of the AMA, the Federation accepted the authority of the AMA when rating medical schools. Re-

[68] The Foundation for the Advancement of Teaching was established in 1905 to improve the status of teachers and to create uniform standards of education in colleges and universities. It was felt that "If the study was done by a presumably neutral and independent agency with no vested interest in the medical field as such, and the study was directed by an educator with no direct ties to the medical field, then much of the sectarian criticism of the Report would be seen as mere partisanship and help to complete the unfavorable image of the competing sects" (Berliner, 1975:589).

markably, all of these licensing reforms moved forward solely at the behest of a small circle of private interests. Government agencies were reduced to bystanders. "Even though no legislative body ever set up either the Federation of State Medical Boards or the AMA Council on Medical Education, their decisions came to have the force of law" (Starr, 1982:121).

Following the popularization of these basic reforms across U.S. medical schools, major philanthropic foundations stepped in to further this agenda. It was widely recognized (by both medical schools and foundations) that few, if any, medical schools possessed the resources to implement the needed capital-intensive reforms absent outside financial assistance. As a consequence, private corporate foundations were able to link funding to specific reforms and thereby exercise considerable influence over the reshaping of U.S. medical education. One example of this influence was the campaign by foundations to reduce the independence of physicians within medical schools by creating full-time clinical positions that eliminated the faculty's opportunities for private practice and thereby subordinated the interests of physicians to the interests of private industry. "The full-time plan was adopted by [Rockefeller's] General Education Board as its central policy in medical education to help bring the medical profession to heel and subordinate its practices to the needs of industrial capitalism for fully accessible medical care, or, as board member Jerome D. Greene put it, to abate 'commercialism in the medical profession'" (Brown, 1979:158). By 1936, Rockefeller's General Board of Education had provided medical schools with $91 million for the purpose of reshaping their programs to reign in physician independence and to promote research over medical practice.[69]

The shift in emphasis toward science and research (away from clinical issues) was the cardinal feature of U.S. medical school reforms that had begun decades earlier at Johns Hopkins. In 1907, Johns Hopkins created full-time clinical professorships. This pitted the interests of physicians (as private professional contractors) against the interests of those corporate sponsors of reform who sought to harness physicians to the discipline of capital. A full-time Johns Hopkins faculty member could earn an annual salary of $3–4,000, whereas a part-time faculty member with a private practice could expect to earn at least $10,000 a year (Brown, 1979:159). Prior to 1907, only the laboratory sciences were taught by full-time faculty. Clinical medicine had always been taught by physicians who maintained a private practice. Rockefeller's General Education Board fought vigorously for this move to full-time clinical faculty. However, owing to growing resentment from physicians forced to

[69] The total amount given by all foundations to medical schools by 1938 was $150 million. However, two-thirds of this money went to seven flagship medical schools.

give up their private practices, this requirement was dropped as a formal contingency for receiving Rockefeller money after 1925.

Science and research were increasingly valued over clinical training by major foundations who invested in U.S. medical schools. It was, after all, in the form of scientific research that biomedicine was most susceptible to commodification (such as pharmaceuticals, equipment, biotechnology). "As American medical education became increasingly dominated by scientists and researchers, doctors came to be trained according to the values and standards of academic specialists . . . The foundation-sponsored victory of the Johns Hopkins model prevented American medicine from remaining as practical in its orientation as might have been its natural tendency" (Starr, 1982:123). This emphasis on full-time research and teaching over clinical practice was premised, in part, on the notion of biomedicine as a science in which bedside diagnosis and care was secondary to laboratory research that advanced the medical sciences.[70] Reducing private practice could also create a sense of common purpose and mission among all members of the medical school community. It was hoped that "Elite practitioners would now have to choose either a grand income or a respected teaching and research position" (Brown, 1979:163). Not surprisingly, among elite medical schools, only Harvard was initially able to ignore this movement to create full-time clinical faculty. This was due to its strong reputation as an exemplary scientific medical school as well the faculty's connections to the social elite of Boston. This struggle over full-time clinical appointments, thus, provides further evidence of the central role of social power relations as a defining feature of biomedicine.

Ultimately, in a rather transparent display of biomedicine as an expression of social power, these early 20th-century "reforms" were designed to solidify biomedicine's privileged stature vis-à-vis alternative medical practices in the United States and to shrink the pool of competing physicians by closing the few existing opportunities for aspiring women, African American, and working-class physicians. The basic goal of biomedicine's proponents was twofold. On the one hand, they sought to define medical care strategically in a fashion that narrowly limited its scope to those beliefs and practices associated with profit-based, Western, scientific medicine. This created a monopoly for biomedicine. On the other hand, the goal was to create

[70] Shryock observes that there was, in fact, a significant gap in expectations between physicians and laboratory scientists that was linked to the historical origin of each. "In the case of physical science, there was no large and ancient guild whose organization or vested interests might retard an effective pursuit of new science. It was far otherwise in medicine. Consider, for example, the situation in the United States during the 19th century. In this country, by guild tradition, there were rarely any full-time professors in medical faculties before 1900. Within the universities, professors of physical science could give all their time to teaching and investigation; but medical instructors were selected from among the best known—and therefore the busiest—practitioners" (1953:223).

the conditions for further reducing competition by severely circumscribing who could become a biomedical practitioner. As detailed below, these biomedical reforms resulted in the systematic exclusion of women, African Americans, and working-class whites and immigrants from opportunities to practice medicine that had previously been available to them. This created a monopoly for wealthy white males. The U.S. system of biomedicine that evolved through the first half of the 20th century was, therefore, as much the product of social exclusion and elite privilege as it was of advances in bacteriology and immunology.

Biomedicine, as a social institution, reflected the deep racial disparities endemic to U.S. society. The pursuit of a medical career had always been greatly restricted for African Americans, however following the licensing and medical school reforms, the paths for African Americans were made even more difficult. Prior to the reforms, a formal system of discrimination had denied African Americans the opportunity to attend white medical schools. African American medical schools were among the poorest and most neglected in the United States. Nonetheless, Flexner held these medical schools to the same criteria as any other. As a consequence, following his report, most were closed. The cost of these developments for African American communities was stark. By 1910, only two of the seven (pre-Flexner) African American medical schools (Howard and Meharry) remained open. In that same year, there were 2,883 African Americans for every African American doctor—for whites the ratio was 684:1. By 1942, it decreased to one African American doctor for every 3,377 African Americans. In the rural south these disparities were compounded. Mississippi had one African American doctor for every 14,634 African Americans. "Consistent with the racism of his period, Flexner argued that 'the practice of the Negro doctor would be limited to his own race.' However, 'self-protection not less than humanity' should encourage white society to support improved training for Black physicians: 'ten millions of them live in close contact with sixty million whites'" (Brown, 1979:148).

For women, too, the Flexner-era reforms signaled significant setbacks. Women had gained access to male medical schools just prior to the start of the 20th century.[71] By 1900, there were seven thousand female physicians in the United States.[72] One effect of reducing the number of medical schools was to increase competition among students for fewer spots. Male medical school officials considered the female applicants for increasingly scarce medical school slots to be weaker than males in two respects. On the one

[71] Johns Hopkins accepted women in 1890 only after a half-million dollar donation from a group of wealthy women.

[72] By contrast, for the same year, there were a mere 258 female physicians in England and just 95 in France (Starr, 1982:117).

hand, it was simply presumed that men were intellectually superior to women. This was seen as purely a matter of natural law that, just coincidentally, worked to the advantage of the male officials. On the other hand, as mothers and wives, women had important roles to play in society. A medical career was seen as a tremendous burden, therefore, not only on a woman's intellectual faculties but on her family hearth as well. Consequently, with the exception of wartime, U.S. medical schools imposed a strict quota that limited female students to about 5% of all medical student admissions between 1910 and 1960 (Starr, 1982:124).

Those of modest means were also effectively cut off from medical careers following the licensing and medical school reforms. The high cost of a medical education after the reforms and the need to forego a steady income for five or six years of study and apprenticeship severely limited participation by anyone from the lower social classes. Prior to these reforms, the prospect of a working-class youth pursuing a medical career, though uncommon, was at least feasible. "It was entirely conceivable [at the turn of the century] that a working class youth disenchanted with factory life could, by saving up a little money, enroll in one of the many proprietary medical schools" (Berliner, 1975:584). The cost of a medical education now required an exorbitant sum of money up front with a commitment to several years of little or no income as a student. Like African Americans and women, the poor were systematically denied access to a medical career, as wealthy white males took full control of biomedicine as a social institution—a blatant advertisement for the underlying social power relations.

The U.S. case thus illustrates biomedicine as an expression of social power and thereby exposes a third side of biomedicine as an ontological whole. From this perspective, the scientific content of biomedicine is linked to the interests of industrial capitalism and its symbolic-cultural forms are mined for the hidden power relations they obscure. Rather than reflexively celebrating the promotional tale of biomedicine as a cascade of scientific discoveries and breakthroughs in realization of a universal scientific ethos, biomedicine as an expression of social power highlights the wars of position between advocates of competing social interests who sought to reap the rewards of a budding biomedical industry, as capital absorbed biomedicine within the logic of capital accumulation. "Because it is, of historical necessity, in harmony with the general philosophy of capitalism, i.e., classical liberalism, the clinical paradigm is overwhelmingly concerned with the individual and neglects the study of collectivities" (Turshen, 1977a:58). Biomedicine is simultaneously a source of physical remedies as well as a source of stupendous financial profits. The contemporary U.S. biomedical industrial complex is thus an outgrowth of this marriage of science and capitalism that is held together by an array of self-justifying symbolic-cultural forms.

The Analytical Premises of Biomedicine in Africa

The developments described above in the second half of the 19th century exemplify the imbricated nature of transformation across biomedicine's ontological spheres. This was a period of dynamic change and solidification in the life history of biomedicine, an era of significant material, ideological, and political consolidation for each ontological sphere across all spatial-temporal locations. At the level of middle-range episodes, there was a dramatic cascade of interrelated developments that later came to define Western biomedicine in the modern era. For biomedicine as a scientific enterprise, this was the era of spectacular bacterial discoveries. The revolutionary breakthroughs of Koch and Pasteur wiped out a host of ancient deadly scourges that disappeared practically overnight. Following an exciting four-decade period—punctuated by a series of cumulative short-term events, such as Pasteur's accidental rabies' vaccine—the field of bacteriology was firmly established and the germ theory of disease achieved unrivaled status within medicine. In light of these discoveries, the principles of scientific medicine, now the exclusive domain of biomedicine, defined the criteria by which the most modern and progressive medical practices were judged. In combination with the colonial imperative, these medical discoveries would help legitimize the so-called white man's burden in Africa.

At the same time, for biomedicine as a symbolic-cultural expression, the second half of the 19th century was a period of strategic popularization. The primary vehicles for this growing public adulation were the remarkable new technologies that promoted an ideology of scientific rigor and professional detachment, while ushering in the machine metaphor. The popular identification of biomedicine with a neutral scientific objectivity followed both from a spate of short-term events in the form of new inventions (such as the sphygmograph, sphygmomanometer, and electrometer) and from the emerging techniques and specializations that identified specific diseases with certain parts and functions of the body. Elevating the precision of medical observations and measurements to that of the other physical sciences was essential for creating the proper scientific imagery both for rival scientists and among the general public. These developments allowed Koch and Pasteur to stand alongside Michael Faraday and James Clerk Maxwell. At the same time, the symbolic-cultural content of the world opened up by bacteriology inspired a reductionist etiological rationale that limited disease to phenomena within the natural world and that came to dominate the belief system of biomedicine. This was a myopic cultural trait that African medical practitioners would later view with considerable skepticism.

For biomedicine as an expression of social power, this was a period of remarkable economic and political consolidation that has continued up to the present day. As the details of the U.S. experience indicate, the potential for biomedicine as a source of prestige as well as profit was first fully exploited in the second half of the 19th century. This coincided, more generally, with the transition from competitive to monopoly capitalism. A number of powerful elites from industry and commerce brought the same business acumen and sensibilities that had built railroad, mining, and oil empires to the task of restructuring U.S. medicine. Investors seized on the opportunity further to commodify biomedicine and to reorganize medical practice and medical research better to comply with the logic of accumulation. Whereas breakthroughs in chemistry and physics had long had direct applications in various industries, the value of medical innovations were generally limited to treating individuals' maladies. The stunning rush of major medical discoveries in a brief span of time, in combination with an emerging popular medical ideology that venerated technology and innovation, suggested that biomedicine itself could be industrialized. Biomedicine's consolidation of economic and political power in the latter 19th century is, therefore, as salient a feature of its development in this era as the germ theory or the machine metaphor. By the time it reached the African shore, of course, the notion of biomedicine as an expression of social power was not especially well hidden.

This depiction of Western biomedicine in the second half of the 19th century thus chronicles an era of remarkable transformation, shaped by a collection of colorful events and dramatic episodes whose profound consequences survived long into the 20th century. However, when these developments of biomedicine as an ontological whole are further recast against the backdrop of the *longue durée* and a single, global unit of analysis, one begins to catch a glimpse of the reciprocal potential of global cultural flows set in motion when biomedicine later traveled to Africa. As a scientific enterprise, biomedicine attaches itself, across the *longue durée,* to a heroic and revolutionary saga of linear and cumulative scientific progress that dates from the 16th century forward. As such, the discoveries in the field of bacteriology are framed as contributions to this heroic narrative and biomedicine is self-consciously identified with the mythical traditions steeped in utilitarian progress. The principles of biomedicine that resulted were believed no less universal than the immutable laws of physics. Thus, transported to Africa or anywhere else, they would surely apply with equal utility and vigor. As a symbolic-cultural expression, biomedicine safeguards the ideological edifice identifying knowledge and truth with the cultural norms of practicality and a stoic objectivity. In this regard, the flurry of technological advances that stamped the public image of medicine in the second half of the 19th century represented a period of spectacular triumph for the guardians of reason. The resulting precision of medical observations and measurements allowed the mantra of science-based progress to colonize yet another domain. Lastly, as an expression of social power, the latter 19th-century evolution of biomedicine contributed to processes of endless accumulation across the *longue durée* via its commodification and monopolization. Nonbiomedical competitors were effectively vanquished and the practice of medicine itself was routinized and restructured in accordance with the rational principles of efficiency, calculability, and predictability.

The analysis of biomedicine to this point has been limited to Europe and North America. Even restricted across space in this manner, biomedicine remains in motion through time. When the element of movement across space is brought in, however, then the dynamics of biomedicine achieve still greater degrees of inventive complexity. As outlined in Chapter 1, simultaneously conceptualizing biomedicine as an ontological whole and as a singular historical-cultural formation is a basic prerequisite for analyzing the reciprocal nature of global cultural flows between Africa and the West with respect to biomedical values, beliefs, and practices. Each ontological sphere contains its own set of embedded levels of abstraction, corresponding to varying spatial-temporal locations across the capitalist world-system. This suggests two things for biomedicine in Africa in particular and for historical-cultural formations more generally. First, biomedicine is never static. It contains its own internal processes of dynamic change, vis-à-vis ongoing interactions between elements across these spatial-temporal locations. Hence, that which Africa seeks to absorb and domesticate continues to retain the drive for still further change. African biomedicine itself evolves. Second, biomedicine is ever-adapting. Adaptation is an inherent feature of biomedicine based on the mutually defining relationships between ontological spheres. Thus, as one sphere evolves (such as the consolidation of social power), the other spheres accommodate and adjust to these developments. The African adaptation of biomedicine, therefore, follows in part from the fact that biomedicine itself, as an ontological whole, is held together by a set of relationships premised on permanent reconstitution.

Thus, just as biomedicine had been fundamentally transformed during the decades between 1850 and 1900 without leaving Europe or North America, biomedicine's journey to Africa would, likewise, radically and irrevocably alter the purportedly universal content of its multiple, embedded ontological spheres. The pretext for biomedicine in Africa was European colonial subjugation in the service of incorporating Africa into the expanding capitalist world-system. Consequently, biomedicine was both a tool for European conquest and a means for aligning African sociocultural beliefs and practices with the global structures and processes that comprised the capitalist world-system. Suddenly seated on the world stage, biomedicine represented a singular historical-cultural formation that was destined, on the one hand, to transform Africa and, on the other hand, to be transformed *by* Africa. It is to this journey that we now turn.

3
Biomedicine's Civilizing Mission

A surprisingly brief period of continent-wide colonial rule in the late 19th and early 20th centuries provided the pretext for the introduction of biomedicine into Africa. The European Scramble for Africa highlighted an era of unprecedented imperialist expansion when the 19th-century rise of industrial capitalism undermined the lucrative sinews of mercantile colonialism. The major industrial powers moved aggressively to carve out territorial claims and the armies of Western imperialism established new exploitative relationships between distinct cultures and peoples based on explicit forms of racial-cultural domination.[1] Colonial rule embodied a naked policy of the Western powers to secure the raw materials and coerced labor that fed capital accumulation in a small circle of advanced capitalist nations. It was a form of economic exploitation based on the projection of political-military power that defined the core-periphery relationship across the capitalist world-system at this time. The Berlin Congress of 1884–1885, therefore,

[1] Given the admixture of empire, global capitalism, and European racism, Balandier suggests that colonial society represented a type of "dual reality." "[H]e is misguided who thinks that a present-day study [1951] of this society can be made without taking into account this dual reality, 'the colony,' a global society within which the study must situate itself, and the colonial situation created by 'the colony.' This is especially true of any study whose avowed purpose is to set forth the facts resulting from 'the contact' and the phenomena or processes of evolution" (1966:55).

signaled the formal entry of the African continent as a pawn in an accelerated land-grab to establish Western dominion over the globe's remaining unclaimed resources. A confident sense of racial superiority justified Western rule over non-Western peoples, as Europeans took on the white man's burden to bring civilization, Christianity, and material progress to the world's savage and backward peoples. In this context, the introduction of Western biomedicine assumed the pretense of a selfless gift that could ultimately justify the harsher aspects of colonial rule. As the architect of French colonial medical services, Hubert Lyautey, famously sermonized, "*La seule excuse de la colonisation, c'est la médecine.*" The remarkable curative powers of biomedicine thus offered both comfort for African afflictions and solace for the Western conscience.

A series of calculated biomedical advances, in the guise of "tropical" medicine, prepared the path for Western expansion.[2] The field of tropical medicine was the conscious, political creation of the Western industrial powers to combat disease among European colonial soldiers, administrators, and settlers. In a sudden burst of scientific zeal between 1895 and 1912, nearly all the colonial powers established their own specialized schools of tropical medicine. Over the next few decades, the Western powers selectively shared the benefits of tropical medicine with strategic sectors of the colonized populations. Laborers in key industries and civil servants, for example, were among the first to receive care. Women, children, and the vast peasantry were another matter. Just as arbitrary colonial borders, cash-crop production, and Christian missionaries had disrupted and transformed social patterns of organization, the introduction of biomedicine undermined longstanding sociocultural practices and transformed collective worldviews.[3] In this sense, biomedicine in Africa served as an essential instrument of colonial rule and subjugation and thereby earned the Africans' understandable skepticism. However, beginning with a number of successful and highly visible public health campaigns—such as the anti-yaws programs in East Africa in the 1920s—African suspicions and mistrust gradually lifted and biomedical beliefs and practices began to take root.

---

[2] As many have noted, the term tropical medicine is inherently misleading (Worboys, 1996). The deceptive reference to a geographic descriptor shifts attention from a host of underlying social and political conditions that support and perpetuate diseases regardless of climate. "The label 'tropical' reinforces the impression that natural conditions like climate rather than economic conditions or political circumstances are responsible for the persistence of these diseases in the Third World" (Turshen, 1984:14–15).

[3] Feierman (1985) notes the strong link between control over healing and social power. "The person who controls therapy serves as a conduit transmitting general social values, but is also capable of reshaping and reinterpreting those values in the healing process" (p. 75).

As outlined in Chapter 1, the story of biomedicine in Africa involves a singular historical-cultural formation across multiple social times. In this sense, biomedicine's arrival is a middle-range episode embedded in the longer history of European colonial rule in Africa. This era of colonial rule, of course, is itself an episode in the development of the capitalist world-system over the *longue durée*. The analysis of biomedicine in Africa is thus premised on developments at each level informing developments at the other levels. The analysis of biomedicine in Africa that emerges is both shaped by and helps to shape the interactions between European colonialism and biomedicine as a singular historical-cultural formation. This, therefore, requires a manner of presentation that entails the overlapping, multiple levels of analysis that structure the story. For instance, from one angle of vision, biomedicine in Africa is a creature of European colonization and the expanding capitalist world-system. As such, the Scramble for Africa—and its attendant sociocultural transformations—is a pivotal epoch that is defined by the longer history of Western global expansion. However, from a second angle of vision, biomedicine in Africa reflects the combined influences of tropical medicine and African medical campaigns, which gave form to African colonization and conditioned Africa's incorporation into the capitalist world-system. These intersecting interpretations, across multiple spatial-temporal levels of analysis, thus inform and organize the present analysis of biomedicine's civilizing mission to Africa.

African Colonization and the Expanding Capitalist World-System

Western Global Expansion

The non-Europeans' encounters with the West of the past five hundred years is conventionally divided into two major eras. The first period, the late 16th century through the mid-18th century, was an extended period of mercantilist colonial rule premised on maritime military power.[4] In this period, the Dutch, British, French, Spanish, and Portuguese empires were built on the buying and selling of slaves, spices, sugar, and precious metals, as Europeans used colonial networks to secure access to these resources. With the notable exception of the Americas, there was little interest in territorial expansion (such as settler colonialism) in this era and few significant efforts to alter established patterns of social organization. "However disruptive these changes may have been to the societies of Africa, South America, and the isolated

[4] See Magdoff (1978), Rodney (1981), and Wallerstein (1976).

plantations of white-settler colonies, the social systems over most of the earth outside of Europe nevertheless remained much the same as they had been for centuries" (Magdoff, 1978:18). By the 1750s, much of the non-European world was dotted with a patchwork of Western trading posts and forts to guard commerce and project European power.

The second colonial period, the mid-18th century through the mid-20th century, ushered in the industrial revolution and growing European rivalries that resulted in a world map overlaid with Western (and Japanese) colonies, protectorates and spheres of influence.[5] The economic and strategic rationale for colonization changed at this time. Colonies were increasingly the buyers of Western manufactured goods and the producers of raw materials (for example, cotton, wool, rubber, tin, copper, vegetable oils, jute) and food (such as wheat, tea, cocoa, meat) for urban, industrial Europe. "[T]he major fact about the 19th century is the creation of a single global economy, progressively reaching into the most remote corners of the world, an increasingly dense web of economic transactions, communications, and movements of goods, money, and people linking the developed countries with each other and with the undeveloped world" (Hobsbawm, 1989:62). As the rationale for the colony turned increasingly on its ties to industrial capital, the nature of colonial rule was transformed as well. The importance of trading posts and forts was surpassed by the need for mines, plantations, warehouses, factories, refineries, and railroads. Between 1840 and 1910, global merchant shipping increased from ten million tons to thirty-two million tons. Between 1870 and 1914, railroads increased worldwide from two hundred thousand kilometers to one million kilometers (Hobsbawm, 1989:62). Massive social disruption followed. Colonial powers moved from the coastlines to the interior, overturning age-old land and property customs, creating alienable land, and developing various forced labor systems for mining and commercial agriculture.

Beyond the economic rationale of colonial policy in this second period, there was the growing chauvinistic rivalry among Western powers[6] that drove European expansion. "[C]olonies came to have an intangible but momentous value in symbolism and prestige. To have colonies was a normal criterion of greatness. It was the sign of having arrived as a Great Power"

---

[5] Colonies, protectorates and spheres of influence were all administrative strategies to establish exclusive access to a territory. Each differed with respect to the degree of direct administrative control. In general, colonies had the most elaborate and extensive administrative units while spheres of influence had the least. Special commercial treaties presented a fourth strategy. These were agreements with nations with whom other nations also traded (e.g., China) and did not imply exclusive administrative control.

[6] By the late 19th century, Japan was included among the Western powers following the Meiji Restoration and its conscious and deliberate strategy of westernization for purposes of geopolitical advantage (M. Jansen, 2000; Sugiyama, 1988; Beasley, 1981).

(Palmer, 1963:622). A number of mercantile-era powers were on the decline throughout this era—Portugal, Spain, and to a lesser extent the Dutch. Meanwhile, by the late 19th century, several newly industrializing powers were on the rise—Germany, the United States, Japan, Belgium, and Italy. The era opened with the British exercising unmatched global power and influence. The Treaty of Paris of 1763, following victory in the Seven Years' War, granted Britain extraordinary control over the South Pacific, Far East, South Atlantic, and African coastline.[7] "In 1763 the first British Empire was primarily focused on North America. By 1815, despite the loss of the thirteen colonies, Britain had a second empire, one that straddled the globe from Canada and the Caribbean in the Western Hemisphere around the Cape of Good Hope to India and Australia" (Magdoff, 1978:24).

Due to the scale and accelerated nature of colonial acquisition and global Western competition, the final decades of this period (the 1870s through 1914) constituted the age of imperialism. At the turn of the 19th century, Europe and its colonies had comprised 55% of the world's land surface (Europe, the Americas, India, and the coast of Africa)—though it is estimated that effective control was exercised over only 35% of this area, primarily Europe (Magdoff, 1978:29). By 1878, control increased to 67% and, by World War I, it reached 85%. Germany, the United States, Italy, Japan, and Belgium had joined ranks with the older colonial powers (Britain, France, the Netherlands, and others) to increase significantly the number of Western nations prowling the globe in search of further colonial possessions (and access to labor, raw materials, and cash crops) to feed their nation's industrial needs. The age of imperialism gave definitive form to a new international division of labor in which industrial nations produced and sold manufactured goods while colonial territories produced and sold raw materials and food. The 19th century was, therefore, a period of unrelenting European expansion, culminating with the partition of Africa and the opening of China. It was a time of heightened inter-rival competition and intermittent wars between Western powers and non-Europeans, as colonizers moved more deeply inland from their coastal colonial holdings.

The crumbling Ottoman Empire, Asia, and Africa were the major arenas of colonial expansion in the 19th century.[8] The Ottoman Empire, though

---

[7] In Africa, the British took control of the coastal areas of Sierra Leone (1808), Gambia (1816), and the Gold Coast (1821). These primarily served as bases for suppressing the slave trade.

[8] In light of the Monroe Doctrine (1823) and its growing industrial muscle, the Americas were increasingly recognized as a U.S. sphere of influence and thus less subject to colonial competition. The U.S. strategy was twofold: (1) Territorial expansion proceeded via annexation and war—e.g., Texas (1845); Hawaii, Puerto Rico, and the Philippines (1898); (2) Regional control was pursued through protectorates (Panama), treaties (the Platt Amendment in Cuba), direct invasion (Haiti), and the Dollar Diplomacy of the early 20th century.

greatly weakened by growing independence movements and Pan-Slavic nationalism (along with periodic Russian incursions), still stretched across an enormous land mass over several continents from Eastern Europe into portions of North Africa and the Middle East. The empire's gradual demise picked up pace in the 1850s and continued through its formal dissolution and the establishment of a Turkish Republic in 1923.[9] With Britain and Russia poised for war over the control of Ottoman land following the Treaty of Stefano in 1877, Bismarck hastily organized a congress of European powers in Berlin to discuss the brewing conflicts over claims to Ottoman territory. The resulting Treaty of Berlin in 1878 allowed European powers to share in the spoils of the Ottoman Empire's dissolution. Britain retained control of Egypt[10] and gained Cyprus, France expanded its hold on Algeria, Tunisia, and later Morocco, and Russia compromised on its spoils from the Treaty of Stefano.[11] Subsequent wars further decimated the Ottoman Empire.[12] Not surprisingly, while most of the European territory lost in this period (Serbia, Bosnia, Montenegro, and others) became nominally independent states, most Arab areas (Algeria to the Persian Gulf) were grafted onto European colonial holdings before becoming mandates of Britain and France following World War I. By the end of that war, the centuries-old Ottoman Empire was no more.

European imperial expansion in Asia resulted in a hodgepodge of territorial holdings. The Dutch East Indies and the British in India were long-standing colonial powers in the region. However in 1815, the Dutch occupation amounted to little beyond the island of Java. To guard against rival powers, Dutch control was systematically spread across the entire Indonesian archipelago over the course of the 19th century, sparking multiple revolts in 1830, 1849, and 1888. Following the 1857 Indian Mutiny, the British expanded their territorial hold on India and tightened their direct rule through the expanded use of Indian surrogates. The British also captured Singapore, the Malay Pen-

---

[9] Already by 1850, Russia controlled parts of Crimea and the Caucasus, Serbia was semi-autonomous, Romania was self-governing, the Sauds ruled Arabia, Mohammed Ali controlled the Nile Valley, and France occupied Algeria.

[10] The French had completed the Suez Canal in 1869. Given the canal's enormous strategic value, the British moved swiftly to become its majority owner by 1876 and Egypt was made a protectorate of Britain shortly thereafter, in 1882.

[11] Though gaining no territory directly from the Treaty of Berlin, Germany was able to establish itself as an influential force in the Middle East. Toward this end—and much to the consternation of Russia, France, and Britain—between 1878 and 1914, Germany was nearly able to complete a railroad linking Berlin with Baghdad.

[12] The Turco-Italian war (1911–1912) gave Libya and the Dodecanese Islands to Italy, and the Balkan wars (1912–1913) cost the Ottomans the remainder of its European territory.

insula, North Borneo, Burma, and Sumatra. France meanwhile took Indochina (Vietnam, Laos, Cambodia) in the 1860s and Germany annexed eastern New Guinea and the Marshall and Solomon Islands in the 1880s.[13] Russia's defeat in the Crimean War (1853–1856) briefly blocked its expansionist aims in the Near East, while the emancipation of serfs in 1861 led to massive migrations to Siberia and Central Asia.[14] Russia and Britain continued to battle over Persia from the 1860s through World War I, while Japan, following the Meiji Restoration, emerged as a late-industrializing colonial power. Japan moved quickly to annex a number of contested neighboring islands, including the Ryuku Islands, Kuril Islands, Bonin Islands, and Hokkaido.

China remained the major prize in Asia. For centuries, China had frustrated European attempts to establish commercial pacts until finally, by the 19th century, China was threatened by a combination of colonial powers advancing from all sides. To the north sat Russia. From the south and west beckoned the British via India and Burma. French-controlled Indochina lay to the south, and China remained vulnerable to the United States via the Philippines and to Japan from the east. The West's imperial aims in China provoked a series of wars. The first Opium War in 1841 and the resulting Treaty of Nanking in 1842 provided Britain with commercial access to China. The United States, France, and Russia soon secured similar treaties. The second Opium War between 1856 and 1860 led to the Tientsin Treaties, granting Britain, France, Russia, and the United States extensive commercial access to China's interior.[15] As competition grew among Western powers for spheres of influence within China, the United States promoted the Open Door Policy designed to restrict exclusive commercial privileges. Attempts by the Chinese to curtail commercial access met with swift and ferocious opposition. In 1900, the joint forces of Britain, France, Italy, Russia, Germany, the United States, and Japan crushed the Boxer Rebellion. Japan's rise as a global power, meanwhile, became evident when war broke out with China in 1894. The resulting Shimonoseki Treaty in 1895 gave Japan control of Korea, Taiwan, the Pescadores, and the Liaotung Peninsula (with access to Manchuria).[16] By

---

[13] By 1914, there were no independent states left in the Pacific. All fell under British, French, German, Dutch, or U.S. control.

[14] Russia mounted several imperial campaigns in Siberia, Central Asia, the Caucasus, and the Far East. A continuing quest for a warm water port resulted in Russia's founding Vladivostock in 1860 on the Sea of Japan.

[15] China was subsequently forced to sign a series of similar treaties with Germany, Italy, the Netherlands, Denmark, Spain, Belgium, and Austria-Hungary.

[16] Shortly thereafter, Russia, Germany, and France intervened to force the return of the strategic Liaotung Peninsula to China, with assurances of international access.

the time of the Russian-Japanese War (1904–1905), most of China had been parceled out among the Western powers.[17] China ended the age of imperialism weakened and defeated. The competing powers had largely succeeded in opening China to the global economy.

Africa represented a third region of colonial expansion at this time. As noted above, the partition of Africa in 1884–1885 was preceded by a lengthy mercantilist period (1500–1750). Over the period of 1750 to 1880, however, trade had increasingly centered on slaves and goods destined to feed the growth of European industrialization, as parts of West Africa were pulled within the outer orbit of the expanding capitalist world-system, followed by much of East Africa by the end of the 19th century (Wallerstein, 1974; 1976). The slave trade expanded, for example, on both the west and east coasts between 1750 and 1810. Indeed, by 1810 the East African Atlantic slave trade equaled that of West Africa at its height. Importantly, by the time of the partition of Africa, a single, global division of labor had emerged across the capitalist world-system based on production for an integrated world market. This global order, organized around the logic of capital accumulation and feeding expanded reproduction, experienced growing polarization between those in the industrial manufacturing core and those in the raw materials-producing colonial periphery.[18] As the colonial powers settled in to divide up Africa's riches, this represented, therefore, as much an expansion of the capitalist world-system as an expansion of European power. "Late-nineteenth-century imperialism in Africa was the final sortie by which the world capitalist system captured the last continent to remain partially beyond its pale" (Lonsdale and Berman, 1979:487).

In 1878 Henry Stanley, of David Livingston fame, persuaded Leopold II of Belgium to create the International Congo Association, a private enterprise designed to explore the central African Congo basin for productive resources. At roughly the same time, Karl Peters, a private German adventurer, was busy pursuing treaties with various leaders in East Africa, and a French naval officer, Savorgnan de Brazza, was exploring routes to the Congo River from the west coast. The British, Portuguese, French, and others already held a string of territories along the coastlines.[19] Britain held parts of Gambia, the Gold Coast, and Sierra Leone on the west coast. Zanzibar in the east and the Cape Colony had passed from Dutch to British control in 1795. France held

[17] Victory allowed Japan to regain the Liaotung Peninsula and to establish a protectorate in Korea—until its formal annexation in 1910. Japan also gained the southern portion of the Sakhalin Islands.

[18] See Amin (1972), Emmanuel (1972), Frank (1967), Rodney (1981) and Wallerstein (1976).

[19] Other European powers with coastal possessions included the Netherlands, Denmark, Sweden, and Brandenburg.

coastal sections of the Ivory Coast, Dahomey, Gabon, and Senegal.[20] Portugal held Angola, Mozambique, Guinea, and São Tomé e Principe. By the eve of the Berlin Congress in May 1884, the competition for African territory had reached a fever pitch. Two major issues galvanized the remarkable gathering of fifteen nations[21] in Berlin—the contested legal status of the International Congo Association and the details of partition itself.

After a series of negotiated agreements, the Congo Association became the Congo Free State under the dominion of Leopold II (with no state involvement)[22] and the area of the Congo Free State was expanded to include the mineral-rich Katanga region. The Congo River was internationalized and declared open to all imperial powers. Slavery was outlawed and tariffs were barred for any exports—though the enforcement of such provisions was rarely effective. Delegates to the Berlin Congress next crafted a legal framework that specified the procedures for the European powers to lay claim to African territory. By the conclusion of the Congress in February 1885, a basic plan for partition among the imperial powers had been drawn up. The resulting boundary lines created a collection of territories that haphazardly crisscrossed established African kingdoms and territorial units. As John D. Hargreaves observes, however, haphazard did not always mean arbitrary. "Since European claims were often based upon treaties with African rulers, there were many cases where the new frontiers coincided with traditional ones; other things being equal, the colonial powers preferred to follow chiefdom boundaries, where these were known" (quoted in Wallerstein, 1970:404–405).

As the Scramble for Africa proceeded, the continent's map underwent radical re-shaping. In West Africa, the French established French West Africa (Senegal, Mali, Burkina Faso, Benin, Guinea, Ivory Coast, and Niger) along with its possessions in French Equatorial Africa (Gabon, Chad, the Central African Republic, and portions of the Congo). The Germans grabbed Togoland and Cameroon, and the British held Nigeria and the Niger region. In Central Africa, the British captured northern Rhodesia (Zambia), southern Rhodesia (Zimbabwe), Nyasaland (Malawi), and Bechuanaland (Botswana). Germany held onto South West Africa (Namibia), and South Africa was given the Republic of the Transvaal. Britain retained control of the Cape Colony and annexed Zululand. The Boer War (1899–1902) eventually gave Britain control of the Transvaal and the Afrikaner Orange Free State. In East Africa, the 1890 Anglo-German Treaty granted Germany Tanganyika (Tanzania),

---

[20] France also had a long-standing presence in Algeria (since 1830) and Tunisia.

[21] This included the United States. Switzerland was the only European nation not to attend.

[22] It was not until the death of Leopold II in 1909 that the Congo Free State became the possession of Belgium.

Rwanda, and Burundi, and gave Uganda, Kenya, and Zanzibar to Britain. In Northeast Africa, Britain and France fought for control of the strategic upper Nile. Eastern Sudan was ruled jointly by the British and Egypt, and France was given the rest of the Sudan from the Congo to Lake Chad to Darfur. Meanwhile, Italy moved into Eritrea and Somaliland (Somalia) before their defeat at the hands of Ethiopia in the Battle of Aduwa in 1896.[23]

Germany was forced to renounce most of its colonial holdings at the Treaty of Versailles in 1919, and the League of Nations Covenant created three categories of mandates. Class A mandates referred to those areas soon to become independent. This did not include any African territory. Class B mandates included those colonies that were to be transferred to a new European power with the stipulation that they could not be combined with existing colonies to create larger territories. In Africa, these included Cameroon (transferred to France), Togoland and Tanganyika (transferred to Britain), and Rwanda and Burundi (transferred to Belgium). Class C mandates were areas where the new owners could integrate the territory as they saw fit. This included South West Africa, which was given to South Africa. In a remarkably brief span of time, all of Africa came under foreign rule and this would last, for most, through the 1960s.

Colonial Rule and Social Transformation in Africa

European colonial rule in Africa was remarkable for both its totalizing impact and its surprising brevity. Large-scale direct European colonial rule in Africa lasted little more than a single lifespan, beginning in the 1880s and ending with decolonization in the 1960s and 1970s.[24] In this brief period, however, almost all of Africa's political, economic, and sociocultural institutions were radically restructured. "The colonial state in Africa lasted in most instances less than a century—a mere moment in historical time. Yet it totally reordered political space, societal hierarchies and cleavages, and modes of economic production. Its territorial grid determined the state units that gained sovereignty and came to form the present system of African politics" (C. Young, 1994:9–10). European languages, religion, science, habits, and customs were introduced in the context of global commerce, forced labor, and political subjugation marked by extreme violence and systematic

[23] Ethiopia had been an Italian protectorate from 1889 to 1896 and was later reconquered by Italy in 1935.

[24] "[I]t is a surprising fact that in most parts of Africa the entire experience of colonialism, from original occupation to the formation of independent states, fits within a single lifetime—say that of Winston Churchill (1874–1965)" (Hobsbawm, 1989:79).

exploitation.[25] Africa was treated as a bountiful reservoir for industrial raw materials, precious metals, and a variety of cash crops. Africans were treated as a pliable labor force and an untapped market for European consumer goods, resulting in a combination of compulsory labor systems, migrant labor, and pass systems. "[The colonial system's] *raison d'être* was the ruthless exploitation of the human and material resources of the African continent to the advantage of the owners and shareholders of expatriate companies and the metropolitan governments and their manufacturing and industrial firms" (Boahen, 1987:62). The first obstacle for Europeans was other Europeans. This was largely resolved with the Berlin Congress. The second obstacle for Europeans was the Africans. The story of European colonial rule in Africa largely hinges on how the different European powers adopted a variety of strategies to assure effective control over large populations across often enormous territorial claims.

European colonial rule required a comprehensive strategy that combined political, economic, and sociocultural instruments of control. Colonial rule (the continued control and manipulation of people and land) required administrative structures that promoted a sustainable "peace" and a social order that facilitated the development of an integrated infrastructure along with basic medical services for Europeans and African laborers and a western educational system for civil servants and low-level administrators. A contrast is conventionally drawn in this regard between British and French rule. Following Lord Lugard's successes in northern Nigeria, the British developed a system of "indirect rule," whereby local African leaders were co-opted to assist and advance the colonial mission. While the British then established administrative systems for each colony based on the model of indirect rule, Cartesian logic persuaded French colonial officials to create massive, centralized colonial administrative units that were professionally staffed and formally linked with France's other colonial holdings. There was less reliance on local rulers given this arrangement and a greater role for professionally trained Africans. While these Anglo-Franco differences may reflect general tendencies, the colonial powers adopted a range of nuanced policies to fit specific situations. In the British case, for example, Wallerstein observes that, "[T]he sharp line between direct and indirect rule was thereby blurred. In fact the line was seldom sharp in Africa; all the colonial powers evolved a pragmatic policy which emerged, in one way or another, working with or through chiefs but always within the framework of overall colonial rules and values" (Wallerstein,

[25] The population of the Belgian Congo, for example, fell by 50% during colonial rule. The population of the Herero people (of Namibia) fell by 80%. Indeed, the Herero (along with the Khoikhoi and Zulu of South Africa and the Maji Maji Rebellion in Tanganyika) provided Europeans with some of the most fierce opposition to colonial rule (Davidson, 1968).

1961:41). France, likewise, made exceptions to the use of Western-trained African leaders in the case of certain ethnic groups with powerful chiefs such as the Mossi in Upper Volta (Burkina Faso) and the Lamidos in northern Cameroon. Ultimately, administrative policies were much more a matter of pragmatic adjustment than rigid, ideological orthodoxy.

Profit remained central to the European motives for the colonization of Africa. For the purposes of colonial rule, each colony became part of an international economic network in which trade occurred within a single economic unit (such as the British empire) rather than between units (such as between Nigeria and Britain). Each network was itself linked to other networks via the capitalist world-system.[26] A cardinal feature of European colonial rule was prohibitions barring industrialization, manufacturing, or the processing of raw materials—the very activities that could have provided a degree of economic independence for later development. Prior to colonization, Africans had produced their own building materials, pottery/crockery, soap, beads, iron tools, cloth, and gold. Predictably, underdevelopment and technological backwardness were the result of colonial rule at the time of African independence (Amin,1972; Rodney, 1981).

Following land confiscation, much of African agriculture was reorganized around export cash-crop production, based on white settler farms and a large African small-holding peasantry.[27] The pricing of exports (and European imports) remained in the hands of the colonizers. Prior to colonial rule, Africans were able to control the access to most raw materials and thereby to exercise greater control over pricing.[28] Palm oil, used in the production of soap and as a lubricant for machinery, is a case in point. As Europeans gained greater control of the palm oil market, the traditional role of Niger traders was eliminated. Previously, "the price of palm oil was kept un-

[26] Beginning with the Congo Free State, private companies played a critical role in the economic development of colonies. British companies included the Royal Niger Company (1886), the British East Africa Company (1888), and the British South Africa Company (1889).

[27] White settler colonies were most prominent in Kenya, southern Rhodesia, South Africa, and Algeria. By contrast, there were very few settlers in western and equatorial Africa where the land proved less fertile. The major African agricultural exports included sisal in Tanganyika; cotton in the Congo, the Sudan, and Uganda; rubber in the Congo; wine in Algeria; peanut oil and palm oil throughout West Africa; cocoa in Ghana; coffee in the Ivory Coast; tobacco in southern Rhodesia; and cloves in Zanzibar.

[28] A thriving regional and intra-regional trade within Africa was interrupted by colonialism. "The most immediate effect of colonial rule was its impact on the African traders, whose ability to play their traditional late 19th-century 'monopolistic role as middlemen' was drastically curtailed. The merging of European trading firms into large-scale enterprises capable of mobilizing vast amounts of working capital, commanding superior or exclusive credits with European colonial banks, and having direct access to a European commercial network, put the African traders at a great disadvantage from the outset" (Wallerstein, 1970:407).

reasonably high by the Niger delta middlemen who brought it to the coast" (Headrick, 1981:73). The resulting monocultural export economies were fully integrated into the world economy via the colonial powers. The fortunes of African producers, therefore, increasingly rose and fell with the vicissitudes of the capitalist world-system, and the commercialization and alienation of private and communal land left large masses of Africans homeless and impoverished.[29] Displaced populations soon crowded into shantytowns that circled the growing cities.

Large-scale industrial mining was perhaps the West's most profitable economic activity in the colonial era. It is estimated that two-thirds of the value of all of Africa's colonial output originated in the mining regions of South Africa, the Congo, and northern Rhodesia (Wallerstein, 1970:407). African laborers mining for precious metals and diamonds produced a massive transfer of wealth from Africa to Europe. "Availability of African labor was crucial to the accumulation imperative. Virtually all operations, vegetable and mineral, were labor intensive" (C. Young, 1994:137). Gold flowed from South Africa and Ghana, diamonds from South Africa and the Congo, tin from the Congo, and copper from northern Rhodesia (Zambia and parts of Zaire). Oil and rubber were also major products from the Congo. Trade unions emerged after World War I, as labor recruitment efforts and patterns of European land settlement created an enormous cash-crop peasantry and a conventional working class. By 1935, there were an estimated nine hundred thousand peasants involved in compulsory labor on cotton plantations in the Belgian Congo (Boahen, 1987:77). Indeed, Lyons (1988a) documents how one of the primary motives for the aggressive Belgian response to the Congo sleeping sickness epidemic in the early 20th century was to address growing criticism of colonial abuses. "[Leopold] intended to make the most of this opportunity (to address sleeping sickness) to combat the increasingly effective anti-Congo Free State propaganda campaign being waged in England. In March 1900, E. D. Morel, an Englishman who had worked for Jones' shipping line since 1891, wrote a series of articles exposing the scandal of 'Red Rubber' in the Congo Free State" (Lyons, 1988a:250).[30] Notwithstanding these developments, it is important to recall that throughout the colonial era, most African peasants retained a semisubsistent livelihood with only limited contact with the market economy.

[29] See Austen (1987), Brett (1973), and Bowles (1979).

[30] "[D]uring the early 1940s Zande District [in southern Sudan] was selected for the operation of a pilot scheme designed, ultimately, to fit this and other remote African peoples into the world economy. The Zande Scheme was essentially concerned with growing cotton for the world market" (Gillies, 1976b:xvi).

Alongside coercive administrative mechanisms and extractive economic schemes, European colonial rule was premised, above all, on the racial oppression of Africans. The denigration of African cultural forms was an integral aspect of colonial rule. A common tactic of European conquest was to target cultural symbols of African authority and power. "Sacralized symbols of African power were a special target: the gold stool of the Ashanti state, the 'long juju' of the Aro Chuku in eastern Nigeria" (C. Young, 1994:93). European cultural norms, values, and languages were promoted over African via the church, the schoolhouse, and the health clinic.[31] For example, European powers introduced an ethic of individualism with a strong patrilineal emphasis that disrupted established communal social orders, which often valued matrilineal lineages. Christianity and Western science further eroded African authority structures and governing belief systems. "The colonial regimes ruthlessly suppressed practices that were incompatible with the Christian traditions of the western society . . . In doing so, they shook people's confidence in the old gods and the older social order; they encouraged a scientific disbelief in the direct intervention of supernatural forces in human society, and in this destroyed faith in the traditional sanctions that held society together" (Ajayi, 1968:195). The sudden loss of sovereignty only heightened the impact of these European cultural exports.

Cultural change was, of course, nothing foreign to precolonial Africa. Africa had long experienced large-scale migrations with ongoing interethnic exchanges and conflicts. In these interethnic exchanges different peoples were exposed to competing cosmologies and varying social beliefs. Therefore, at the time of European subjugation, Africans were accustomed to evolving belief systems and contrasting social values. Indeed, ongoing cultural change was the norm of African society and a common experience. Furthermore, the adoption of cultural values, beliefs, and practices from foreign peoples was an established pattern of social development and a recognized historical precedent.

> [I]n any long-term historical view of African history, European rule becomes just another episode. In relation to wars and conflicts of people, the rise and fall of empires, linguistic, cultural and religious change and the cultivation of new ideas and new ways of life, new

[31] As explored below, the introduction of health care into colonial settings was initially a matter of pragmatism. Its purpose was to treat Europeans and essential members of the African labor force. In 1920, Dar es Salaam boasted one hospital bed for every ten Europeans compared to one bed for every 400 to 500 Africans. By the 1930s, Nigeria had 12 hospitals for 4,000 Europeans and 52 hospitals for 40 million Africans (Boahen, 1987:106).

> economic orientations and so on, in relation to all these colonialism must be seen not as a complete departure from the African past, but as one episode in the continuous flow of African history. (Ajayi, 1968:194)[32]

In the context of African colonial rule, biomedicine represented both a valuable tool of Western science to combat disease and an ideological set of sociocultural beliefs and practices suitable to civilize and Westernize the Africans. Many, such as H. C. Trowell, a medical officer in colonial Kenya in 1935, were rather blunt in this regard. "[T]he combined forces of scientific invention, materialistic philosophy, philanthropic humanism, Christianity, education and economic enterprise are breaking down this primitive philosophy, and the greatest of these is the ruthless energy of modern economic enterprise which in every plantation, every market and every wayside stone is throttling out the life breath from the primitive philosophy of magic" (quoted in Beck, 1970:139). In light of such colonial "philanthropy," Africa's rich, fluid and ever-developing collective worldviews were abruptly to reach the "end of time," as logical complexity, ambiguity, and overlapping belief systems were challenged by a form of singular, unchanging truth hailed by the West. Scientific reason was presented as the sole guardian of truth (within the physical world) and one of the primary sources of evidence for this were the benefits of biomedicine. In this way, biomedicine became one of the most powerful weapons for imposing Western cultural values, beliefs, and practices on African peoples and, thereby, for furthering the colonial mission of conquest and economic exploitation.

In light of these European aggressions—political, economic, and cultural—African resistance remained a significant challenge for colonial rulers throughout their stay. This resistance was heavily infused with a collective supernatural sensibility that largely prefigured African attitudes toward biomedicine and other European cultural offerings. The period from the 1890s through World War I was a time of continual rural rebellion and insurrection led by local leaders, resulting in tens of thousands of African deaths.[33] Suppression of Algeria's numerous rebellions in 1871, 1876, 1879, and from 1881 to 1884 ultimately required more European troops than the

[32] Ajayi argues that colonial rule was ultimately less a matter of cultural "disruption" and more a matter of cultural "adaptation." "I think that the really significant question which emerges from the little we know is not whether colonial rule disrupted African institutions or whether or not the institutions have shown continuity, but rather how they have been adapted to the changing circumstances" (Ajayi, 1968:198).

[33] Among the many rebellions were the 1898 Sierra Leone Hut Tax Rebellion; the 1900 Ashanti rebellion against taxation, forced labor, and Western education; the Nigerian Ekumeku rebellion between 1893 and 1906 in defense of traditional authority; and the numerous Zambezi Valley uprisings

British conquest of India.[34] Popular priests and spirit mediums commonly played key roles in planning and leading African resistance. In Kenya, where the Kitombo movement of 1896 was followed by the Kathambi movement—named after the female Kamba water-spirit—in 1910, colonial officials reported that, "The new types of possessing spirits and frenzied dances, drumming and promise of deliverance associated with these cults served to focus Kamba frustrations and their opposition to colonial rule" (cited in C. Good, 1987:80). The Tonga priest Maluma led a rebellion in Nyasaland in 1909. A Mbona priest led the Massingire rebellion in 1884. Maria Nkoie, a priestess in the Congo, led the Ikaya Rebellion from 1916 to 1921. Shona spirit mediums periodically led rebellions in the Zambezi Valley in 1897, 1901, and 1904. In Kenya, the Mumbo religious leader Onyango Dande led a revolt in 1913, and the Akamba priestess Siofume led a rebellion in eastern Kenya in 1911. Finally, the prophet Kinjikitile Ngwale led one of the largest African revolts, the Maji Maji rebellion in 1905, to drive the Germans out of Tanganyika. Over seventy-five thousand Africans were killed in this rebellion alone. Charles Good (1987) drew comparisons between these early anticolonial messianic movements and the 1950s Mau Mau rebellion in Kenya with respect to the role of pluralistic-medical beliefs and practices.

> Conditions in the mid-1950s seem to have paralleled those that gave birth to the messianic and cult movements that convulsed [the region East of Nairobi] during the 1890s and the first two decades of the 20th century. The fact that the "witchcraft" aberrations occurred during the tumultuous Mau Mau years, and were quite possibly an outgrowth of the political turmoil following the oathings that took place in Mbitini, seems a plausible link and a fruitful line of inquiry. (C. Good, 1987:98–99)

Insurrection was only one method of African resistance to colonial rule.[35] Various forms of organized and semi-organized social disruption and lawlessness—generically referred to as social banditry—fit within a long tradition of subaltern resistance across colonized peoples.[36] Social banditry in

---

(including the Manjaanga insurrection in Lower Congo) between 1890 and 1905 to protest labor recruitment.

[34] African resistance campaigns also led to significant migrations. Over 2,000 fled Ivory Coast for Ghana between 1916 and 1917. Another 14,000 left the Misahohe District in Togo for Ghana in 1910 (Boahen, 1987:66).

[35] Importantly, efforts to organize via trade union activity were widely suppressed in the early colonial period. Nonetheless, strike activity was fairly common (Boahen, 1987).

[36] See Guha (1999), Hobsbawm (2000), and Scott (1985).

colonial Africa represented a common tactic. Its primary purpose was to sabotage administrative control and frustrate the colonial powers. Typically, social banditry attacked strategic and symbolic targets of colonial rule, such as plantations, warehouses, shops, and tax collectors. Mapondera, a renowned social bandit in southern Rhodesia, harassed British and Portuguese officials from 1892 to 1903 with celebrated attacks on a range of colonial interests. Alongside calculated forms of social banditry, Africans practiced passive resistance. This took many forms including the refusal to adopt Western cultural practices (such as languages, religion, or medicine) or undermining elements of the colonial system such as labor slow-downs. "[T]he rural and illiterate people resorted to such passive resistance as refusal to comply with orders, absenteeism, feigned illness, loafing, and work slow-downs, refusal to cultivate compulsory crops, and above all, rejecting all 'civilized' innovations introduced by or connected with the colonial system or the foreign presence, whether schools, churches or the colonial languages" (Boahen, 1987:67).

Africans developed further forms of resistance to colonial rule by drawing from their local cultural traditions to mock colonial officials and undermine colonial authority. Janzen (1982) depicts the activities of the Lemba healing cult in Central Africa, for example, as an informal collective response to the encroachments of disruptive external trade patterns. African art and dance commonly provided powerful communal weapons of unity and struggle that could galvanize community-wide sentiment, while passing undetected by the Europeans. These activities fed anticolonial anger, while reinforcing African traditions and cultural forms as alternative sources of leadership and authority.

> A strategy resorted to more and more during this period, especially in the rural areas of East and Central Africa, was the use of the cultural symbols of dance, song, and art, which were often unintelligible to colonial officials. In many East African colonies, dance associations were organized, and the associations created dance forms in which colonial officials were ridiculed. Not only did these associations become popular throughout eastern Africa, but they spread from there into the Belgian Congo after the First World War . . . The Chope of southern Mozambique also developed a whole repertoire of songs in which the colonial regime in general and the hated tax officials in particular were denounced. Makua and Makonde artists ridiculed state officials in their carvings, in which they deliberately distorted their subjects' features. (Boahen, 1987:80–81)[37]

[37] Iliffe (2006) provides a contemporary example of Malawi performers who use dance to "satirize doctors equipped with camera and portable telephone reporting that they had found wasted villagers sick with AIDS" (p. 91).

The period between 1919 and 1935 was a time of further European territorial consolidation. By 1935, the few remaining areas of resistance were brought under colonial control.[38] As a result, though resistance to colonial rule continued in this period, rebellions were mostly localized in scope, and anticolonial struggles shifted strategies from violent confrontation to a combination of national (and Pan-Africanist) political tactics and symbolic-cultural resistance. Clubs and associations advocating greater African self-determination sprang up, especially among Western-educated Africans.[39] Most of these associations ostensibly organized for the reform, not overthrow, of the colonial system. Their demands focused on abolishing the pass system, reducing the hut tax, ending forced labor, and building more schools.

The Export of Biomedicine to Africa in the Context of Western Colonization

The Emergence of Tropical Medicine and African Medical Campaigns

As in the case of biomedicine more generally, efforts to capture the full complexity of tropical medicine must approach it as an ontological whole, comprised of multiple, embedded ontological spheres. As a scientific enterprise, tropical medicine is a unique branch of biomedicine designed to identify and treat a specific category of "tropical" diseases. By the time of tropical medicine's arrival, bacteriology was a well-established field in biomedicine and parasitology was still struggling to make its mark. Notwithstanding their distinct disease sources, the basic criteria by which parasitology sought to stake its rightful claim within biomedicine, a narrow notion of etiology based on parasitic vectors, paralleled that of bacteriology. Consequently, the histories of tropical medicine are replete with the heroic pursuits of Patrick Manson, Ronald Ross, and others to link this or that insect or worm to a specific ailment. As a symbolic-cultural expression, tropical medicine in Africa promoted the benevolent virtues of Western science and a funda-

[38] These included the Rif areas of northwest Africa, eastern sections of Kenya, the Darfur area of Sudan, the Lunda homelands of Quico (in Angola), the Makonde highlands of Mozambique, and the Obbia districts of Somalialand.

[39] In East Africa, the Young Baganda Association was organized in Uganda in 1919. The Tanganyika Territory African Civil Service Association was formed in 1922, and the Tanganyika African Association in 1929. [This became the Tanganyika African National Union (TANU) in 1954.] In Kenya, the Young Kavirondo Association was established by a group of teachers in 1921, while the Young Kikuyu Association and the Kikuyu Central Association were formed in 1921 and 1924, respectively.

mentally utilitarian worldview. The manner by which the Europeans presented tropical medicine was no less important than its actual curative powers with respect to symbolic-cultural influence. Tropical medicine was designed to convince Africans first of the superiority of the European's medicine and second of the need to treat "medicine" as an ends-driven, purely scientific matter—unrelated to supernatural or interpersonal concerns. As an expression of social power, tropical medicine in Africa supported and legitimated European colonial rule and persistently marginalized African pluralistic medicine. The benefits of tropical medicine for treating age-old scourges provided a benign rationale for European activities in Africa. At the same time, the "scientific" methods behind tropical medicine were purposely portrayed in a manner to denigrate and belittle African pluralistic medicine. Each of these ontological spheres interacted with the others in a dynamic and reflexive fashion and the analysis of tropical medicine in Africa, therefore, must incorporate these reciprocal and overlapping spheres, as each was shaped by (and helped to shape) the others.

The export of biomedicine to Africa coincided historically with the formal development of "tropical medicine" as a biomedical subspecialization.[40] The underlying logic (and scientific content) of tropical medicine mirrored the narrow etiology of biomedicine in general, while the agenda of tropical medicine advanced the colonial drive for Western conquest.[41] The explicit purpose of tropical medicine was to transform those colonies from "the white man's grave"[42] into productive regions (most especially across Africa and India) where Europeans could thrive while developing new colonies.[43] The British assault on the Ashanti Empire in 1874 provides a convenient starting point for the history of modern tropical medicine in Africa (Bynum,1994; Curtin, 1996). Six major British expeditions to West Africa between 1805 and 1841 had met with an average mortality rate of 50%. Similar expeditions into the Gold Coast (Ghana) and Nigeria between 1881 and 1887 suffered

---

[40] The literature tends to use the terms "colonial" medicine and "military" medicine interchangeably with tropical medicine.

[41] Inseparable from European conquest was the role of mission medicine (C. Good, 1991). John Vanderkemp, a Dutch physician, is generally credited with establishing the first medical missionary in Africa in 1799. Medicine in the hands of the missionaries became a vital instrument for Christianizing colonial peoples.

[42] There was an estimated fatality fate of 77% among Europeans sent to West Africa in the early 19th century (Headrick, 1981:63). Of the 1,843 European soldiers in Sierra Leone between 1819 and 1836, 890 perished. The likelihood of surviving travel to Sierra Leone between 1808 and 1850 was less than 50% (Bruce-Chwatt and Bruce-Chwatt, 1980:47).

[43] See Bynum (1994), Denoon (1988), MacLeod (1988), Porter (1997), and Worboys (2000).

mortality rates of 5-8% (MacLeod, 1988:7). In the 1874 expedition, twenty-five hundred British troops were given quinine to ward off malaria and sent into the interior of West Africa to battle the intransigent Ashanti people. When the troops triumphantly returned with minimal loss of European life, a new era of colonial rule opened for the Western powers in Africa. From its inception, therefore, tropical medicine was recognized as an essential instrument for Western expansion. "European medicine, and its handmaiden, public health, served as 'tools of Empire,' of both symbolic and practical consequence, as images representative of European commitment, variously to conquer, occupy or settle" (MacLeod, 1988:x).[44] In the context of colonial rule, the Western powers deployed tropical medicine first to protect European soldiers and administrators from tropical diseases, second to protect settlers, civil servants, and laborers in key economic sectors, and third as an ideological weapon to demonstrate the superiority of Western culture (Baer et al., 2003b). One professor of parasitology from the Liverpool School of Tropical Medicine was especially transparent regarding the link between capitalist profit and the health of colonial workers.

> My whole argument goes to show that a very large part of the potentially productive areas of the tropics is stagnant as a market, solely because of the ill-health of the people. Such an outpatient clientele is not likely to prove a remunerative one for the exchange of commodities: the wretched people must be restored to moderate health, so that they can produce their raw materials for your trade and thus obtain purchasing power for the manufactured articles which they wish to buy and to sell. (quoted in D. Ferguson, 1979:332)

Western efforts to treat tropical diseases spanned the long history of European colonialism from the 16th century forward (Marks, 1996; Porter, 1997).[45] The field of tropical medicine was not formally organized, however, until the latter 19th century, and the first reference to tropical medicine did

---

[44] See also Brown (1978) in this regard.

[45] The major tropical diseases of concern to Europeans by the 19th-century included kala-azar (leishmaniasis) in India and Africa; bubonic plague in Asia and the Near East; yellow fever in West Africa, the Caribbean, and Central America; leprosy in Asia, Africa, the Pacific Islands, and parts of the Americas; malaria in Asia, Africa, Central and South America, and the Mediterranean Basin; bilharzia (schistosomiasis) in Africa and Asia; sleeping sickness (trypanosoma) in sub-Saharan Africa; pneumonic plague in India; dengue in the Caribbean, Africa, Asia, and Australia; Chagas' Disease in South America; beriberi in Asia; filariasis in China; hookworm (ankylostomiasis) in the Southern United States and Central America; and nagana (a cattle disease) in sub-Saharan Africa. Of these, kala-azar, sleeping sickness, and bilharzia were primarily confined to indigenous populations.

not appear until 1897. "In October 1897, [Patrick] Manson opened his series of lectures at St. George's Hospital with a plea for 'The Necessity of Special Education in Tropical Medicine.' This appears to be the first use of the term 'tropical medicine'" (Worboys, 1976:85). The original rationale for tropical medicine lay in the common belief (and racial stereotype) that some diseases were specific to tropical climates and other diseases to temperate climates (Aidoo, 1982; Lyons, 1988a).[46] Europeans, for example, frequently contracted malaria, yellow fever, or dengue when entering tropical climates and this often impeded further European ambitions. Prior to the discovery of its mosquito-borne origins in the 1890s, yellow fever had halted French construction of the Panama Canal and was the leading cause of death in the Spanish-American War. As recited in Chapter 2, by the 1870s biomedicine was in the midst of major medical discoveries in the field of bacteriology. It was hoped that this work would provide tropical medicine with valuable insights, though in point of fact, "the professional study of parasitic organisms predated the era of Pasteur and Koch" (Farley, 1992:34). Both Robert Koch and Louis Pasteur, the esteemed pioneers of bacteriology, personally headed cholera expeditions to India and Egypt in the 1880s and 1890s.[47] Koch, in fact, spent time between 1897–1898 and 1906–1907 in German East Africa studying malaria and sleeping sickness. As it turned out, however, the major breakthrough in tropical medicine did not come from a bacteriologist but a British medical researcher investigating parasitic vectors for disease transmission in China.[48]

Tropical medicine's modern scientific impetus thus began in China with Patrick Manson's discovery of a link between elephantiasis and the *Filaria* (a nematode worm) in 1877. This was the first time that Western medicine had established the role of an insect in the natural history cycle of a disease and

---

[46] Increasing trade and travel between distant regions of the world also brought tropical diseases to the West. An 1890s outbreak of the bubonic plague in China spread quickly to India, eventually setting off an epidemic in San Francisco, California, in 1900. The occasional epidemics in the West, of course, could not compare with the devastating epidemics suffered by those in the colonies from diseases (such as syphilis and smallpox) introduced by Westerners (Kunitz, 1994).

[47] Of course, cholera, bubonic plague, and leprosy are all bacterial in nature and, at different times, have been prevalent across Europe. At the time of colonial conquest, however, they remained endemic to areas of the tropical world.

[48] The relationship between bacteriologists and parasitologists remained strained. "Important parasite-related discoveries made in the mid-nineteenth century did not enter into debates over the etiology of infectious diseases and had little if any impact on the genesis of germ theory. Similarly, after the germ theory became generally accepted, parasitologists continued to exclude bacteria and viruses from the organisms they studied. The two groups remained intellectually and institutionally unwed" (Farley, 1992:34).

this greatly advanced medical research in the evolving area of parasitology.[49] Manson was later appointed Medical Advisor to the Colonial Office in 1895 by Joseph Chamberlain, the Secretary of Britain's Colonial Office between 1895 and 1903. Understanding the important relationship between disease control and imperialism, Chamberlain created the School of Tropical Medicine in London. Shortly thereafter similar institutions were established in Boston (1900), Hamburg (1901), Paris (1901),[50] New Orleans (1902), Berlin (1905), Brussels (1906), and Amsterdam (1912). These schools were instrumental in documenting the association between certain diseases and specific classes of organisms (parasites). For example, schistosomiasis was linked to *trematodes Bilharzias* (a class of worms), sleeping sickness to a *Trypanosoma* protozoan, and malaria to *Plasmodium* (a protozoan). These chains of infection based on parasites proved even more complex than the food-, water-, milk-, and air-borne diseases prevalent in the temperate climates. Given the link between military campaigns and tropical medicine, the colonial powers were able to use these discoveries in parasitology as opportunities for further conquest. In the late 1890s two Italian researchers, Giovanni Batista Grassi and Amico Bignami, and a disciple of Manson, Ronald Ross, simultaneously discovered the role of the *Anopheles* mosquito in the transmission of malaria. Soon thereafter, the U.S. Army Yellow Fever Commission identified the *Aedes aegypti* mosquito with the transmission of yellow fever. Based on these findings, colonial administrators rapidly completed mosquito eradication campaigns leading to further settlements in Africa and completion of the Panama Canal.

Whatever the inherent links between climate and tropical diseases, it soon became evident that the pattern of European colonization was itself further exacerbating the spread of disease.[51] Colonization had been largely justified on the basis of bringing modern medical practices to backward peoples to combat epidemics and improve the general health of the population. Colonial authorities convinced themselves that they could, on the one hand, conquer, exploit, and colonize peoples while, on the other hand, cultivating the scientific understanding and social conditions leading to advances in health and epidemic control. In point of fact, the origin and spread of disease was often a direct function of the disruption to settled patterns of social organization and

---

[49] Manson's 1898 textbook, *Tropical Disease: A Manual of the Diseases of Warm Climates*, played an integral role in the popularization of parasitology.

[50] A chain of Pasteur Institutes spanned France and the French colonies.

[51] See, for example, Kramer and Thomas (1982), Lyons (1988a), Patterson (1981), Porter (1997), Prins (1992), Ranger (1988), and Vaughan (1991).

daily life introduced by colonial structures.[52] "[T]he 1880s and 1890s in Tanzania were decades of social dislocation, the cumulative effects of the slave trade, rebellions, foreign exploration and wars of conquest. People moved around on a scale and at a rate never before experienced in East Africa. Epidemics spread rapidly in these unsettled circumstances" (Turshen, 1984:134).

Widespread wars hastened large migrations as hundreds of villages and small towns were abandoned upon word of the advancing European armies. The evolving colonial infrastructure of roads and railways further accelerated the movement of people into unfamiliar regions and large-scale contact between previously separated populations. Clearings, settlements, encampments, and other ecological disruptions created opportunities for insect-borne diseases to flourish. "Deforestation allows sunlight to reach pools of water, creating favorable breeding conditions for *Anopheles gambiae*, the major vector of falciparium malaria" (Patterson, 1981:8). Meanwhile, monocultural, cash-crop economies based on coercive labor regimes took their toll on Africans' nutritional needs and general physical health. "The ecological transformation and social proletarianization created by Ross' 'pioneers of civilization' triggered massive epidemics, in particular sleeping sickness, while the planting of coffee, cocoa, rubber and other cash-crop monocultures led to decline in the nutritional status and general well-being of natives" (Porter, 1997:466). Sleeping sickness in the Belgian Congo is a case in point. In the aftermath of Leopold II's slash-and-burn economic development of the Congo basin, sleeping sickness spread out from the region. Whole villages were abandoned in the disease's wake. As missionaries carried the ill to nearby mission stations, the infected zone grew and fatalities climbed. Between 1896 and 1906, recurrent epidemics killed half a million people in the Congo and over two hundred fifty thousand in the Lake Victoria region.[53] Colonial developmental patterns thus played a direct role in the deterioration of the African population's overall health.

> [P]art of the cost of a switch to cash crops in eastern Tanzania is paid in increased perinatal mortality, itself a result of increased demands on women's time, with resultant stress; colonial "development" projects in northern Ghana and increased pressure to use river-valley land carried a price of increased onchocerciasis (river blindness); part of the cost of power and irrigation dams is paid in increases in schistosomiasis; a heavy part of the cost of gold-mining in South Africa was the

---

[52] See Feierman (1985:96–99), for example, for a detailed discussion of the links between colonial social development in Africa and sleeping sickness and malaria.

[53] Paul (1978) similarly details the plague and cholera epidemics that followed the 25-year French pacification campaign in Morocco and the introduction of monocultural cash crops.

> wholesale introduction of tuberculosis into African recruiting-grounds. (Prins, 1989:165)

As an extension of the European colonial agenda, tropical medicine reflected a racist, utilitarian logic that consistently prioritized European health and profits over native wellbeing. The Dutch, British, French, and Belgian medical services were modeled after the military, and its physicians—however benevolent their care—were plainly viewed by colonized populations as agents of colonial rule.[54] "[I]t was not uncommon for the doctor to arrive in an area accompanied by armed soldiers and an administrator, and then to begin a systematic examination of the people, who were obliged by show of force to present themselves" (Lyons, 1988b:117).[55] The emphasis on epidemics over endemic diseases and curative rather than preventive measures allowed the health of the masses of colonized people to deteriorate while the conditions of colonial rule (cash crops and forced labor regimes) remained beyond the scope of medical matters. When preventive measures were offered, a basic utilitarian logic drove this. "Preventive measures and reduction of mortality (in the Ivory Coast) were put forward as a means of strengthening and increasing the pool of productive labor, and curative services were expanded to those who worked in the colonial economy" (Lasker, 1977:285). Thus, as was often the case in the field of bacteriology in 19th-century Europe, the narrow focus of tropical medicine on "magic bullets" and disease eradication resulted in a general neglect of the more mundane, though fundamental, issues of sanitation, nutrition, and ecological deterioration (Arnold, 1988a; MacLeod, 1988).

> Tropical medicine was fraught with ambiguities. Based in the metropolitan centres of colonial or neocolonial powers rather than in the infected countries themselves, the specialty inevitably reflected white priorities and attitudes. Funds were channeled into high-profile laboratory research, though critics claimed problems could better be managed by investing in things of little interest to scientists—drinking water, sanitation, food. Not least, tropical medicine was vulnerable to characterization as the tool of colonial powers or post-colonial multinationals,[56] mopping up the mess created by the "develop-

[54] See Césaire (1972), Fanon (1967), Vaughan (1994), and Worboys (2000).

[55] See Fanon (1967) for the fullest treatment of this aspect of tropical medicine.

[56] Worboys (2000) observes that, following independence, medical systems in the former colonies were even more tightly linked to the advanced industrial nations. "Paradoxically, as colonial medical institutions gained greater formal autonomy they were drawn into international medical and

> ment" which imperialism and capitalism produced. Medicine also seemingly set itself at the service of empire by providing justifications for racial dominance. Colonial doctors often portrayed "savages" as ignorant, filthy, childlike and stupid, sometimes out of real contempt, sometimes prompted by "rescue" motives, or to raise money in the mother country for hospitals and education. (Porter, 1997:480)

Chamberlain and others well understood the essential role of tropical medicine in the context of growing imperial competition among the advanced industrial powers to control vast regions of the globe. Tropical medicine was not merely a matter of scientific discovery, it was a source of power and dominance. "If medicine could tame the diseases that were rampant in the tropics, it had undoubted political force as a tool of empire, and the country with the most advanced medical capabilities stood the greatest chance of success in the hostile environments of Africa, Southeast Asia and the Caribbean" (Bynum, 1994:148). Consistent with these immediate aims of the Western colonial powers, the health of the masses of colonized people was, at best, of secondary concern for the engineers of tropical medicine.[57] This focus shifted over time as patterns of European settlement and colonial labor regimes developed. However, even as medical care expanded to indigenous laborers or civil servants, it systematically continued to neglect most women, children, and rural peasants (Marks, 1996; Worboys, 2000). Nonetheless, over time it became evident that it was not always possible to separate the health concerns of the larger masses of indigenous inhabitants from those of Europeans and their allies (Marks and Andersson, 1988). This was especially the case in colonies with significant settler populations.

Over time, as the benefits of tropical medicine were extended to indigenous populations, Western conquest and subjugation remained foremost on the agenda. In this respect, tropical medicine fit well with the popular Western justification of colonial rule as a humanitarian gesture, an arm of its civilizing

---

science networks which meant that rather than setting their own priorities, they were drawn to the priorities of the North and its approach to disease control" (p. 68).

[57] Bilharzia, for example, had been long recognized as a devastating disease for Africans and Asians. However, "Unlike malaria, it was almost exclusively a 'native disease' rarely touching the lives of colonial administrators" (Farley, 1988:189). It was not until U.S. personnel began acquiring bilharzia in the Philippines after WWII that serious steps were first taken by the West to seek a long-term, effective treatment (Porter, 1997).

mission.[58] It was the burden of advanced Western cultures to bring civilization to the backward peoples of the colonies. Chief among these civilizing gifts was scientific medicine. Medicine was seen by Westerners as an apolitical source of rational, scientific thought that could supplant local superstitions and serve as an effective weapon against witchcraft and other backward practices.[59] "Western medicine was cited as indisputable evidence that colonial rule stood for rationality and progress, while indigenous society foolishly cherished superstition and witchcraft, was ruled by ignorance and cruelty, and held beliefs and practices Europe had left behind in the Dark Ages" (Arnold, 1993:1406). Colonial agents, and Westerners in general, fervently believed that demonstrations of tropical medicine's benefits would translate into widespread acceptance of Western civilization, more generally, as an unqualified good among colonized peoples.

> In treating medicine as scientific objectivity rather than as a political construct and cultural artifact, it has conventionally been seen as a panacea, a means of liberation, not a regulatory or repressive device. Even at a time when European colonialism itself was in decline, many scholars still held to the idea that medicine was one of colonialism's nobler and more redeeming features, evidence that whatever the "political disadvantages" of colonialism, it had brought real benefits to the people of Africa and Asia. (Arnold, 1993:1393)

The racialized ideologies that fueled tropical medicine frequently depicted disease simply as an inherent feature of indigenous cultural practices. Colonial authorities in India, for example, regularly attributed cholera outbreaks to various aspects of Hindu pilgrimage (Arnold, 1988a). As such, colonial health campaigns—such as those against the plague in India in 1890, sleeping sickness in Uganda in 1901, or malaria in Malawi in 1912—served, in part, as thinly disguised attacks on indigenous customs and lifestyles (Lyons, 1994; Marks, 1996). Indeed, tropical medicine was instrumental in devising campaigns to suppress local, pluralistic-medical practices. Colonial officials imposed prohibitions on variolation—the inoculation of individuals with the smallpox virus to produce immunity to the disease—in parts of

---

[58] See Lyons (1988a), MacLeod (1988), Porter (1997), and Worboys (2000).

[59] At the same time, somewhat anticipating the notion of "African biomedicine" developed here, Arnold (1996) suggests that the transfer of medical knowledge was not entirely one-sided. "[T]ropical medicine was often the result of a 'synergetic relationship between core and periphery' rather than, as has often been assumed in the past, a simple transference or imposition of European ideas and techniques" (p. 13).

India in the second half of the 19th century. In Nigeria, British authorities outlawed the Sopona smallpox cult in 1917 before imposing sweeping anti-witchcraft ordinances across all their African colonies in the 1920s and 1930s (Arnold, 1993; Porter, 1997).[60] At the same time, given that the majority of the colonial population relied upon African pluralistic-medical practices, they were generally tolerated (Worboys, 2000).

Given the realities of colonial rule, as well as the dual roles of physicians in the colonies,[61] Africans remained acutely skeptical of Western "humanitarian" medicine. Frequently, different forms of biomedicine (such as the vaccination) were interpreted as tricks to enslave or convert the people. Indeed, medical services were often used to collect population data in the colonies and create statistical profiles as tools for even greater social control (Arnold, 1988a). It was difficult, at times, for Africans to ignore the self-serving rationale of tropical medicine to expedite colonial subjugation by developing "cures" for epidemics that were themselves largely attributable to patterns of colonial conquest and disruption. "From the late 1870s, this tropical medicine—its ideology European, its instrument the microscope, its epistemology the germ theory of disease—served the interests of the dominant economic groups and obscured the relationship of disease to social structure" (MacLeod, 1988:7). The introduction of biomedicine into colonial East Africa well illustrates this fundamental relationship between biomedicine, colonial rule, cultural disruption, and the social order.

---

[60] Antiwitchcraft ordinances were commonplace across Africa at this time. Chavunduka (1978) cites the language from an 1899 edict in Rhodesia. "Whoever imputes to any other person the use of non-natural means in causing any disease in any person or animal or in causing any injury to any person or property, that is to say, whoever, names or indicates any other person as being a wizard or witch shall be guilty of an offence and liable to a fine not exceeding two hundred dollars, to imprisoning for a period not exceeding three years or to a whipping not exceeding twenty lashes or to any two or more of such punishments" (p. 101). Prins (1992) observes that continuing colonial efforts to root out witchcraft and sorcery occasionally took a toll on the work of Western scholars, as well. "The witch-hunt has also left a specific technical problem for the historian fieldworker because it is popularly believed that the real cause of the witch-hunt was an anthropologist who asked questions about African therapeutics in the 1940s and then gave lists of names to colonial authorities" (p. 358).

[61] For physicians there was a constant overlap between their medical and military roles in the colony (Fanon, 1967; Levy, 1978; Onoge, 1975; Paul, 1978; Turshen, 1984). "In British India, mainly for want of any alternative agency, colonial doctors were pressed into service as prison superintendents and forestry officers. There, the relationship between the army and the medical profession was typically close. Members of the Indian Medical Service combined military and medical rank, and in times of war, were likely to be switched from civilian posts back to military duties" (Arnold, 1993:1398).

Colonial East Africa and the Arrival of Biomedicine

The introduction of biomedicine into colonial East Africa took place gradually and somewhat disjointedly over seven decades of British rule.[62] Biomedicine was initially reserved for colonial officials and their local agents. Over time, however, a loose confederation of government dispensaries, medical missions, and local pluralistic-medical practitioners (who were generally tolerated though not encouraged) combined to create an eclectic range of health care options for East Africans. In the first few decades of colonial rule, rural-based medical missions were the primary source of contact with biomedicine for the vast majority of East Africans. Treatment was generally limited to particular medical conditions for which biomedicine had proven effective, such as yaws. Beginning in the 1920s, the colonial authorities began developing a system of rural dispensaries to reach the wider population and the primary medical priority remained curative rather than broad-based preventive measures.[63] This was, in part, due to a belief that the more immediate and visible nature of curative measures would more quickly hasten the African adoption of biomedicine than long-term, less dramatic preventive programs. As noted, notwithstanding the occasional and lightly enforced prohibitions, pluralistic-medical practices remained commonplace alongside biomedical services throughout the colonial period. Consequently, biomedicine in Africa evolved throughout the colonial era as a complementary form of medical care alongside—and never as a substitute for—African pluralistic medicine. Africans continued in pragmatic fashion to draw from a combination of medical beliefs and practices up to the time of independence.[64]

The Early Decades

East Africa was cobbled together over several decades of British trade and conquest. In 1888, Britain granted the Imperial British East Africa Company (IBEA) a royal charter to explore and exploit the region of Uganda. After only five years, the IBEA turned administrative functions over to

---

[62] See M. Gelfand (1976) for a description of parallel events in British-ruled Southern Rhodesia and Patterson (1981) for developments in Ghana.

[63] This mirrored the 19th-century public health campaigns in Europe that sought quick cures rather than more sweeping social reforms. "The government and physicians chose the cheap solution for delivering [medical] care. Rather than raising the living standards of the rural population (prevention), the colonial authorities tried to cure the population of yaws with injections of a drug of uncertain properties" (Dawson, 1987a:343).

[64] This was true throughout much of Africa. In the Ivory Coast, for example, Lasker observes that "Western medicine was and continues to be one of a variety of therapeutic options used by Ivorians" (1977:294).

Gerald Portal, the British commissioner, and the Foreign Office took formal control of Uganda in 1894. One year later, the East African Protectorate (Kenya) was established. It was not until 1905, however, that the Colonial Office took over Uganda and Kenya as separate colonies. To the South, Germany had claimed the colonial territory of Tanganyika[65] in 1891. Large parts of Tanganyika were added to British-ruled colonial East Africa in 1917 after Germany's hold had been weakened on the eve of World War I. Following World War I, all of Tanganyika became a British mandate.[66] While many of the major health issues presented common challenges across all three colonies, with the exception of a brief unified health policy between 1903 and 1908, there was little effort to create a single, integrated medical system. Thus, despite overlapping health needs and policies, each colony administered its own health care system. Nonetheless, whether in Kenya, Uganda, or Tanganyika, it was well understood, especially in the early years, that the health of European soldiers, administrators, and settlers was the top priority. The health of their Indian and African colonial agents was a secondary concern, while the health of all other Africans (especially those on the African reserves[67]) was a distant third. For this reason, the thinly scattered network of Catholic and Protestant missionary stations provided the vast majority of Africans with their first introduction to biomedicine. Mengo Hospital was a missionary hospital established by Dr. Albert Cook in Kampala, Uganda, in 1897. Along with Sewa Haji, a very poorly resourced government hospital (see description below) built in Dar es Salaam in 1893, these were the only Western hospitals initially available to East Africans.[68] By 1901, Mengo Hospital had 70 beds and treated 1,070 inpatients and 76,840 outpatients.

The first decade of British rule was primarily a period of medical neglect and indifference toward Africans. This followed, in part, from British geopolitical interests. Initially, the acquisition of Uganda and Kenya was of greatest value as a strategic point within a larger colonial network rather than as

[65] Tanganyika officially became Tanzania in October 1964, three years after independence.

[66] There were many running battles between German and British troops across the region throughout WWI. The British called upon a combination of British, South African, East African, and Indian soldiers. The outmatched German General von Lettow-Verbeck led an unconventional guerrilla war and the final German surrender came on November 25, 1919.

[67] *African reserves* refers to a landholding system that developed primarily in Kenya. Colonial Kenya received far more settlers than Uganda or Tanganyika, especially after 1919. By 1920, Uganda had a European population of 350 (Hopwood, 1980:148). Kenyan officials developed a reserve system whereby 31,000 square kilometers of prime land was set aside for European settlers. That land beyond these 31,000 square kilometers was referred to as the African reserves.

[68] An Indian merchant, Sewa Haji, provided the funds for the hospital built in his name specifically to provide medical services to Africans, Indians, and Arabs (Iliffe, 2002:29).

colonies in and of themselves (Beck, 1970:11). As in most of colonial Africa, official segregation was imposed as a "health policy" to protect Europeans from possible disease (Marks and Andersson, 1988). The disparities in medical care that resulted were stark. A medical officer in Dar es Salaam just after WWI compared the hospital facilities available to Europeans with those set aside for Africans.

> We have inherited from the Germans some medical buildings which compare favorably with any in Tropical Africa. The European Hospital, Dar es Salaam, is capable of accommodating fifty beds easily . . . It has a separate maternity section, well-fitted X-ray room and photographic dark room, and room for the examination of eye cases, spacious operating theatre, outpatient department and quarters for nursing staff and Medical Officer. It faces the Indian Ocean and receives the benefit of the sea breeze . . . At the other end of town near the Gerezani Creek is the Sewa Haji hospital for Indians and Natives, a curious rambling collection of buildings of which the administrative block is the outstanding feature. Its capacity is also about fifty beds, a number which is insufficient for the needs of a native town with a population estimated at twenty or twenty-five thousand, as well as for the K.A.R. Garrison, civil police, prisoners, railway and other Government Native and Indian employees. (quoted in D. Ferguson, 1979:326)

By 1903, the colonial medical services for Africans were staffed by a small number of doctors, nurses and hospital attendants (mostly Indians). Resources were woefully inadequate. Between 1894 and 1919, there were never more than twenty-five doctors for three million Africans in Uganda (Hopwood, 1980:147). The medical budget for all of East Africa in 1900–1901 was £4,712. This compared to a military budget of £38,005 for the same year (Beck, 1970:14).

In the first few decades of colonial rule, medical missions were, therefore, the primary source of biomedicine for Africans in East Africa.[69] "Medical missionary memoirs abound with stories of the early African dispensers, and the value of their work was readily recognized. In particular, they were the vanguard of the 'battle against superstition and witchcraft,' persuading recalcitrant patients and skeptics of the superiority of Western medicine" (Vaughan, 1991:65). There were four major medical missions in East Africa in the early 20th century. The Church Missionary Society (CMS) established

---

[69] See Beck (1970), C. Good (1987), Iliffe (2002), and Vaughan (1991).

Mengo Hospital in 1897 and by 1903 CMS had three doctors and thirty-two stations throughout Uganda. A Protestant mission, CMS began work in the Kikuyu region of Kenya in 1907 under the direction of Dr. John Arthur and built a hospital there in 1914. The other significant medical missions were the White Fathers, the Mill Hill Fathers, and the Church of Scotland Missions.[70] Though they initially had no doctors, these three missions dispensed medicine, dressed wounds, and offered minor diagnoses. While tacitly acknowledged by colonial officials as a critical supplementary resource, mission medicine was not a part of formal medical services. It was the CMS hospital in Kampala, in fact, that proved essential in the early diagnosis of the sleeping sickness epidemic in 1901.

Colonial officials understood the extension of biomedicine to Africans both as a utilitarian need and as a device to introduce Western scientific norms. Missionaries viewed biomedicine as a means to introduce Christianity. Missionaries often found that even when many Africans rejected them as evangelizers there was still an interest in their medicine.[71] It was invariably saving souls, however, rather than relieving suffering that motivated mission medicine. In 1897, Archdeacon Walker of the CMS in Mengo, Uganda, declared that, "I regard the medical work from its missionary aspect . . . I consider how far it is likely to aid our work, not how much suffering will be relieved" (quoted in D. Ferguson, 1979:319). One result of the overriding proselytizing agenda was an emphasis on curative measures over preventive measures. "The interest in the conversion of Africans inevitably biases missionary medical work toward curative treatment" (Turshen, 1984:140).

The advances of tropical medicine elsewhere in the world did not go unnoticed by colonial officials in East Africa, and the period of 1900 to 1914 was a time of protracted health campaigns to combat the plague, malaria, sleeping sickness, and later yaws. The growing European community in East Africa increasingly understood that health epidemics among Africans were very difficult to isolate and limit to the African population. At the same time, in the case of certain epidemics such as the plague, the links between disease and the deteriorating living conditions stemming from colonial rule were quite evident.[72] Long endemic to Uganda, the plague made its first appearance in Nairobi in 1902 within the Indian community before spreading to other parts of Kenya. Plague, in fact, proved a continuing problem, with further outbreaks in Nairobi in 1902, 1905, 1906, 1911, 1912, and 1913. The crowded

[70] See Iliffe (2002:19–27) for a detailed overview of the various medical missions in East Africa at this time.

[71] See Clyde (1980), Dawson, (1987a), and C. Good, (1987).

[72] See Swanson (1979) for a discussion of similar efforts to combat the plague in South Africa in the early 20th century.

and unsanitary conditions conducive to the plague were only exasperated by strictures of colonial rule.[73] In Tanganyika, a sanitary authority modeled after the *Gesundheitskommission* in German cities was created in 1901 to address worsening conditions.

One example of the link between colonial policy and deteriorating health conditions was the imposition of the hut tax. At the start of colonial rule, overcrowding had not been a significant problem in Nairobi. It was local custom for one adult to occupy a hut with young children. Once the hut tax was introduced, however, it became necessary for more than one adult to live in a hut to afford payment.[74] Furthermore, the need for cash payments forced males into the labor force and out of subsistence agriculture.[75] The resulting systems of labor migration impacted the health of both the men traveling great distances to labor for cash incomes on plantations and the women and children left behind (Turshen, 1977b). The plantation system in Tanganyika grew from five thousand wage-laborers in 1900 to ninety-two thousand by 1913 (D. Ferguson, 1979:320). By the start of World War I, twenty thousand registered laborers passed through Kisumu in western Kenya (Dawson, 1979:248).[76]

Many of the advances of tropical medicine regarding malaria were inspired by the 19th-century experiences of the British in India. By 1900, health officials certainly understood what needed to be done to alleviate the spread of malaria. As noted, the celebrated Robert Koch visited East Africa three times between 1897 and 1907. However, given that malaria was not considered a major health threat to Europeans, efforts to control malaria in East Africa proceeded very slowly and with few resources. Additionally, due to scant public education, those antimalarial measures that were taken were generally seen as yet another burden, and many peasants adopted creative strategies to circumvent the new rules.

---

[73] In a similar fashion, Dawson (1979) suggests that in the case of the famine in central Kenya in 1897–1900, it was the social reaction to the famine—mass population movements into crowded areas with food—rather than malnutrition that left the population susceptible to the rapid spread of smallpox. See also Marks and Andersson (1988) and Turshen (1984) in this regard.

[74] By 1935, African taxes provided one-third of the total revenue in colonial Tanganyika (Turshen, 1977b:13).

[75] Patterson (1981) describes the health impact of this practice in colonial Ghana. "With an increasingly mobile population came enhanced risks of disease transmission. People entered unfamiliar disease environments, where they encountered new pathogens or new strains of familiar ones" (p. 5).

[76] Lasker describes similar developments in Ivory Coast. "The development of cash crop plantations represented a major change in mode of production for the African population. The growing of products for export served to spread the money economy, and labor migration, created largely by the forced labor system, assumed significant proportions" (1977:282).

> As with any regulations, individuals sought to evade them. In Tabora, for example, two years before Independence, the health officer stuck signposts into the ground in several parts of a wet valley. The signs proclaimed "Cultivation is forbidden here." In a few weeks' time, when the whole valley had become a sea of rice, the farmers were summoned to court where they indignantly stated that they had taken the greatest care to comply with the notices and had left at least an inch of ground uncultivated around each and every signpost. (Clyde, 1980:102)

Sleeping sickness received much greater attention from colonial officials who were fearful of its potential for spread as far as India (Lyons, 1988a). Mengo Hospital reported the first cases in February 1901 and within six months two hundred persons had died. When the epidemic began, its cause and treatment presented a major medical mystery, though sleeping sickness itself was not new to the British, who first encountered sleeping sickness in 1734 in Guinea. By 1903, the cause had been traced to a *Trypanosoma* and the tsetse fly had been identified as its means of transmission to humans. Given that tsetse flies numbered in the tens of millions in the vast Lake Victoria region, their eradication was considered all but impossible. Consequently, the only practical solution was to resettle large segments of the African population in areas far removed from the threat of sleeping sickness. A combination of limited resources and stagnant policy debates stalled action for several years until 1907 and an estimated two hundred fifty thousand Africans perished in the interim (Duggan, 1980:22). Like the European sanitation campaigns of the 19th century, the effort to relocate whole ethnic groups required both sympathetic persuasion and paternalistic coercion (Lyons, 1988b). Beck argues that this marked a shift in colonial attitudes toward the treatment of African populations. "In the brutal campaigns which accompanied the 'pacification' of certain areas, officials justified their disregard of human rights by the necessity of civilizing a district . . . Strange as it may sound, in the case of sleeping sickness, they felt at first that they could not justify compulsion" (Beck, 1970:244). By 1908, almost everyone from the northern Uganda shoreline of Lake Victoria had been moved north.

Beginning in the 1930s, sleeping sickness policies reflected a genuine evolution in the relationship between Europeans and Africans. When there was a need to move people from Mwanza, a small village on the Tanganyikan side of Lake Victoria, the local population was allowed to participate in the selection of a relocation site. "[The villagers] asked in how many other countries [relocations] had been instituted to check disease and other dangers. If they were sure that the [relocations] would eventually extend everywhere, they would be agreeable and willing to do as the others had done. But, they said, they wanted only the place they chose" (Beck, 1970:123). In the case of sleeping sickness and other epidemics, therefore, it was biomedicine as a scientific enterprise and as an expression of social power that most directly contributed to social transformation in the first few decades. Advances in identifying the etiology of "tropical" diseases pinpointed the potential sources of infection and dictated the necessary measures to avoid them. Biomedicine at the service of the colonial mission determined how these medical campaigns would be carried out. Biomedicine as a cultural-symbolic expression, meanwhile, provided the general rationale for forcing compliance. After all, breaking Africans of the cultural superstitions behind various pluralistic-medical practices was thought to strengthen the African body and rectify the mind.

Unlike the slow and disappointing results from campaigns to control the plague, malaria, and sleeping sickness, the yaws eradication campaign of the 1920s met with a great deal more initial success and the stricken East African population experienced rapid and dramatic improvement. Given this success, many believed that the yaws eradication campaign held much promise for a more profound impact on African attitudes toward biomedicine than the earlier health campaigns.[77] The 1920s yaws eradication campaign was the first major health initiative targeting a disease exclusively impacting Africans. In addition, because the primary treatment involved an injection, the role of the syringe created a mystique of healing power that became associated with biomedicine. In fact, medical officers explicitly viewed the yaws campaign as an opportunity to popularize biomedicine and turn Africans away from local traditions.

> [T]he popularity of injections with the African population would forward the long-range goals of the [Medical] Department. [J. L.] Gilks (Kenya's principle medical officer) and others felt that the anti-yaws therapy would show the population the value of Western biomedicine and turn them away from using "native medicine and witchcraft." They also believed that the clinical success of the anti-yaws campaigns would both make the administration of rural reserves easier and make other public health campaigns more popular. (Dawson, 1987a:420–421)

Prior to World War I, medical missions were the primary source of biomedical care for yaws.[78] In southern Tanganyika, for example, large camps

[77] See Clyde (1980), Dawson (1987a), and Ranger (1981).

[78] Primarily a childhood disease found in rural, tropical areas with poor sanitation, yaws progresses from a primary lesion to secondary infections and relapsing skin eruptions.

sprang up around medical missions in Masasi and Luatala. "'The hospital at Luatala is a wonderful sight,' wrote Miss Andrews (a mission nurse) in July (1914), 'a great camp of some 220 people and 50 or 60 little fires at night'" (quoted in Ranger, 1981:266). Beginning in 1920, colonial authorities initiated a formal yaws eradication campaign based on the system developed by the Church of Scotland mission at Tumutumu in Central Kenya. A series of satellite dispensaries staffed by African dressers were built around a central hospital with European physicians and nurses. This was a prelude to the rural-based dispensary system discussed below.

Initial reticence for injections was overcome by the positive results and the demand for treatment grew exponentially as sprawling campgrounds began to sprout up along the edges of medical stations. Between 1920 and 1931, 712,228 Africans were treated in Kenya alone (Dawson, 1987a:425).[79] By 1929, another five hundred thousand plus had been treated in Tanganyika (Clyde, 1980:104). Given the novelty of the treatment mode, an injection, tremendous faith was placed in the healing power of the syringe. Ranger interprets African reverence for injection-based treatments as an extension of local healing traditions. "The fame of the needle—*sindano*—spread far and wide; people came for very long distances; and so soon as a dispensary was opened in a new part of the district there were at once crowds of yaws patients. The atmosphere was very clearly that of the spontaneous and intense movements of mass cleansing" (Ranger, 1981:266). The popularity of the injection-based 1920s yaws eradication campaign contrasts sharply with the occasional smallpox vaccination campaigns prior to 1920, which encountered skepticism and hostility. Rather than leading to popular demands for treatment, the smallpox campaigns relied upon force and coercion (Dawson, 1987a:432).[80] Both Clyde (1980) and Dawson (1987a) argue that the 1920s anti-yaws campaign created the first significant public demand for biomedicine in East Africa. "Despite the broadening of health-care measures in the early decades of this century, it took the dramatically effective campaign against the widespread and crippling disease of yaws to engender public demand rather than, at best, passive acceptance" (Clyde, 1980:103).

Alternatively, Ranger (1981) suggests that the nature of the medical care that Africans experienced fit well within the established African tradition of "indigenous healing cults." "In its intensity, its periodic and spasmodic character, and in its isolation from general notions of misfortune and healing, the movement of yaws victims to the mission clinics resembled nothing

[79] This reflects only the number of persons treated at government facilities and does not record the number treated at mission sites.

[80] See Arnold (1988b) for a discussion of British efforts to control smallpox in colonial India.

so much as an indigenous healing cult, of which there had been a succession in [the Masasi region of southeast Tanganyika]" (Ranger, 1981:265). Because of the complementary nature of biomedicine with certain local African practices, Ranger argues that the yaws eradication campaign ultimately led to only a negligible number of African converts to Western medical practices.[81] Rather, following the yaws eradication campaign, a resilient and pragmatic attitude prevailed in which biomedicine was seen as appropriate for certain afflictions and local pluralistic medicine for others (Orley, 1980; Ranger, 1981).[82]

These views reflected a more general African sentiment regarding the utility of biomedicine. At one level, there was a general acceptance of biomedical practices for certain diseases. This was based on practical, empirical experience. As patients improved, community skepticism waned and biomedical beliefs and practices were accepted and found compatible with African collective worldviews. At the same time, given the failure of biomedicine to treat other illnesses, it was naturally concluded that biomedicine was inadequate for other medical conditions. This was, in part, a simple matter of contrasting etiological frameworks. As was freely conceded by colonial officials, biomedical treatments were restricted to those diseases with causes found in the natural world. Insofar as biomedicine was useless to treat those afflicted by diseases linked to the supernatural or social worlds, it was accepted by Africans within these limitations. The British had encountered this attitude of pragmatic empiricism early on during the introduction of missionary medicine in Uganda. Witness Dr. Wright's arrival in Mengo.

> After his arrival at Mengo, Dr. Wright seemed to have the support and trust of the African community. Apparently the Africans expected "miracles" from him along the lines performed by the witch doctors and they expected that he could bring them immediate relief

---

[81] There were, likewise, few conversions to Christianity resulting from yaws treatment, as reflected in a mission doctor's lament. "Dr. Taylor wrote in 1929 'from the missionary point of view this part of our work (yaws treatment) at first sight seems of very little direct value, for the patients rarely stop long and often come from great distances, so that it is useless to try to teach them the Faith'" (Ranger, 1981:267). See also Ranger (1988) for a similar analysis of the 1918 flu epidemic in Southern Rhodesia. "[T]he pandemic of 1918 with its atmosphere of crisis and with the effective failure of all medical treatment, powerfully assisted and legitimated the emergence of African anti-medicine" (p. 186).

[82] Patterson (1981) documents similar attitudes and practices in colonial Ghana. "Many people took an eclectic approach, seeking the best elements of various medical systems. Advised or directed by family and friends, they might consult a colonial physician and a local practitioner simultaneously or, more likely, go to the clinic after the village healer had failed" (p. 28).

> for their sufferings. When the doctor did not perform the "miracles" the Africans expected, they went back to their witch doctor. (Beck, 1970:18)[83]

The Later Decades

World War I exposed many weaknesses of the medical services in East Africa and opened the opportunity for Africans to be trained as medical workers for the first time. As standards of medical care for Africans rose, the role of mission medicine declined. Beginning in 1914, colonial officials first gave serious consideration to providing medical services to populations beyond Europeans and their African and Indian colonial assistants. This required replacing medical missions in the African reserves and elsewhere with government medical stations. Recruitment efforts and battlefield experiences during World War I served as major catalysts in this regard. In East Africa, World War I involved battles between German- and British-backed troops over several years, requiring territory-wide recruitment efforts. The large number of Africans rejected as physically unfit (as high as 50%) alarmed officials who attributed this to more general health problems across the population. Additionally, an essential component of the British forces was the East African Carrier Corps, created in 1914 to deliver provisions to soldiers. Over the course of the war, the Carrier Corps suffered over forty-two thousand deaths due to illness, compared with just over forty-three hundred deaths among Ugandan and Kenyan troops (Beck, 1970:63).[84] The high mortality rate among the Carrier Corps along with the number of unfit recruits thus led officials to investigate the dire health conditions of the larger population.

Parallel to these developments, Africans were recruited to join the African Native Medical Corps. There were two categories of recruits. Stretcher bearers required no education and performed basic manual labor. Better educated recruits were given brief training in basic first aid. The success of the African Native Medical Corps during the war later persuaded officials that Africans should be trained to provide skilled medical services. "[I]n addition to its achievements in a real medical emergency, was the example the Corps set. It clearly dispelled doubts held by many administrators that African youth could not be trained for independent and advanced work" (Beck, 1970:69). By 1919, colonial officials were moving away from their established practice of relying on African elders and other leaders within a structure of

---

[83] By contrast, Prins (1992) describes a mission hospital in Bulozi, Zambia, in 1977 that was inundated with patients, both local and distant, who abandoned the local government hospital following news of dramatic successes attributed to a newly arrived physician (p. 351).

[84] D. Ferguson (1979) details how large-scale troop movements across rural East Africa also contributed directly to the spread of disease.

indirect rule and increasingly trained Western-educated African leaders, as a new generation of Africans emerged. Lastly, because the Carrier Corps and Medical Corps combined Africans from a variety of ethnic groups across Uganda and Kenya, one of the indirect effects of their creation was to further expose many Africans to the world beyond their isolated villages and to stoke nascent nationalist politics (Rotberg, 1966).

By the end of World War I, a number of further factors combined to reshape colonial medical services significantly throughout East Africa. Tanganyika was officially included in British-ruled East Africa with League of Nations mandate status. In theory, mandate status implied greater reporting responsibility with regard to the welfare of Africans in Tanganyika and greater international scrutiny. This coincided with a large influx of new settlers who entered East Africa as Kenyan officials actively recruited Europeans. With the arrival of new settlers, the demand for cheap and productive labor increased, requiring further medical services to maintain a basic level of health for the African labor force. At the same time, African anger and resentment over colonial land and labor ordinances festered and a new generation of young, educated Africans began to challenge African elders for leadership and the first nationalist political movements emerged.[85] These political agitations put further pressure on colonial officials to address the dire medical needs of the African population.

As noted, settlers were unevenly distributed across the three colonies in East Africa. While Kenya had a large population of settlers concentrated in the central Kikuyu region, Uganda and Tanganyika had far smaller and more dispersed settler communities. Following World War I, many British veterans were promised opportunities as settlers in Kenya and labor recruitment became a major priority for the growing settler population. Given that there was little reason for Africans to work the settlers' land (wages were meager), colonial officials enacted a number of compulsory labor policies (Leys, 1975; Rodney, 1979). The most notorious of these was the *kipande*, a pass system for Africans traveling outside their home reserve, for the purpose of limiting mobility. In response to these developments, new political movements arose. Among the Kikuyu, Harry Thuku helped form the Young Kikuyu

[85] The rise of national liberation struggles coincided in ironic fashion with the popularization of biomedicine. Nationalist politics was premised, in part, on the weakening of local, ethnic identities and consequently on the decline of local traditions and customs. Western medicine tended to facilitate this process. Thus, on the one hand, the Western physician was linked to the modernist spirit that fed nationalist aspirations of breaking with the limitations of local ethnic identities. On the other hand, the Western physician symbolized the tyranny and racial supremacy of foreign colonial authority (Fanon, 1967). The ambivalence of Africa's anticolonial leaders toward biomedicine continued into the early decades of independence.

Association,[86] demanding more educational opportunities for Africans and economic development plans that included the entire population.

In this context, colonial officials finally made the first serious efforts to update and expand medical services. In Kenya, for example, the Public Health Ordinance of 1921 expanded health concerns from the colonial staff to the entire population. The anti-malaria campaign in Kenya, and later in Tanganyika, was expanded in this regard. Previously, such campaigns were limited to eradicating breeding grounds for mosquitoes and providing quinine. It was now recognized that anti-malaria programs touched on a range of health and sanitation issues beyond the immediate malady (Beck, 1970:107). Initial efforts to transform the East African Native Medical Corps for civilian use were slow and frustrated by many funding delays. East African provincial commissioners met in 1919 and plans were made to create a system of local dispensaries with an emphasis on curative care staffed by trained Africans.[87] Health improvements, in general, were seen as a matter of cultural education rather than compulsion. "Through education, through constant reminders of the dangers of the threat of infection to the lives of the sick as well as their families, the natives were to be weaned off customs which contributed to infection and disease" (Beck, 1981:10). After further delays, training began in 1922 with the assistance of the medical missions who had the most experience working with Africans in this regard. Two years later, an Annual Report from Uganda indicated that much remained to be done in the area of rural medical care.

> We are confronted with a difficult but essential task of extending the scope of medical work so as to embrace all tribes and all provinces with a population of over three million spread over an area of 107,000 square miles. All are similarly afflicted and all merit similar treatment. I am more than ever convinced that the extension of sub-dispensaries in charge of trained native attendants under the supervision of inspecting medical officers and based on good permanent district hospitals throughout all populous districts of the Protectorate represents a successful solution of this difficult problem of affording adequate medical treatment for the massive native population,

[86] This later became the Kikuyu Central Association.

[87] The British East African curative medical emphasis contrasted with French West African medical policy. In 1915, the French conducted a series of rural health surveys to assess medical needs before creating a mobile preventive health service. "Mass campaigns to seek out and combat the most debilitating endemic diseases were undertaken as the most efficient means for dealing with so many people" (Lasker, 1977:283).

the vast majority of whom are still inaccessible to hospital aid. (quoted in Hopwood, 1980:150)[88]

At the same time, there was a significant change in government policy toward medical missions. Prior to World War I, the government left medical care on African reserves and throughout the countryside to the missions. After World War I, the government continued to subsidize these missions on a temporary basis until the government could take this over.[89] Considerable confusion and growing friction resulted between colonial officials and medical missions. One of the major areas of conflict concerned the practice of female circumcision among the Kikuyu. Though abhorring the practice, colonial officials chose to proceed slowly with their objections to promote goodwill. The missions, on the other hand, called for its complete abolition in 1928, in part, objecting to certain presumed sexual mores associated with female circumcision.[90] For the Kikuyu Central Association, it was a matter of ethnic pride. Efforts to end female circumcision were interpreted as the repression of African culture. Ultimately, medical officials opted to remain detached from the debates, preferring to work for gradual change through further education.

By the 1920s, the demand for medical services among Africans was palpable. In Uganda, 62,405 Africans received medical care in 1920. This grew to over two hundred fifty thousand by 1924 and signaled an urgent need for more medical staff. In 1925, the systematic medical training of Africans began in Uganda. Prior to this, Africans were trained as dressers who were limited to treating minor afflictions and providing first aid. By 1929, 247 dressers were treating over 190,500 persons in Tanganyika (D. Ferguson, 1979:327).[91] One of the major developments in East Africa in the 1920s, therefore, was the opening of Makerere College in Kampala. This was the first university for medical training in East Africa, though it was not until 1938 that the first

---

[88] The three-tiered medical structure depicted in this account was common across East Africa. Typically, the first tier included a chief medical officer and his staff located in central headquarters. Provincial medical officers (senior medical officers) and their staff comprised the second tier and district-level medical officers, based in regional hospitals, made up the third tier.

[89] Nonetheless, as late as 1979, missionaries operated 21% and 45% of all biomedical healthcare facilities in Kenya and Tanzania, respectively—as well as 40% in Malawi, 34% in Cameroon, and 29% in Ghana (C. Good, 1987:66, 67).

[90] Beck (1970:96) explores a seeming contradiction between the missionaries' zealous opposition to female circumcision compared to their more flexible attitudes toward other non-Christian and equally dangerous beliefs and practices.

[91] Beyond the modest medical care they provided, colonial officials also viewed the African dressers as optimal vehicles for popularizing Western scientific principles (Iliffe, 2002:49).

Africans were trained to become medical doctors.[92] Against this backdrop, a formal dispensary system was developed throughout East Africa in the 1920s. These African-staffed, local dispensaries became the primary source of biomedicine throughout the colonies. The dispensaries offered both inpatient and outpatient care. Services were provided by dressers and other assistants under the direction of a medical resident assistant who was an African trained in medical care.[93] Periodically, a colonial medical officer would visit for consultation. Because dispensaries were locally financed and administered, they were largely under the control of local ethnic groups—through local councils established by the 1924 Native Authority Ordinance—who were responsible for building, staffing, and equipping the dispensaries. As a consequence, the quality of medical care varied considerably across East Africa (C. Good, 1987). Tanganyika, for example, faced unique challenges with its vast territory, poor roads, minimal supervision, and the remoteness of its dispensaries. Its dispensary staff began with next to nothing and grew slowly. Tanganyikan dispensaries had no dressers in 1926, 90 in 1927, 147 in 1928, and 288 by 1930 (Beck, 1981:17). Notwithstanding significant advances in East Africa, by the 1930s, the quality and standards of care in rural dispensaries had become a significant concern among colonial officials.

> One District Medical Officer visiting a particularly remote dispensary reported that the building was clean, the man in charge neatly dressed, and the confidence the local people had in him was obvious from the large numbers awaiting treatment. But when asked to produce his records, he explained that none had been kept since the dresser had gone sick two months before; he himself was only the untrained sweeper who could neither read nor write. (Clyde, 1980:110)

By 1940, with the growing popularity of the dispensary system among Africans, rural-based biomedicine was well established throughout East Africa.[94] However, after two decades of building up the rural dispensary system across East Africa, World War II proved a major drain on staff and resources, which were rerouted to the war effort. Over time, resources were built back up and the period from the late 1940s through the 1950s was a time of significant growth with respect to biomedical resources across East Africa. In 1945, Kenyan dispensaries treated 1,029,860 patients. By 1948, this grew to 1,457,873

[92] Makerere College trained Africans from across East Africa and later became the University College of East Africa in 1950. See Iliffe (2002) for a detailed account of the development of Makerere College.

[93] In 1934, a further position was created between the dressers and the medical resident assistant.

[94] See Beck (1970), C. Good (1987), and Iliffe (2002).

(Beck, 1970:154). Kenyan medical officials urgently sought to develop new rural health centers[95] and to establish a new medical training school to complement Makerere College in Uganda. In 1949, Kenya had only fifteen trained African doctors (C. Good, 1987:35). Given their even larger territory, the equally understaffed and underresourced Tanganyikan dispensaries had the additional challenge of communicating and traveling over great distances. The immediate Tanganyikan priority was building more dispensaries and recruiting more staff. The 1950s and 1960s was a period of significant growth in this regard for Tanganyika. By 1960, there were 425 doctors in Tanganyika (twelve of whom were African),[96] ninety-nine hospitals, twenty-two rural health centers, and 990 dispensaries (Turshen, 1984:193). The rate of hospital beds per one thousand population grew from 1.1 in 1951 to 2.2 in 1966 (Clyde, 1980:101). Uganda, meanwhile, with 174 rural dispensaries by the close of the colonial era, suffered from many of the same general deprivations. The total number of medical staff in Uganda grew from 1,451 in 1948 to over five thousand in 1960 and the number of persons treated in hospitals rose from five million to seven million for those same years (Hopwood, 1980:157). At the same time, the percentage of Ugandan government expenditures for health care fell from 11% to 7.3% between 1949 and 1956 (Iliffe, 2002:101).

For all these impressive developments in the area of biomedical services in these decades, long-standing colonial policies based on racial exclusion proved highly destructive during the decade of independence in the 1960s. The rapid withdrawal of Uganda's expatriate medical staff, for example, dealt a severe blow to Uganda's post-independence medical system precisely due to the fact that under colonial rule Africans had been systematically excluded from positions of responsibility within the medical establishment. The period of independence in East Africa coincided, meanwhile, with a growing sentiment across the Third World that access to health care was a fundamental right of the people.[97] By 1978, this ferment resulted in the politically charged Alma Ata international conference, held in the Kazakhstan region of the Soviet Union, to discuss the state of health care among impoverished peoples. The resulting Alma Ata Declaration proclaimed health care to be a basic human right, marking a highpoint in Third World cross-border solidarity. The precipitous abandonment of postcolonial East Africa by the former colonial rulers, however, left Kenya, Tanzania, and Uganda with few

[95] Kenya's 25 rural health centers in 1957 mushroomed to 140 on the eve of independence.

[96] Africans could not be licensed as medical doctors in Tanganyika before 1953.

[97] Tanganyika achieved independence in December 1961, Uganda in October 1962, and Kenya in December 1963.

means to follow through on the principles embodied in the Alma Ata Declaration. Thus, in 1975, nine decades following the Berlin Congress and eight decades after the birth of tropical medicine, the World Health Organization described the abysmal state of health in Africa:

> If you happen to be born to grow up on the African bush, you are liable to have four or more disease-producing parasites simultaneously . . . In your village every child at times suffers the paroxysms of malaria fever and your wife will mourn the death of one or two children from this disease. The snails in the village pond carry schistosomiasis . . . If you live near a river black flies breed, one in two of your friends and neighbors will be blind in the prime of life. You know that waves of killing diseases like measles and meningitis and perhaps sleeping sickness are liable to strike your village. But, lacking effective remedies, you tend to philosophize in the face of sickness. You may make an effort to walk the ten miles to the nearest dispensary when you or your child is ill, but there may be no remedies, and it may be too late. (quoted in Beck, 1981:46)

African Pluralistic Medicine and Colonial Attitudes and Policies

Throughout the colonial era, pluralistic medicine remained a pivotal sociocultural institution across East Africa, shaping health beliefs and practices. Pluralistic-medical practitioners (referred to variously by Westerners as witch doctors, sorcerers, medicine men, diviners, and such) predominated in the rural hinterland and were generally ignored by colonial officials so long as they were not perceived to interfere with colonial rule (Iliffe, 2002). "[T]he medical department—interested primarily in the good will of Africans living in the few urbanized centers—did not care to inquire into the living habits of the vast masses of the rural population. Therefore, the African traditional healer was left alone to exercise an important function of healing among his own people" (Beck, 1981:62). While most pluralistic-medical practitioners were content to persist quietly in their remote work, many also assumed key roles in fomenting and organizing anticolonial struggle. Indeed, the role of pluralistic-medical practitioners as instigators and leaders during popular insurrections presented colonial authorities with some of their most serious challenges. The 1905–1906 Maji Maji Revolt in German East Africa was rumored to have gained its strength from the popular belief that certain occult powers protected Africans in their attack on German colonial forces. The lasting impression of the power of pluralistic-medical practitioners to galvanize revolt was evident when, over half a century later in

1957, a colonial government report persisted in the belief that—rather than popular opposition to colonial rule—the revolt was "touched off and spread by witchdoctors who duped the people with 'magic water' and when this failed to protect them from the German bullets, drove them again to their deaths by lies and excuses. The Germans were certainly ruthless, but the high casualties during the revolt were in no small measure due to the deceit of the witchdoctors" (quoted in Turshen, 1984:147). It was evident to colonial officials that the position of pluralistic-medical practitioners as interpreters of—and mediators within—the broader African cosmological order granted them considerable power and influence.

It followed that, at least for a period, the colonial authorities felt compelled to tolerate pluralistic-medical practitioners and a pragmatic balance of biomedicine and local medical practices remained a cardinal feature of rural life. British officials combined this attitude of indifference toward policing local healing practices with a pernicious belittling of local beliefs and customs.[98] The prohibitions against female circumcision were rarely enforced and the witchcraft ordinances of 1909, 1918, and 1925 did not lead to any major effort to police the activities of pluralistic-medical practitioners. Thus, unlike other parts of colonial Africa, such as the Belgian Congo, in East Africa there was little systematic effort to prohibit the practice of pluralistic medicine. In fact, many colonial officials developed an appreciation for such practices and endeavored to understand the underlying cosmology that organized African life. For example, a 1929 Tanganyikan witchcraft ordinance distinguished between the exercise of benevolent magic (*uchawi*) and the practice of malevolent magic (*uganga*). While the line between *uchawi* and *uganga* was not always precise, the attempt to draw such distinctions, nonetheless, suggests that colonial officials recognized differences among the pluralistic-medical practitioners whose key social role was undeniable.

At the same time, the European colonial powers brought with them an unshakeable faith in those modern scientific principles born of the Western Enlightenment, and the colonial order they established in Africa was, in part, premised upon the promulgation of, and a respect for, these basic principles. Thus, when an illness was attributed to supernatural forces and a pluralistic-medical practitioner was consulted to interpret the origin of the problem, the colonial authorities labored to frame these beliefs and practices within a familiar set of epistemological premises. From this encounter emerged a number of crude dichotomies intended to distinguish between European and

---

[98] Notably, colonial medical officials did not view pluralistic-medical practitioners as a supplement to their efforts—as they did, for example, with missionaries. Their general efforts went toward weakening the influence of pluralistic-medical practitioners and this was given as an explicit rationale, for example, by those advocating the expansion of dispensaries in Tanganyika in 1955 (Beck, 1981).

African mindsets—for example, modern/primitive, logical/illogical, rational/irrational, civilized/uncivilized, backward/progressive. Colonial officials in East Africa generally thought of pluralistic-medical practices as combining rational and irrational elements and this was dutifully confirmed by legions of Western anthropologists throughout the colonial era. L. F. Gerlach, a British anthropologist, represents a case in point with his study of the health practices of the Digo from northern Tanganyika.

> In a study on the Digo of East Africa, Gerlach concerned himself with the contradiction of logical conclusions and magic in his presentation of Digo conceptions of health and disease. Diagnosis, he wrote, proceeded in a logical manner, but it was based on the unscientific Digo premises as to the cause and effect of illness. The fact that logical conclusions were drawn from non-logical and non-verifiable assumptions caused many misinterpretations of the relationship between magic and natural treatment in traditional medicine. The average Digo would first determine whether illness was natural or God-sent and treat it with herbs, roots or patent medicine available in stores. If improvement did not come, he would consult the [pluralistic-medical practitioner] to discover what taboo had been broken, what particular treatment was required, whether sorcery was the cause . . . One finds a combination of first searching for a logical explanation and then resorting to supernatural revelation. (Beck, 1981:68)

Of course, the purpose of such anthropological work was not greater cultural understanding between peoples. The ethnographic goal was to wield cultural sensitivity as a weapon of subjugation, whereby one culture could subsume another.[99] In this regard, the colonial authority's relentless rhetorical demonizing of African pluralistic medicine invariably framed European cultural values and rationalist traditions in even starker relief. Through its depictions of biomedicine as "scientific" and African pluralistic medicine as "primitive" it was made clear to Africans that the continued practice of pluralistic medicine was a sign of shameful backwardness.[100]

With respect to African pluralistic medicine, the colonial project embodied a difficult tension, balancing both its civilizing mission (the introduction of Western, scientific medicine) and its need for stable governance (the appeasement of local populations). Overturning long-standing cultural prac-

[99] See Baronov (2004) for a contemporary example regarding public health educators in Puerto Rico and U.S.-sponsored HIV/AIDS prevention campaigns.

[100] See Fanon (1967), C. Good (1987), Memmi (1965) and Vaughan (1994).

tices and social institutions wholesale was rarely conducive to pacification. However, perpetuating local customs that were an anathema to the colonizer's understanding of the world would merely sustain an unbridgeable gulf between European and African. Most Europeans assumed that, ultimately, the steady advance of biomedicine in East Africa would invariably erode the influence of local cultural beliefs and practices.[101] Judging by the strong retention of pluralistic-medical beliefs and practices throughout the colonial era, such notions clearly proved mistaken. At the same time, whatever their competencies in the realm of medicine, colonial medical officials were hardly trained or qualified to negotiate the breach between the sacrosanct traditions of the Western Enlightenment and East African collective worldviews. Conflicts over female circumcision and the link between these conflicts and the rise of Kenyan nationalism, for example, were well beyond the expertise of medical officials. Furthermore, given the danger of violent rebellion—and the central role of pluralistic-medical practitioners in this regard—such issues were clearly as much political concerns as medical matters.

Thus, biomedicine's dramatic advances across East Africa notwithstanding, African pluralistic medicine ultimately survived and generally thrived throughout the era of colonial rule and this continued after independence. "[Pluralistic medicine] was an aspect of African life that had not been eliminated by the building of roads, ports, railways and a few cities in Kenya and Tanzania. Even dispensaries operated in the bush by young African helpers coexisted with the traditional healer" (Beck, 1981:70). Many independence leaders, however, considered biomedicine to be integral to progress and development and, in the period just after independence, pluralistic medicine was an area of major interest for governments. It was beginning with the Arusha Declaration in 1967, and its call for the mobilization of all available national resources, that pluralistic medicine came to be seen as a valuable asset in Tanzania and elsewhere to assist development—especially given the dire shortage of rural medical staff.[102] By the 1970s there was a growing international awareness of the need for less developed nations, such as Uganda, Kenya, and Tanzania, to make greater use of pluralistic medicine and a mounting skepticism towards an over-reliance on capital-intensive, high-tech medicine (Baer et al., 2003b; Thomas, 1975). In Tanzania, Julius Nyerre took the lead in such efforts, launching a research initiative in 1974 into the benefits of pluralistic medicine and the role of pluralistic-medical practitioners in Tanzanian society.

---

[101] See Beck (1970), C. Good (1987), and Olumwullah (2002).

[102] See Harrison (1974), Janzen (1976/77), and Oyeneye (1985).

The colonial experience in East Africa and the cascade of sociocultural dislocations that accompanied the introduction of biomedicine thus offers a glimpse into the peripheralization of an African region within the capitalist world-system. Colonial rule in East Africa exemplified a series of binary tropes—civilized/uncivilized, rational/irrational, primitive/modern—that informed the expansion of the capitalist world-system (and Africa's simultaneous peripheralization) and represented an ideological fixture of European/non-European contact. Incorporation into the capitalist world-system came to imply a concomitant transformation of underlying sociocultural values, beliefs, and practices as a precondition for non-Europeans to join the civilized world. In this sense, biomedicine was no mere benign gift from the civilized to the uncivilized, but a veritable Trojan Horse with which, over time, Western cultural values and beliefs could inundate East Africa and transform the region into a compliant peripheral zone within the capitalist world-system. "So long as biomedicine remained integral to colonialism's political concerns, its intents and cultural preoccupations in colonial Africa ceased to be merely a matter of scientific interest" (Olumwullah, 2002:286).

It is no small irony, therefore, that with the advance of Western influences in East Africa, the role of long-standing African sociocultural forms, such as pluralistic-medical beliefs and practices, likewise grew in importance. Within the brief span of one or two generations, the admixture of biomedical beliefs and practices with elements of African pluralistic medicine began to redefine medical care and reshape collective worldviews. As a singular historical-cultural formation, however, biomedicine itself proved equally susceptible to the transformative influences of African beliefs and practices that followed from this encounter. We turn next, therefore, to those elements of African pluralistic medicine that, subsequent to Africa's incorporation, began to radically reshape biomedicine, as a singular historical-cultural formation across the capitalist world-system.

4

African Pluralistic Medicine and Its Biomedical Antecedents

The analysis of biomedicine in Chapter 2 began with a critique of the distortions introduced by its conventional depiction as a set of discrete phenomenal forms—those associated with biomedicine as a scientific enterprise, as a symbolic-cultural expression, and as an expression of social power—before positing its necessary constitution as an ontological whole. In the case of "premodern" and "prescientific" African pluralistic-medical systems, the matter is otherwise. This follows, in part, from traditional Western descriptions of social development and modernization as a linear, multistage process in which individual societies are analyzed in the context of specific nations or regions rather than across a single capitalist world-system, as discussed in Chapter 1.[1] The three pillars of this modernization narrative are social differentiation, specialized interdependence, and scientific progress—the hallmarks of advanced, Western societies beginning in the late 19th century. By contrast, premodern and prescientific societies are thought to exhibit low levels of differentiation and specialization, and appeal to magic, superstition, and mysticism for explanations of events in the natural world. Consequently, the boundaries between the natural, supernatural, and social worlds are inherently fluid and, in contrast with biomedicine, African pluralistic-medical sys-

[1] Among the seminal modernization works in this regard are, Germani (1975), Hirschman (1958), Huntington (1968), Inkeles (1969), Lerner (1958), and Rostow (1971).

tems appear to constitute implicitly integrated systems.[2] Our analysis of African pluralistic-medical systems, therefore, necessarily follows a different strategy than that for biomedicine and proceeds both as a detailed review of Western efforts to describe these systems and as a critique of the conceptual categories that organize such efforts. To begin, it is helpful to identify those general features of African pluralistic-medical beliefs and practices that Westerners have emphasized in a conscious effort to frame differences between African pluralistic medicine and biomedicine as categorical dichotomies (for example, primitive/modern).

Beginning in the late 19th century, with the advent of tropical medicine and riding the crest of a new spirit of imperialism, Western anthropologists set out to scour the African continent and bring back detailed ethnographic studies of exotic, prescientific medical beliefs and practices linked to witchcraft, sorcery, ancestral spirits, and magic. In parallel fashion, historians of advanced Western societies reconstructed records of primitive medical beliefs and practices in the West prior to the modern scientific age, and comparisons were drawn with contemporary backward peoples from less-developed societies (Bakx, 1991; Hudson, 1983). Consequently, African pluralistic-medical systems came to be regarded as either in transition to biomedical norms or in a static, precontact phase.[3] The retention of premodern beliefs and practices is attributed to either a lack of resources to fully exploit biomedicine or a delayed, but inevitable, generational change. By such accounts, pluralistic medicine represents an outdated and backward mode of health and healing that, with time, will be supplanted by the superior results of scientific Western medicine. To the extent that pluralistic medicine fulfills any social role such as preserving and perpetuating collective cultural values these are characterized as atavistic vestiges that merely retard social development and modernization (Huntington, 1968; Lerner, 1958).

As detailed in previous chapters, the present analysis takes issue with such incomplete and self-serving portrayals of pluralistic medicine. The effort here is to interpret African pluralistic-medical systems as dynamic social

---

[2] Morley's analysis is typical in this regard. "In traditional societies medical knowledge is more closely integrated with the institutions and all-encompassing cosmology of the society as a whole than is the case in more differentiated industrial societies" (Morley, 1979:16). See Leslie (1974) for a discussion of modernization and medical systems in the Asian context.

[3] As detailed in Chapter 2, others view biomedicine itself as just another ethnomedical system (Hahn, 1995; Kleinman, 1980, 1986, 1995). Like the exotic premodern beliefs and practices, biomedicine is thought to contain a set of beliefs, practices, and rituals. Such studies, however, generally reveal far more about biomedicine than about pluralistic medicine, while doing little to challenge directly the underlying stagist teleology of the first approach. For example, it is generally presumed that once pluralistic medicine is set in competition with biomedicine much of biomedicine, over time, will crowd out the less developed pluralistic-medical beliefs and practices.

orbits that continue to evolve and develop. In this regard, two cardinal features of the standard Western interpretation of African pluralistic medicine are rejected. First, those exotic beliefs and practices that are stumbled upon by Western powers are not pristine and static self-contained medical systems, untouched and unaffected by other peoples and societies. Each medical system has evolved over time, borrowing liberally from others and constantly recasting purportedly primordial beliefs and practices. "There is, then, no essential medicine. No medicine that is independent of historical context" (Kleinman, 1995:23). Importantly, therefore, among practitioners of pluralistic medicine, respect for tradition and custom is invariably combined with an affinity for change and pragmatic adaptation.[4]

> [Pre-colonial African] societies had certainly valued custom and continuity but custom was loosely defined and infinitely flexible. Custom helped to maintain a sense of identify but it also allowed for an adaptation so spontaneous and natural that it was often unperceived. Moreover, there rarely existed in fact the closed corporate consensual system which came to be accepted as characteristic of "traditional" Africa. (Ranger, 1983:247–48)

Second, beginning in the late 19th century, pluralistic medicine was increasingly subsumed within the expanding capitalist world-system and its marauding agents of social change, including biomedicine. In this context, biomedicine was not merely a contrasting set of medical beliefs and practices. It was introduced alongside other instruments of Western power that devoured land, labor, and productive resources. From its initial introduction, the benign pretensions of biomedical science were severely compromised by its paramount political agenda. The African retention of pluralistic-medical beliefs and practices is, therefore, in part, a response to Western aggression—an alternative understanding of health and illness[5] that partially borrows from the colonizer without wholly abandoning fundamental African organizing principles and beliefs.

---

[4] Akerele (1987), Feierman (1979), and Katz and Katz (1981), for example, document continuing efforts within African pluralistic medicine to evolve and develop. Herskovits and Bascom (1959) provide an early analysis of African society as dynamic and subject to changes.

[5] Use of the term "illness" points to a lingering imperfection of Western idiom. Conventionally, the term "disease" refers to health-related afflictions linked to biological pathologies and "illness" refers to how individuals experience various infirmities (Hahn, 1984; Kleinman, 1995). Here, a variation of this distinction is observed. Use of "disease" is restricted to health-related afflictions recognized by biomedicine and, given the broader etiological premises of African pluralistic medicine, "illness" refers those afflictions identified and treated by it.

It is true that over the past century biomedicine has gained increasing acceptance across Africa and that, in the course of these developments, certain fundamental beliefs and practices have been radically challenged. Emerging from this encounter have been many novel medical beliefs and practices. The basic features of the resulting medical systems, however, are neither uniform nor universal across African societies and ethnic groups. Rather, a heterogeneous collection of pluralistic-medical systems has evolved that are greatly influenced by—but not reducible to—Western biomedical beliefs and practices. Notwithstanding such variation across contemporary African pluralistic medicine, it is argued here that a number of common elements permit certain guarded generalizations.[6] To disentangle these evolving African pluralistic-medical systems from the obfuscating web of modernization narratives it is necessary to identify that which is unique to African pluralistic medicine most broadly—a constellation of common elements that cut across the heterogeneity of African pluralistic-medical systems. Having first distilled a set of broad features characterizing African pluralistic medicine, four widely cited ethnographies representing distinct regions and eras then allow us better to detail the contrasting and unique manifestations of these elements across diverse communities at different times. The cryptic images that emerge from the fog of these inherently fluid developments provide our first glimpse of the crude outlines of "African biomedicine" and, thereby, point toward Africa's contributions to biomedicine as a singular historical-cultural formation.

African Pluralistic Medicine and the Origins of African/Western Dualism

Each African pluralistic-medical system is firmly embedded in a more general cosmology whose purpose—as with all cosmologies, considered primitive or otherwise—is to construct broad explanatory narratives that logically incorporate varied interpretations of reality.[7] At the most general level, for purposes of deciphering pluralistic-medical beliefs and practices as symbolic

[6] In reference to African pluralistic medicine, Frankenberg and Leeson (1976) observe, "There is no written body of knowledge or beliefs, no systematic means of instruction; they are in fact a heterogeneous collection, with no unanimity of theory or practice, although of course they share some common features" (p. 239).

[7] See Sindzingre (1985) in this regard when analyzing African pluralistic medicine among the Fodonon in northern Ivory Coast. More generally, see Horton's seminal essay (1967) regarding the similarities and differences between Western scientific thought and African cosmologies, along with the related commentaries by Finkler (1994), Gyeke (1997), Pearce (1986), and Wiredu (1984). In a related analysis, Argyle (1969) distinguishes between the dualistic categories of "tribe" and "nation."

artifacts of premodern cosmologies, medical anthropologists in the West commonly distinguish between natural (or impersonal) explanations of health and illness and supernatural (or personal) explanations.[8] Simply put, natural explanations identify phenomena and forces within the physical world as the cause of illness and supernatural explanations identify phenomena and forces beyond the physical world (such as witchcraft, sorcery, and magic) as the cause of illness. This natural/supernatural divide operates as a heuristic device for highlighting certain differences between biomedicine and pluralistic medicine.[9] However, such dualistic taxonomies tend to conflate the unique contributions of phenomena from the supernatural and social worlds—whereby, explanations linked to social relationships are simply subsumed within the category of supernatural (Westerlund, 1989a). Accordingly, for purposes of exposition, consideration of African pluralistic medicine has been organized around forms of explanation in the natural, supernatural, and social worlds—as three distinct yet overlapping spheres. Beyond the roles of natural, supernatural, and social explanations there are several further elements that, broadly speaking, characterize Western depictions of African pluralistic medicine. These include holistic frameworks, pragmatic attitudes toward alternative medical systems (including biomedicine), the role of empirical-rational methods of investigation, and the hybrid nature of health-related services as both a profitable commodity[10] and a social obligation.

This constellation of elements provides the West with a conceptual language to describe and interpret specific African pluralistic-medical beliefs and practices—depicted as primordial and unchanging cultural features. These elements also provide a framework for placing specific beliefs and practices within a broader cosmology that reveals the dynamic contours of African collective worldviews. Therefore, before considering each of these elements in greater detail, several general comments are in order regarding their origin as products of Africa's encounter with the West. Colonial-era caricatures of African cosmologies were artfully drawn to stain the Western

---

[8] See Foster (1976), Green (1999) and Last (1993).

[9] Foster (1976) and Murdock (1980) provide typical dualistic taxonomies. Murdock divides pluralistic-medical explanations into two areas. Natural explanations are comprised of five subtypes—infection, stress, organic deteriorization, accidents, and overt human aggression. Supernatural explanations constitute three broad categories—mystical explanations, animistic explanations, and magical explanations. Such taxonomies are helpful for highlighting certain key features of pluralistic medicine. However, as with any effort to catalogue and categorize, idiosyncratic differences are often emphasized at the expense of more fundamental similarities.

[10] Iliffe (2002) describes pluralistic-medical practitioners in East Africa as "entrepreneurial, competitive, and often mercenary, especially among full-time specialists with wide reputations" (p. 11).

image of the African as savage and primitive.[11] The civilizing mission, in fact, begins with a depiction of the African mind, or the African worldview, as a prison whose walls and chains must be shattered. It follows that the West's representation of these elements is specifically designed to draw contrasts with Western worldviews. The essential rationale informing Western characterizations of African pluralistic-medical beliefs and practices is to highlight differences with enlightened, scientific medicine and, thereby, to establish the necessary preconditions and premises for modern change across the continent. African pluralistic medicine represents an alternative worldview and the resulting language, concepts, and frameworks provide an African image of the world that stands in sharp relief against Western notions. The basic elements shaping Western portrayals of African pluralistic medicine thus reflect contrived dualistic categories that are creations of the West, fostering the image of African primitiveness and justifying its civilizing mission.[12]

The first three elements of African pluralistic medicine follow from the natural/supernatural divide and correspond with explanations of illness—as a subcategory of misfortune in general—that are attributed to forces within the natural, supernatural, and social worlds.[13] Explanations of health-related misfortune associated with the natural world identify physical phenomena in the environment (for example, infection, contagion, and pollution) as the cause of an illness and rely on physical substances (for example, medicinal herbs, roots, and plants) for treatment. Such illnesses are depicted as naturally-occurring events that originate in harmful environmental conditions. Explanations of health-related misfortune linked to the supernatural world detail the manner by which supernatural forces (that is, witchcraft, sorcery, magic, and spirits) are present and operate within the natural world. The events attributed to supernatural phenomena cannot be explained by appeal to the dynamics of the natural world and, therefore, require an understanding of the forms of interaction between the natural and supernatural worlds. Explanations of health-related misfortune tied to social networks focus on fractious social relationships at the individual and community levels as the cause of illness. Hostilities within the social world may make individuals susceptible to illnesses that are willed upon

[11] In his penetrating analysis of the "invention of tradition in colonial Africa," Ranger remarks that, "[M]any African scholars as well as many European Africanists have found it difficult to free themselves from the false models of colonial codified African 'tradition'" (1983:212).

[12] See Mamdani (1996) for a more general analysis of this process and of the African internalization of this dualism.

[13] Framing illness as a specific manifestation of the more general category of misfortune is, of course, not unique to African pluralistic-medical systems. In his overview of non-Western medical traditions, Worsley observes that, "(B)odily ills are commonly taken to be mere epiphenomena: themselves material outcomes of immaterial force and agencies which inflict punishment for social misdeeds" (1982:327). See also Whyte (1989).

one person by another. Given the capacity of individuals and groups to command supernatural forces (such as witchcraft or sorcery), there is considerable overlap between supernatural explanations and social network explanations of illness.[14]

Importantly, though the phenomena and forces within the natural, supernatural, and social worlds are here treated as separate forms of explanation for purposes of exposition, in general, African pluralistic medicine invokes such explanations without drawing any sharp distinctions between them. This follows from a fourth element of African pluralistic medicine, the role of holistic frameworks. Holism represents a core organizing principle that provides an understanding of social reality in which phenomena across the natural, supernatural, and social worlds are necessarily interrelated and conceptually inseparable. The notion of the three as distinct realms is a contrivance of the West for the purpose of understanding a contrary cosmological order. The everyday operating logic of African pluralistic medicine requires this holistic framework which is viewed in the West, by and large, as a relic of prescientific, pre-Enlightenment thought. It is this holistic framework, for example, that complicates efforts to proceed in the reductionist manner of biomedicine to isolate the specific cause of an illness in the natural world. As noted, African pluralistic medicine is anything but static and tradition-bound. Appropriately, therefore, a fifth and long-established element of African pluralistic medicine concerns its receptive attitude toward other medical systems. African ethnic groups constantly borrow from one another and today nearly all African pluralistic-medical practices are amalgams of a great many other traditions. This pragmatic disposition extends to the acceptance and incorporation of biomedicine as a duly respected, alternative medical system.[15] The notion of interchangeable and evolving beliefs and practices, however, does not suggest the wholesale replacement of one medical system for another based upon the ethnocentric Western premise of inherent incompatibility. Rather, over time, a mix of medical beliefs and practices emerge.

As follows from the role of explanations within the natural world, empirical-rational methods are a sixth element of nearly all African pluralistic-medical systems. Observation, experimentation, and prediction, for example,

---

[14] Explanations of illness and misfortune generally follow a consistent logic. In his study of the Ndembu of Zambia, for example, Turner (1967) noted that the role of logic did not provide a clear distinction between pluralistic medicine and biomedicine. He observed, in fact, a high level of systematic logic, though this was based on explicitly supernatural premises. See also Young (1979) in this regard with respect to the role of practical logic within Amhara pluralistic medicine.

[15] Based on fieldwork in eastern Uganda, Whyte (1988) documents the extensive experience and training of Nyole pluralistic-medical practitioners outside Nyole society and concludes that, "In Africa, the power of foreign medicines was already established long before Western pharmaceuticals began to circulate on a large scale" (p. 227). See also Last (1981).

are the bases for the prevalent use of botanical treatments. Over the past half century the Western pharmaceutical industry has learned and profited a great deal from the extensive African botanical pharmacopoeia that has resulted from decades of rigorous African study and trial-and-error experimentation.[16] This widespread African adherence to the basic principles of empiricism further complicates Western efforts to reduce African pluralistic-medical beliefs and practices to mindless concoctions and senseless superstition. In fact, extensive professional training and apprenticeships are generally required before African pluralistic-medical practitioners are considered sufficiently knowledgeable and competent to provide care. Finally, with respect to the delivery of African pluralistic-medical services, a seventh element concerns the manner by which such services take the form of both a commodity and a social obligation. African pluralistic-medical practitioners quite frequently collect fees that can turn their practices into modest if not quite profitable enterprises. Practitioners clearly view their work as something to be protected—primarily from competing practitioners—and as a source of income not merely for basic survival but, when possible, for amassing significant personal wealth. At the same time, given their position within the community, providing pluralistic-medical services is often considered a social obligation— especially to members of one's own ethnic group. As a rule, however, while fees are almost always imposed, adherence to social obligation is less strictly enforced. Notably, with respect to prevailing moral economies, even when services are treated as a profitable commodity, fees are often based on a person's ability to pay.

As previously discussed, characterizing the nature of biomedical beliefs and practices across the various advanced capitalist nations requires prudent caution with respect to overgeneralizations. Arguably, even greater care must be taken when attempting to characterize pluralistic-medical beliefs and practices across hundreds of heterogeneous African societies. The effort here is merely to highlight certain features that characterize Western depictions of African pluralistic medicine across these societies. The elements discussed in this regard, though common across most of Africa, are thus not universal and *do not* apply in the same manner in all places. At the same time, given the historic link between efforts to characterize African pluralistic-medical systems and the West's civilizing mission, a series of dualistic categories continue to influence its consideration in a fashion that can be more confusing than illuminating. Thus, it bears repeating that the beliefs and practices analyzed here are not the primordial features of different African societies, somehow frozen in time. African pluralistic-medical beliefs and practices

[16] See Beaujard (1988), Bibeau (1979), Chhabra et al. (1990), Etkin (1981), Flint (2001), Gbeassor et al. (1989), Keharo (1972), Prins (1992), and Rowson (1965).

are, in fact, constantly evolving and changing. "African healing methods and theory have not remained frozen in a timeless ethnographic present, but have changed and adapted with the times" (Schoepf, 1992:232).

Lastly, the use of terminology when describing those who practice African pluralistic medicine presents a number of challenges. Some terms (such as witch doctor or medicine man) are outdated at best and strikingly ethnocentric at worst.[17] Others, such as *nganga* or *mundue mue*, are too specific to a particular ethnic-linguistic group—KiSwahili and KiKamba, respectively. For purposes of clarity, therefore, specific practitioner roles provide useful categories. Most pluralistic-medical practitioners perform one of four roles: (1) Diviners attempt to identify the cause(s) of an illness attributed to the supernatural and social worlds; (2) Herbalists treat illnesses with a range of local botanicals; (3) Pluralistic healers simultaneously treat the physical symptoms of an illness while addressing its underlying supernatural cause(s); and (4) Priests and prophets work to reconcile individuals or communities with offended spirits through purification rites and exorcisms. A significant number of practitioners specialize in one or more of these roles, with many performing all four. For this reason, when referring to a specific practitioner role, the name of that particular role has been adopted (for example, diviner, herbalist). More commonly, however, it is necessary to refer to the broad class of all such practitioners as a whole or to persons who engage in more than one of these roles. In such cases, the acronym for pluralistic-medical practitioner (PMP) has been adopted. It is hoped that this will clarify more than it confuses, but no choice with respect to terminology is without its shortcomings.

Natural Explanations

The link between natural phenomena and illness is a fundamental aspect of African pluralistic medicine that guides the diagnosis and treatment of conditions linked to infection, contagion, or environmental contaminants. Among the Sukuma in Tanzania, for example, when illness impacts the whole village or community, this is attributed to some form of environmental pollution or contamination (Reid, 1982). Importantly, when an individual falls ill due to natural causes this is not because he or she has been singled out by forces within the supernatural world, but simply because he or she happens to come in contact with a naturally-occurring, unclean, or contaminated substance. The sources for such substances are many. Among the BaKongo, it is recommended that infants be given three purges in the first months of

[17] See Sindzingre (1985) for a more general discussion of linguistic issues pertaining to African pluralistic-medical beliefs and practices.

life to cleanse the *vumu* (a food substance thought to form in the stomach) (Janzen, 1978). The Zaramo of Tanzania identify certain physical ailments with different forms of contamination that enter the body as poison (L. Swantz, 1990). These are most often food-borne or air-borne contaminants, but illness can also result from inadvertently stepping on *uchawi* (witchcraft) that was meant for someone else.[18] As explored below, the notion of "stepping on" witchcraft suggests that witchcraft itself represents a material substance with physical properties. Even witchcraft, therefore, is susceptible to empirical-rational investigation, to be confirmed or refuted. The Koma in northern Nigeria, for example, practice a forensic, post-mortem technique to identify physical evidence—distinct holes in the skull—to confirm witchcraft suspicions (Paarup-Laursen, 1989). Furthermore, the widespread notion of contamination indicates that the etiological rationale informing many African pluralistic-medical systems is premised on isolating specific physical matter within the natural environment—not unlike biomedicine (Farley, 1992). Given Western fascination with the exotic and supernatural aspects of African pluralistic medicine, the commonplace appeal to natural causes is often elided in favor of detailing the exciting drama of witchcraft, sorcery, and magic. In his review of the literature on contagion and pollution beliefs among ethnic groups in southern Africa, Green (1999) questions the implicit ethnocentrism of Western anthropology in this regard.

> [Robert] Pool suggests that anthropologists who find naturalistic thinking among Africans are projecting or imposing their own "biomedically determined constructs" on Africans. Perhaps Pool does not recognize the implication here: If an explanation sounds naturalistic or scientific, it must be of Western, scientific origin. But why can't non-personalistic explanations of illness be of indigenous, African origin? Westerners seem to have trouble conceding this possibility. (p. 73)[19]

The role of infection[20] or contagion as a cause of illness has been widely documented in Africa.[21] In Tanzania, Harjula (1989) interviewed a Meru PMP, Mirau, who outlined a variety of natural causes. "Mirau regards the patient as

---

[18] Whyte (1997) describes a similar phenomenon among the Nyole of eastern Uganda.

[19] Green refers here specifically to Pool (1994).

[20] See Temkin (1977c) for a discussion of the evolution of the concept of infection in Western biomedicine.

[21] See Buckley (1985a), Mburu (1977), MacLean (1979b), Olsson (1989), Wall (1988), and Wolff (1979).

a complicated 'machine' that can get out of order for many external reasons: dirt and worms cause diarrhea and other stomach troubles, cold rains cough and fever; eating too much fat and sugar results in heart disease, and so on" (p. 133). Worms, insects, and germs are common sources of infection leading to illness and in some cases mental disorders. Among the Yoruba, "there are important indigenous ideas about the injurious effects of certain worms, germs and of impure or abnormal blood. A wide variety of maladies and some psychiatric illnesses, are believed to be due, in whole or in part, to invisible worms" (Westerlund, 1989b:199). Olsson (1989:235) observes that, among the Maasai, "Mosquitoes are known to be carriers of malaria," while Kamba PMPs attribute measles to "a reddish brown worm lodged in the stomach just under the spleen" (Mburu, 1977:178). Forms of person-to-person, germ-based contagion are also commonplace. "Most illnesses [among the Yoruba] are said to be caused by germs, and in certain cases these germs are said to be transmitted from person to person" (Buckley, 1985b:195). Among many Zulu, the notion of illness and contagion are combined with supernatural features. Consequently, great care must be taken in safely disposing of items contaminated by an ill person to avoid further contagion.

> Illnesses that are believed to be mystically caused are believed to be cured by taking them out of the body system as a substance that must be thrown away. Since what is thrown away does not dissipate itself but could be dangerous to other people the problem is, where can one throw it away without polluting the environment . . . In an attempt to solve the problem, cross-roads and highways are said to be the most often used areas for disposing undesirable substances, in the hope that these are much more often used by travelers, outsiders or strangers in the community to whom the illness might attach itself and be carried away from the territory. But the problem is not quite solved. Such a stranger may carry away the undesirable element, but he may also introduce dangers which he brings with him from a foreign territory." (Ngubane, 1976:354–355)

Related to infection and contagion is the role of environmental factors. There are strong health concerns within African pluralistic medicine, for example, tied to hygiene and unsanitary living conditions (for example, open sewers and unsafe water) as well as weather-related phenomena. MacLean (1976:304), argues that treatments for smallpox among the Yoruba "comprise a mixture of magic, herbal medicine and specific hygienic measures which might well have been efficacious in reducing the spread of the disease throughout the community," while a study by Foster et al. (described in Green, 1999:43–44) details the role of poor sanitary conditions (the concept of *imótótó*) as a major cause of illness identified by the Yoruba. Strong winds and the hot sun are frequent environmental sources of illness. The Bambara of Mali associate smallpox with contaminants in the wind, reasoning that "only wind has such widespread contact with the body as to cause so diffuse an eruption" (Imperato, 1979:19). It is, likewise, maintained by the Ibo of Nigeria that illnesses are carried by breezes or winds resulting in coughs or yaws (Ezeabasili, 1982). In a fashion that parallels contemporaneous European public health campaigns, Iliffe (2002) describes efforts by the Hehe of southern Tanzania in the late 19th century to isolate plague victims to thwart further contagion among the population. Flint (2001:202) observes that, "When Europeans first arrived, Africans in the Zulu kingdom had, for the most part, minimized health risks by settling outside low-lying malarial areas and requiring multiple dwelling structures for large families."

Villagers in Ogori, Nigeria, describe malaria as a form of sunstroke and attribute guinea-worm infection to drinking impure water (Gillies, 1976a). Buckley (1985a) quotes a Yoruba PMP in this regard: "[Malaria] is caused by standing in the hot sun. I get bitten by mosquitoes many times each day but I only get [malaria] twice a year. If you don't believe the sun causes [malaria], try standing in the sun for an afternoon and see what happens" (pp. 20–21). Reflecting an Islamic influence, Hausa pluralistic medicine in Nigeria places great emphasis on the role of environmental factors. "The most pervasive cause of illness in the Hausa scheme of things are the effects on the human body of variations in the physical environment: heat and cold" (Wall, 1988:187). Some of the most elaborate explanations of environmental factors contributing to illness, however, are offered by the Zulu (du Toit, 1985; Ngubane, 1976). Local regions present variable environmental conditions. Consequently, when a person who is acclimated to the conditions of one local region travels to another region, he or she is at great risk of falling ill.

> The Zulu believe that there is a special relationship between a man and his environment and that plant and animal life somehow affect the environment. As different countries or regions have different types of plants and animals, they therefore have different environmental conditions. The people in each particular region are adjusted to their surroundings, but if they were to go to a completely different region they would become ill as they would not be adjusted to the new environmental conditions. (Ngubane, 1976:323)

Just as African pluralistic-medical etiology attributes various illnesses to infection, contagion, and a host of environmental factors, PMPS' courses of treatment follow a similar logic with respect to the role of natural phenomena and the course of illness. Herbalists prescribe a wide range of botanical remedies based on a presumed link between the medicinal properties of specific plants, roots, and herbs and specific illnesses.[22] Deafness among the Ile-Ife in Nigeria, for example, is treated with an herbal ear drop (Odebiyi and Togonu-Bickersteth, 1987). An enormous range of botanical treatments has resulted across Africa.[23] In fact, there are virtually no examples of pluralistic-medical systems (African or otherwise) that do not incorporate botanical therapies as a routine treatment.

> All human societies have a pharmacopoeia consisting of a wide variety of materials, including plants, animals (including fish, insects and reptiles), rocks and minerals, waters (salt and fresh, surface and subterranean), earths and sands, and fossils, as well as manufactured items. An estimated 25% to 50% of the pharmacopoeia of indigenous peoples has been demonstrated to be empirically effective by biomedical criteria. Various biomedical drugs, including quinine and digitalis, were originally derived from indigenous peoples. (Baer et al., 2003a:314)

The number of illnesses and associated natural remedies is almost without limit. Willis (1979) records numerous Ufipa botanical treatments in southwest Tanzania. Those with constipation receive herbal purgatives and enemas, while ulcers are treated with a preparation of dried herbs, and persons with eye infections are given a special sap drawn from a tree. For the Shona in Zimbabwe, there are herbal remedies for headaches and common colds (Chavunduka, 1978). The Yoruba treat a range of common illnesses, including colds, fevers, and childhood convulsions, with specific herbal remedies (MacLean, 1976). Zimbabwean PMPs have developed herbal treatments for urinary schistosomiasis (Ndamba et al., 1994), and the Bambari in Mali offer herbal remedies for measles (Imperato and Traore, 1979). Harrison (1979) details a litany of Nigerian herbal remedies for many illnesses. "In Nigeria, medicinal plants used by [herbalists] have been found effective for local cases of infective hepatitis, intestinal hurry, hypertension, convulsions, malaria, ulcers, fractured bones and other ailments" (p. 97). Notwithstand-

---

[22] Botanical treatments vary considerably across African societies (Akisanya, 1977; Onyioha, 1977). Nigerian pluralistic medicine is a case in point. "The prescriptions of [PMPS in Nigeria] can be classified into three categories: (i) that which is made up of plant parts, (ii) that which is a combination of plant parts and parts of animals or animal secretions (iii) that which is made up of plant parts, and/or parts of animals in combination with certain incantations" (Akisanya, 1977:237).

[23] For a modest sampling of the relevant literature, see Buckley (1985a), Chavunduka and Last (1986), Chhabra et al. (1990), Frankenberg and Leeson, (1976), Harjula (1989), Keharo (1972), Kramer and Thomas (1982), Mburu (1977), Mume (1977), Odebiyi and Togonu-Bickersteth (1987), Olsson (1989), Onyioha (1977), Paarup-Laursen (1989), Sofowora (1982), Spring (1980a), Westerlund (1989a), Wall (1988), and Wolff (1979).

ing this extensive and systematic approach, many Westerners remain highly critical of the medicinal use of botanicals, as reflected in the remarks of a Western physician observing African pluralistic medicine.

> Irrespective of the doubtful efficacy of tribal medicine in respect of the great health problems in Bomvanaland, the danger lies in the principle lack of self-criticism of the Xhosa practitioners. The medication provided for the patient is administered according to an exactly prescribed dosage. There is no distinction between therapeutic and toxic doses. This total lack of pharmacological insight makes their dispensing of medicines a hazardous matter. (G. Jansen, 1973:136).[24]

The demonstrated efficacy[25] of many botanical remedies has not gone unnoticed, and this has led Westerners to try to learn (and profit) from the sophisticated pharmacological knowledge developed by African herbalists.[26] Such research allows Westerners to recognize a narrow slice of African pluralistic medicine that lends itself to certain Western scientific precepts. "It is much easier for WHO, or any large organization or for national health planners, to countenance a study of herbs, which are visible, tangible, measurable and manageable, than to take account of the spiritual, psychotherapeutic and social dimensions of traditional medicine" (MacLean, 1987:31–32). The exploitative nature of Western pharmacological research in this regard is clearly evident. "The pharmacological research being carried out appears to be a subtle way of robbing [PMPS] of their knowledge; the aim being to give any result of such research to established pharmaceutical companies for their own use" (Chavunduka, 1987:71). This "robbery" is based on an ongoing relation of exploitation between Africa and the West as well as biomedicine's proclivity to treat medical care as comprised of discrete elements that exist outside a holistic framework.

---

[24] Such views fit a long-established colonial pattern of dismissing African, Indian, and Arab medical practices, as discussed by Arnold (1993). "It was characteristic of medicine's colonizing nature that it sought to establish its superior or monopolistic rights over the body of the colonized. The vigorous denunciation of indigenous healers, from the 'witchdoctors' and spirit mediums in Africa to the *vaidyas* and *hakims* of Hindu and Islamic medicine, was supported by claims that their practices were grounded in superstition, or at best mere empiricism, and were often dangerous" (p. 1408).

[25] See Etkin's critical commentary (1988) with regard to efficacy as a "cultural construct." This is further discussed in Chapter 5.

[26] See Bibeau (1979), Etkin (1981), MacLean (1987), Matthe (1989), Onyioha (1977), Rowson (1965), P. Singer (1977), Wall (1988), and Zeller (1979b).

Supernatural Explanations

Consideration of supernatural explanations within African pluralistic-medical systems is fraught with peril. The literature is vast and the debates, themes, and depictions remain hotly contested. Supernatural explanations attribute the cause of an illness to phenomena and forces whose nature cannot be understood by appealing to the physical laws of nature as recognized by the Western sciences. There are two standard interpretations that follow from this notion and the distinctions between these are critical for evaluating the role of supernatural forces within African pluralistic medicine. On the one hand, it is argued that such forces contravene the laws of nature and are, therefore, surely nothing more than the fanciful rantings of a preliterate, uneducated, and primitive mind—however respectfully discussed. On the other hand, it is suggested that such forces pertain to a reality not captured by investigations of the natural world (for example, ancestral spirits) and are, therefore, simply beyond the self-imposed ontological limits of the Western natural sciences. Importantly, the latter position—that of most PMPs—should not be mistaken for half-hearted agnosticism. It is a full-throated affirmation that the reality of the supernatural world is as consequential and as tangible for the lives of individuals as forces in the natural world. In navigating between these two interpretations, most Western depictions are akin to a psychiatrist's clinical notes. The doctor does not interview a delusional patient to understand the patient's world. The doctor's concern is the patient's understanding of the doctor's world.[27] Unlike the psychiatrist, our interest *is* to understand the PMP's world and, thereby, to recast the Western cosmology as an alternative ontological interpretation of reality.

As noted, terminology presents significant obstacles when exploring the supernatural world. By Western convention, discussions of the supernatural world and African pluralistic medicine have adopted the categories of witchcraft, sorcery, magic, and spirits. Unfortunately, these terms today evoke mythical images of fantasy and fable in the West, complete with fire-breathing dragons and hapless damsels. It is difficult, therefore, to escape the distortion and ethnocentrism inherent in this language. Each African ethnic group, of course, has its own terminology for such concepts that, with considerable strain, can be rendered into the generic Western categories of witchcraft, sorcery, magic, and spirits. However, as in the case of specific PMP roles, it would be cumbersome constantly to shift the terminology to match that of each ethnic group throughout the presentation. Therefore, for want of a

[27] For further consideration of African belief systems in light of Western science see Airhihenbuwa (1995), Ademuwagun (1979), Asuni (1979), Horton (1967), Mbiti (1970), Mburu (1977), Mume (1977), Oguah (1984), Quah (2003) and Wiredu (1984).

more suitable nomenclature, the Western linguistic convention has been adopted here.

Witchcraft, sorcery, magic, and spirits all comprise ubiquitous forces within the supernatural world, though the meaning and role of each differs markedly across African pluralistic-medical systems. Western studies of African witchcraft and sorcery are voluminous.[28] Witches and sorcerers are manifestations of distinct, yet related, supernatural forces. In each case, the witch or sorcerer is a human agent who undertakes purposeful actions that are motivated by contentious interpersonal relationships[29] and a social order bound by explicit norms and mores.[30] Generally speaking, a witch must possess an actual physical entity (witchcraft substance) to bring about harm. Working among the Azande in southern Sudan, Evans-Pritchard (1976:15–17) provides an elaborate description of an autopsy following the death of a suspected witch to recover the witchcraft substance and confirm suspicions. This substance is either inherited or somehow passed to individuals by supernatural forces (such as ancestral spirits). Though quite common, the notion of witchcraft inheritance is far from universal. The Koma of northern Nigeria, for example, maintain that "witchcraft is not inherited, but can be practiced by anyone interested who has the necessary abilities. Witchcraft can also be transferred by eating witch-meat bought in the market" (Paarup-Laursen, 1989:63).

Commonly, the witch is portrayed as the passive recipient of the witchcraft substance. A person is responsible for what he or she does with this substance once he or she possess it, but mere possession is not necessarily evidence of nefarious intent. For example, among the Tswana of Botswana, "The witches who prowl at night are said to be normal humans during the day, not even aware themselves of the nocturnal personalities which they have inherited from an earlier generation" (Ulin, 1979:245). Witches are to be feared, therefore, for the power that they possess, although the witch him- or herself may not be seen as a bad person.[31] Sorcerers are another matter. Sorcerers also possess supernatural powers to harm others. Generally speaking,

---

[28] A tiny sample of this literature includes Beattie (1967), Bjerke (1989), Douglas (1963), Epstein (1967), Evans-Pritchard (1976), Gray (1963), Marwick (1967), Middleton and Winter (1963), Nadel (1952), Park (1967), and Winter (1963).

[29] Less commonly, for example in the case of the Kalahari-based !Kung, individuals can become bewitched by wild animals absent any human enemy (Marshall, 1969).

[30] See M. Gelfand (1964a), Gray (1963), Harjula (1989), MacGaffey (1983), Turner (1964b), Wall (1988), Winter (1963), and Whisson (1964).

[31] Significant gender distinctions exist in this regard, especially in the case of female witches who often face far more stigma than male witches, who are generally given greater latitude as figures in the community. See Austen (1993), Goody (1970), or Gottlieb (1989) in this regard.

however, the sorcerer is an individual who has consciously obtained these powers for the purpose of harming others through a combination of special training and the purchase of magical substances. For the Nigerian Hausa, "The human agencies that cause illness can be subdivided into those powers inherent in the individual (witchcraft) and those which are acquired (sorcery)" (Wall, 1988:193). To become a sorcerer, therefore, unlike becoming a witch, requires a measure of malicious forethought and, because of this, the social sanctions for sorcerers are ordinarily far more harsh.

One of the most essential roles of the PMP is to counter witchcraft and the sorcerer's magic with his or her own magical powers.[32] The PMP's magic, the sorcerer's magic, and the witchcraft substance are all vital forces within the supernatural world that take a wide variety of forms across African pluralistic-medical systems.[33] Importantly, these forces remain under the control of human agents (sorcerers, witches, and PMPs) who use them to different ends. As MacLean (1979) observes, this link between medicine and magic refashions the common Western understanding of medical treatment.

> The concept of medicine and its influence extends far beyond the limits which Western usage imposes. It includes remedies or prophylactics which can act at a distance, and charms and counter charms are available for all kinds of ills and misadventures. The idea of preventive medicine is widespread in the sense of magical preparations which can protect an individual from possible dangers. (1979a:162).

At the same time, implicit empirical-rational premises inform the assessment of magical powers. Different forms of magic are experimented with and tested against a variety of threats. For this reason, various features of biomedicine, such as the syringe, have been integrated into African pluralistic medicine for their well-established magical powers. "The attraction of indigenous medicine and biomedicine has created a market for [PMPS] without biomedical training who not only sell herbal medicines but also make pills out of plant substances or inject extractions of their own plant formulas intravenously" (Westerlund, 1989b:195).

---

[32] In addition to the witch or sorcerer who is causing harm, the PMP also possesses a physical substance—this for the purpose of healing. Among the !Kung, for example, "Those who have learned to heal are said to 'possess' *num* . . . *Num* resides in the pit of the stomach and the base of the spine. As healers continue their energetic dancing, becoming warm and sweating profusely, the *num* in them heats up and becomes a vapor" (Katz, 1982:41).

[33] See Chavunduka (1978), Evans-Pritchard (1976), M. Gelfand (1964a), Gray (1963), MacLean (1979a), and Willis (1979).

A further aspect of supernatural explanations concerns the spirit world. The role and nature of spirit forms within African pluralistic medicine are varied and wide-ranging. In general, the spirit world is dominated by ancestral spirits who protect specific ethnic groups and guard cultural traditions. Illness or misfortune attributed to one's ancestral spirits is commonly interpreted as a sign of broken taboos or customs.[34] Among the Thonga of Mozambique and South Africa, for example, forms of magical retribution may strike someone who breaks a taboo or social norm (Green, 1999). Spirits, therefore, represent the influence of ancestors, as supernatural forces, in everyday life. When disenchanted spirits bring about suffering, a priest or prophet may be called upon to perform an exorcism or other purification rite to cleanse the community for its trespass and assuage the ancestral spirits (Turner, 1964b). Such cleansings are among the most common remedies that PMPs prescribe for illnesses attributed to supernatural forces. The Kamba of Kenya, offer a ritual washing and cleansing of the body (*ng'ondu*) in cases of female infertility (C. Good, 1987). As with many such remedies, this practice extends beyond matters of health to the general category of misfortune. Zaramo PMPs in Tanzania, for example, often recommend a "ritualistic outward cleansing" for persons who are seeking work (L. Swantz, 1990).

The spirit world is home for the remains of those who have passed on. When someone dies, his or her soul leaves its body and joins the souls of past ancestors in spirit form. This conceptual distinction between the body and the soul plays an important role in the diagnosis of illness. As in the case of soul-loss in parts of Latin America and the Caribbean, a number of disorders, especially mental illness, are associated with a person physically separating from his or her body.[35] Evans-Pritchard (1976) describes the "soul of the witch" leaving a witch's body to attack the soul of its victim, while Schmoll (1993) describes the rapacious appetite of Hausa "soul-eaters" in parts of Niger whose victim, usually a child, has had his or her soul consumed by the offender. In equally dramatic fashion, the night-long Giraffe dance among the Kalahari-based !Kung involves epic battles to restore someone's soul (R. Katz, 1982). While in a trance-like state, PMPs battle ancestral spirits who seek to steal the victim's soul. This is generally initiated by the afflicted person's erratic behavior. The Koma of Northern Nigeria have developed a delicate process of "negotiation" for the return of a person's stolen soul. "If the diviner/healer finds that an illness is the result of an abduction

[34] See Bibeau et al. (1980), Chavunduka (1978), Ezeabasili (1982), Paarup-Laursen (1989), Ulin (1979), Turner (1964b), Whisson (1964), and Zeller (1979a).

[35] See Horton (1962), Nadel (1952), Paarup-Laursen (1989), Reid (1982), Wall (1988), and Westerlund (1989b).

of the life-soul by nature-spirits, the healer sends his life-soul to negotiate with the nature-spirit" (Paarup-Laursen, 1989:62).

Social Network Explanations

When individuals experience a major or prolonged illness, African pluralistic medicine often attributes this, in part, to developments within the social world, such as interpersonal relationships. When two persons quarrel, one form of retribution may involve a conscious effort to harm the other person. Commonly, this involves eliciting assistance from supernatural forces to inflict illness.[36] For this reason, the boundaries between the social world and supernatural world are generally difficult to draw with great precision and, when diagnosing a person's illness, PMPS give significant consideration to social conflict and the state of interpersonal relationships.[37] To treat the surface-level physical symptoms of an illness without addressing its underlying origin (interpersonal squabbles) would be pointless. Mburu (1977) frames the differences between biomedical and African pluralistic-medical beliefs with respect to social conflict and etiology in philosophical terms.

> The modern medical practitioner often commits the error of complacency, congratulating himself for being so profound and far-sighted without ever knowing that his explanatory variables are primarily and inextricably biomedical, microbial and bacteriological phenomena or in general they are based on natural causality. [This interpretation] is irrelevant to the native African. He sees the ultimate causes as psycho-social agents invested in man. This ultimate causality states that whatever misfortune befalls man it must have been caused by another man or by personal omission of some ritual. This questions the fundamental basis of germ theory.[38] And the query is philosophical. The African wants to know the reason why on earth should a small 'insect,' like the fly, cause discomfort to man and his family and wealth. Why should such a minute creature want to harm a man

[36] For a sampling of the literature, see Apter (1993), Austen (1993), Beck (1985), Bibeau et al. (1980), Buckley (1985b), Chavunduka (1978), Foster (1976), M. Gelfand (1964a), Harjula (1989), Mburu (1977), Simpson (1980), Tanner (1956), Warren (1979b), and Willis (1979).

[37] In support of this link between illness and social conflict, several studies suggest that fewer illnesses are attributed to social conflict among more sparsely settled communities (Westerlund, 1989b; Guenther, 1979).

[38] Onoge (1975), in fact, suggests that given basically no experience with the scientific equipment needed to observe germs (e.g., microscopes), for Africans to accept the Western germ theory would have been a tremendous leap of faith and "an even more fantastic hypothesis than a witchcraft theory of disease causation" (p. 223).

> with whom there is nothing in common? They have no common land boundary. There is no envy on the part of the small creature. If the insect is said to have caused the illness, then it must have been sent by somebody, by a cultural being envious of the culprit's well-being" (pp. 181–82).[39]

The examples of links between social conflict and illness are plentiful across African pluralistic medicine. Marwick (1967) observes that, among the Cewa in Zambia, the link between quarreling and sorcery reveals a clear understanding of social relations, while Willis (1979) details how the diagnosis of an Ufipa patient in southwest Tanzania begins initially with a focus on the state of his or her interpersonal relations so as to discover the underlying cause of illness. "Questioning specifically directed to his client's personal relations, then enables the doctor to identify the posited intrusive agencies (e.g., as territorial or ancestral spirits, or as sorcery)" (Willis, 1979:144). Among the Yoruba in Nigeria, the diagnosis of congenital versus noncongenital deafness hinges on the analysis of possible "strained social relations" (Odebiyi and Togonu-Bickersteth, 1987:647). Likewise, illness among the Meru of Tanzania often results from "broken human relationships and the curse" (Harjula, 1989). In such cases, the attitude of others toward the person who is ill often takes the form of a curse against him or her that then precipitates illness. Gray (1963) discusses a form of class-based witchcraft among the Mgubwe in northern Tanzania whereby wealthy persons are bewitched by the members of the envious poor. Evans-Pritchard (1976) observes similar class-based distinctions between members of the royal Avongara family and commoners within Azande society in Sudan. While the members of the royal family cannot themselves be witches, they remain susceptible to the witchcraft of the commoners.[40]

By extension, community-level conflict can also put individuals (or whole groups) at risk for harmful retribution in the form of illness.[41] For example, in northern Tanzania when Mgubwe chiefs engage in witchcraft, this can have consequences for whole villages. "The acts of witchcraft attributed

---

[39] Similarly, in their analysis of causal reasoning among the Senufo in the northern Ivory Coast, Sindzingre and Zempléni (1992:315) argue that Senufo etiology turns on four questions: Which sickness is it? How has it happened? Who or what produced it? Why did it occur at this moment to this individual?

[40] In a similar fashion, M. Gelfand (1964a) reports that, among the Shona of Zimbabwe, it was believed that Europeans could not be witches. "It is interesting to note that the African does not think that a European can be a witch because he believes that the spirit of the white man operates on a quite different spiritual plane to his own" (p. 52).

[41] See Chavunduka (1978), Conco (1979), Gray (1963), Horton (1967), Katz (1982), Ngubane (1976), Turner (1964a), Ulin (1979), Westerlund (1989b), Whisson (1964), and Willis (1970).

to chiefs usually caused damage or harm to entire neighborhoods rather than individuals, and thus, they provided explanations for misfortunes or calamities which were of epidemic or group character" (Gray, 1963:148). Both Turner (1967), in the case of the Ndembu in Zambia, and Katz (1982), in the case of the !Kung in the Kalahari, describe community-wide healing practices with large numbers of participants. One of the objectives of the healing process for the !Kung during the Giraffe dance is a restoration of proper balance and harmony between the individual and the community (Katz, 1982). Likewise, when Zulu family members quarrel they must perform a ritual that involves "washing each other's hands, symbolizing the washing away of anger in their hearts" (Ngubane, 1976:331). The link between social conflict and illness suggests that a person's body can signal more general, community-wide distress. "Bodily organs are not silent in Africa, they speak about society. Health means collective harmony rather than 'silent organs'" (Hours, 1987:48).[42]

A further aspect of the integral role of social networks within African pluralistic medicine concerns the role of family and close kin throughout the therapeutic process. Biomedical practitioners generally regard the ill person as the primary focus of care and consultation. The patient is the one identifying that he or she is ill and initiating medical assistance. Within many African pluralistic-medical systems, however, the one thought to be ill is often not the one who either first recognizes that he or she is ill or who initiates medical assistance. Occasionally, the ill person is not even capable of describing why it is thought that he or she is ill—as in the case of spirit possession. As a consequence, the focus of treatment and care shifts from the individual to his or her "therapy managing group" (Janzen, 1978). The therapy managing group is a set of family and close kin members who shepherd an ill person through the process of seeking medical assistance. The group mediates between the patient and the PMP to make routine decisions with respect to which medical practitioners to consult and whose advice to ultimately follow.[43] Janzen's (1978) description of this process among the BaKongo in Zaire remains the classic treatment of this phenomenon. Earlier depictions of therapy managing groups within African pluralistic medicine include that of Michael Gelfand (1964a) among the Shona in Southern Africa and that of Price-Williams (1979) among the Tiv in Nigeria. Importantly, the therapy managing group has proven an adaptable and enduring practice even under

[42] Of course, many biomedical interpretations of hypertension among historically-oppressed communities in the U.S. appeal to a similar logic with respect to the role of unresolved social conflict that is allowed to simmer and later result in community-wide illness (Hajjar and Kotchen, 2003; Fiscella et al., 2000).

[43] See Feierman (1985), Janzen (1978), and Last (1993).

conditions of strenuous urban-industrial change. Lloyd Swantz observes, for example, that for the Zaramo in Dar es Salaam the practice of kin assistance throughout the therapeutic process continues, though in modified fashion. In seventeen of the fifty-eight divination sessions that Swantz documented, a member of the patient's nuclear family attended while he or she remained at home (1990:138).

Holistic Frameworks

African pluralistic-medical systems have adopted a broad range of holistic frameworks for interpreting the overlapping relationships between the natural, supernatural, and social worlds.[44] Thus, within African pluralistic medicine, with rare exception, an explanation of phenomena in any one of these three spheres has consequences for developments in the other two. Vecchiato (1998), for example, observes that among the Sidama in Ethiopia there is a particular link between health and maintaining balance and harmony in one's life. This balance concerns various aspects of one's life including physiology (for example, digestion), interaction with natural forces, and harmony with other people.[45] Such holistic notions contrast sharply with Western cultural practices that emphasize discrete ontological spheres and this points to a fundamental divide between those put under the microscope and those wielding the microscope. "One major projection on the part of the medical anthropologist is the very assumption that the object of study is something isolable. Even more fundamental is the assumption that the divisions we draw as scientists, in scientific situations, between the natural and the supernatural is a distinction that is shared by the subjects of anthropology" (Worsley, 1982:326).

When confronted with a person who is ill, the PMP must record the physical manifestations of illness while also placing this person in the broader context of the supernatural and social forces influencing his or her life. As noted above, illnesses attributed to witchcraft implicate a person's interpersonal relationships, while those attributed to spirits suggest aggrieved ancestral spirits. Often, the specific reason for consulting a PMP (for example, stomach pain) will not be addressed in an initial visit. The PMP must first assess the person's fuller state of affairs and perhaps speak with an angry

[44] The literature in this regard is vast. See Airhihenbuwa (1995), Bibeau (1982b), Buckley (1985a), Davis-Roberts (1992), Foster (1976), Gessler et al. (1995), Gillies (1976), Good (1980), Horton (1962), Iliffe (2002), MacLean (1987), Mburu (1977), Ngubane (1977), Paarup-Laursen (1989), Sindzingre (1985), Wall (1988), Westerlund, (1989a) and Whisson (1964).

[45] Prins (1992) describes similar concerns among the Lozi of western Zambia for maintaining a balance between oneself and the physical world.

neighbor or visit a family shrine before turning to the patient's immediate complaint. Consequently, effective treatment for an illness requires a holistic approach that simultaneously addresses the manifold causes of illness located in a person's natural, supernatural, and social worlds.[46] For example, family members are often integral participants in a person's therapy. "Yoruba patients are not treated in isolation from their families and environment. If a psychotic patient cannot be treated at home, the patient is taken to the doctor's compound and his/her relatives stay with him/her there" (Westerlund, 1989b:210). In describing the Giraffe dance in the case of the !Kung, Katz notes that, "The full range of what in the West would be called physical, psychological, emotional, social and spiritual illnesses are treated at the healing dance" (1982:54).

One of the most stark contrasts between African pluralistic medicine and biomedicine follows from the manner by which the former blends across one's everyday lived experiences. Appreciation for this distinction is complicated by the Western tendency to frame African interpretations of the supernatural world within the discrete category of religion. Lloyd Swantz describes the difficulty of discussing Zaramo "religion" as an isolated entity. "Zaramo religion is not a set of doctrines but is rather the total Zaramo way of life—their thinking, believing and living. The Zaramo religion cannot be separated from the social, material and cultural aspects of their lives. It includes the natural order, the spiritual order as well as the *mila*, the traditional order" (Swantz, 1990:141).[47] In the same manner, African pluralistic medicine itself constitutes one facet of an individual's everyday lived experiences and is not a discrete, specialized sphere or social institution. The role of the rubbing-board oracle among the Azande as both an ongoing conversation with supernatural forces and a practical guidepost for everyday activities is an apt example of this false distinction (Evans-Pritchard, 1976). Certain aspects of pluralistic-medical beliefs and practices, therefore, such as concern for ancestral spirits, involve ongoing facets of a person's life regardless of the momentary state of his or her physical health.[48] "The !Kung do not look upon

---

[46] See Bibeau (1982b), Bibeau et al., (1980), Katz (1982), MacLean (1971), Odebiyi and Togonu-Bickersteth (1987), Sindzingre (1985), and Turner (1964a).

[47] Janzen (1989) presents a similar case for South African medical-religious practices. Leslie extends this analysis beyond Africa. "Medical systems use the categories of thought and sentiment common to many occasions and interests, which is to say that they are part of the general culture in a society. For example, the concepts of humoral medicine in Hindu, Chinese and European tradition involve cosmological theories of an equilibrium of forces and elements in nature and of correspondences between the human body and the universe that are used in religious ritual, sorcery, food choices, art and literature" (Leslie, 1978:xiii). See also Kramer and Thomas (1982).

[48] See Bibeau (1982b), Chavunduka (1978), Feierman (1985), G. Jansen (1973), Katz (1982), M. Swantz (1989), Wall (1988), and Willis (1999).

their healing dances as separate from the other activities of daily life. Like hunting, gathering and socializing, dancing is another thing they do" (Katz, 1982:34). For this reason, pluralistic medicine is not narrowly relegated to occasional episodes of illness requiring treatment, as in the case of biomedicine. Rather, within a holistic framework, it is fully incorporated into how one lives his or her life as the member of a family, a community, or a multi-generational clan.[49]

Pragmatic Attitudes Toward Alternative Medical Systems

One of the reasons that it is possible to discuss, however guardedly, a set of common elements across the heterogeneous world of African pluralistic medicine is the widespread practice among PMPs to borrow openly from one another.[50] Basic beliefs and practices, therefore, have become diffused across populations such that the notion of an African pluralistic-medical system in pure form is hardly imaginable. "In the coastal areas of Tanzania the health practices are as many as the cultures which have met there. Each ethnic group has brought its own traditions and has subsequently borrowed freely from others. The Islamic concepts have mixed with pre-Islamic elements and adoptions from other cultures over the centuries" (M. Swantz, 1989:277).[51] Zaramo PMPs in Dar es Salaam frequently receive their medical training from practitioners in other ethnic groups and it is widely believed that other communities possess more powerful medicine (L. Swantz, 1990). Consequently, African pluralistic-medical beliefs and practices undergo constant change and evolution while at the same time retaining and deepening certain fundamental principles and values—such as the holistic relationship between phenomena across the natural, supernatural, and social worlds.

One result of this steady diffusion of African pluralistic-medical beliefs and practices across African societies has been a notably pragmatic attitude toward biomedicine. Feierman, for example, observes that, unlike biomedical practitioners, PMPs make explicit use of elements from competing medical systems, which can include biomedicine. "[Biomedical] authorities

---

[49] The popular media in Africa often reflect this understanding. "Condensing diffuse forms of historical consciousness in plainspoken prose, some Nigerian newspapers make it apparent that witchcraft has come to permeate everyday conversation about politics, the pursuit of power and the complex interdependence of urban rural life" (Comaroff and Comaroff, 1993:xxvi).

[50] See Feierman (1985), Janzen (1985), Katz (1982), M. Swantz (1989), and Wall (1988).

[51] In the mid-19th century, the Shambaa ruler in northern Tanzania maintained his own personal Muslim healer (Iliffe, 2002).

tend not to test alternative therapies for their efficacy. Those who actually manage the process of therapy in Africa, by contrast, move pragmatically from one type of healing to another" (Feierman, 1985:178). Others maintain that African openness to other medical beliefs and practices creates a unique opportunity for biomedicine's penetration into African culture. Westerlund observes that "the plural and flexible character of African disease explanation and therapies may help to explain the great adaptability to biomedical and other 'foreign' etiologies and types of treatment" (1989b:201). In his analysis of collaborative efforts between PMPS and biomedical practitioners in South Africa, Green (1988) observes that "surveys of [PMPS'] attitudes and limited programmatic experience have consistently shown a willingness on the part of [PMPS] to learn more about Western medicine and to cooperate and collaborate with Western-trained practitioners" (p. 1128). Thus, biomedicine is commonly viewed by Africans as complementary with (and not in opposition to) African pluralistic medicine.[52] Whereas biomedical practitioners in advanced capitalist nations have historically treated pluralistic medicine as antithetical (and a threat) to the scientific integrity of biomedicine, PMPS view biomedicine and African pluralistic medicine as simply operating with different but not necessarily contradictory rationales.[53]

Accordingly, PMPS have readily accepted the role of Western biotechnology as a tool for healing and frequently refer people to biomedical practitioners. Buxton (1973) describes the attitude of Mandari PMPS of southern Sudan toward Western medicine and their general recognition that certain therapeutic practices, such as surgery, are sometimes vital for complete medical treatment. Indeed, PMPS commonly view biotechnology as adjunctive to, and not a replacement for, pluralistic medicine.[54] It represents an additional tool to be called upon as needed in combination with pluralistic medicine. "Antibiotics are used [by the Kalahari-based !Kung] sometimes in conjunction with or instead of indigenous medicinal salves" (Katz, 1982:56). Echoing the analysis of Ranger (1981), a 1972 survey among the Kamba in central Kenya found a common belief that "there [are] 'Kikamba' illnesses which are only amenable to traditional forms of therapy and there are 'hospital' illnesses which accord-

---

[52] See Chavunduka (1978), M Gelfand (1964a), Hours (1987), Janzen (1978), MacLean (1979a), Messing (1977), and Westerlund (1989b).

[53] See Asuni (1979), Buxton (1973), Green (1988), and Mburu (1977).

[54] See Bibeau et al. (1980), Frankenberg and Leeson (1976), M. Gelfand (1964a), Gessler et al. (1995), Good (1980), Janzen (1985), Katz (1982), Mburu (1977), Osborne (1972), Paarup-Laursen (1989), Reid (1982), Spring (1985, 1980a), Staugård (1986), Warren (1979c), and Westerlund (1989a).

ingly respond exclusively to modern medicine" (Mburu, 1977:167).[55] This notion of illness as unique to a specific population reflects a prevalent tendency within African pluralistic medicine to distinguish between "African" and "European" illnesses. It thus follows that many consider Western medical traditions more appropriate for certain illnesses and African medicine for others.

Empirical-Rational Premises

It was a basic axiom of thought among the colonial authorities that the chief distinction between African pluralistic medicine and biomedicine was the latter's scientific content. Whereas biomedical beliefs and practices were grounded in the empirical-rational sciences based on experimentation and objective reason, African pluralistic medicine was perceived to be little more than a dubious collection of primitive traditions based on superstition and myth. In point of fact, systematic observation and experimentation, objective reasoning, and hypothetical prediction are cardinal features of African pluralistic-medical systems.[56] In describing African pluralistic medicine, Westerlund (1989b) observes, "In an open search for effective methods, there is abundant empiricism and experimentation" (p. 194). Examples of this abound. Beattie (1967) found that the Ugandan Nyoro often seek a second opinion from another PMP to confirm an original diagnosis, while Gessler et al. (1995) note that Tanzanian pluralistic medicine "contains both a psychosocial component and a rational physiological component" (p. 157).

Arguably, the two areas of African pluralistic medicine that provide the most glaring evidence for the application of empirical-rational methods are the use of botanical medicines based on trial and error and the development of disease classification schemes based on extensive observation. Indeed, many African pluralistic-medical systems extend the use of empirical-rational scientific principles to the investigation of supernatural phenomena, such as witchcraft. Lastly, the extensive use of systematic, professional training and apprenticeship programs that are required of potential PMPs, as well as informal rating systems that discriminate between highly qualified and less

[55] At the same time, as discussed by Oyebola (1986) in the Nigerian context, the adaptation of biomedical techniques by African PMPs cannot be seen as a purely apolitical matter. See also Pearce's (1980) analysis of Nigerian healthcare in this regard.

[56] For a range of examples, see Beattie (1967), Bierlich (1995), Buckley (1985a), Frankenberg and Leeson (1976), Gessler et al. (1995), Gluckman (1968), Horton (1967), Kargbo (1987), Mburu (1977), Morley (1979), Mume (1977), Olsson (1989), Onyioha (1977), Orley (1980), and Westerlund (1989b).

qualified PMPs, suggest a coherent and organized body of knowledge with consistent rules of application and practice.[57]

The use of botanicals for specific illnesses has evolved through a long process of trial and error. Over time, the observed efficacy of certain botanicals for particular illnesses under controlled conditions has resulted in vast collections of effective herbal treatments for many common ailments, such as nausea, headache, or fatigue. Among the illnesses that Mume (1977) observed being treated in Nigeria, for example, were asthma, colitis, constipation, epilepsy, migraine headaches, sterility, gonorrhea, and liver disorders. Buckley documents the extensive empirical-rational research that Yoruba herbalists rely on to test and develop herbal treatments. "My experience of Yoruba herbalists is that they constantly subject their medicinal knowledge to empirical criticism . . . [H]erbalists are constantly aware that not all medicines are equally effective" (1985a:161). Mburu quotes a Kamba herbalist who describes the ordeal of testing medicines. "I have to test everything, individual herb by herb, then I mix one by one in varying quantities, tasting it every time . . . When I have to mix five or so herbs to produce a solution I need, it is neither interesting nor easy to go through the process" (quoted in Mburu, 1977:170). In 1968, the First Inter-African Symposium on Traditional Pharmacopoeias and African Medicinal Plants was held in Dakar. As one participant from the Congo commented, "Traditional medicine is the result of a long heritage of empiricism based upon the close observation of sickness and transmitted orally from one generation to the next" (quoted in Wall, 1988:322).

In combination with experimentation with botanicals and different illnesses, a number of African pluralistic-medical systems have developed complex classification schemes that categorize illnesses by symptom, cause, and treatment.[58] Warren (1982) identifies a thirteen-level taxonomy of 1,266 named diseases among the Techniman-Bono of central Ghana. Such classification schemes indicate a clear familiarity with, and a strong acceptance of, the basic principles that guide scientific thought in the West, moving from recorded observation to the recognition of patterns to the development of general laws. The Meru of Tanzania, for example, are able to treat a great many distinct illnesses with over one hundred types of botanicals. "Within his total repertoire, [the Meru PMP] identifies over 50 different diseases and other ailments for which he prepares remedies from about 120 different plants" (Harjula, 1989:134). The Hausa in Nigeria apply these same principles to psychological disorders which are systematically distinguished from

[57] See Last (1996), Feierman (1985), Chavunduka (1986), Willis (1979), and Twumasi (1985).

[58] See Conco (1979), Harjula (1989), Horton (1967), Maina-Ahlberg (1979), Paarup-Laursen (1989), Mume (1977), Price-Williams (1979), Ulin (1979), and Warren (1979a, 1979c).

different emotional states (Wall, 1988). *Hauka*, for example, implies that someone is disoriented and has experienced a loss of self-control. *Wauta* suggests that someone has poor common sense and is exhibiting a "disregard of Hausa social standards" (Wall, 1988:207).[59]

At the same time, the empirical-rational techniques of African pluralistic medicine are not limited to the natural world of botanicals. As discussed above, the attribution of illness to supernatural phenomena, such as witchcraft, does not preclude empirical confirmation of a diagnosis. Evans-Pritchard's (1976) detailed descriptions of Azande autopsies and the search for witchcraft substance is a case in point. In other instances, supernatural forces are thought to operate by means of physical objects inside a person's body. For example, the San of the Kalahari Desert attribute illness to substances secreted into the body, sometimes by witches or spirits (Baer et al., 2003). Thus, within African pluralistic-medical systems it is completely consistent both to frame medical concerns within a holistic framework in which natural, supernatural, and social worlds overlap and interact and simultaneously to adhere strictly to the basic principles of the Western scientific method when investigating illness, whether examining phenomena in the natural, supernatural, or social worlds.

Finally, as in the case of biomedicine, the systematic content of African pluralistic medicine often requires a practitioner to submit himself or herself to a considerable period of professional training and apprenticeship.[60] Whatever its level of proven efficacy, it is evident that to practice African pluralistic medicine, a prospective PMP must undergo a process of specialized training and study that introduces him or her to an established body of knowledge and techniques. "African witch finders usually acquire their magical powers through lengthy training and the purchase of magical spells and incantations from their tutors" (Foster, 1983:20). This widespread reliance on training and apprenticeship to prepare PMPs underscores the significant empirical-rational content of African pluralistic medicine. In a similar fashion, the lay public's distinctions between PMPs follow from explicit empirical-rational premises. Not all PMPs are considered equal in skill and ability. Community members often identify certain PMPs as superior with respect to their degree of expertise and their level of experience.[61] An individual PMP's stellar reputation is earned through consistent and prolonged demonstrable success.

---

[59] Michael Gelfand (1964b) describes similar practices among the Shona.

[60] See Chavunduka (1986, 1978), Conco (1979), Frankenberg and Leeson (1976), Gessler et al. (1995), Janzen (1992), Katz (1982), MacLean (1979b), Mburu (1977), Mume (1977), Reid (1982), Staugård (1986), Ulin (1979), Spring (1985), Wall (1988), Warren (1979b), and Willis (1979).

[61] See Beattie (1967), Bibeau (1982a), Conco (1979), Flint (2001), M. Gelfand (1964a), Jansen (1973), Katz (1982), MacLean (1987), Mburu (1977), and Spring (1980a).

Based on her work among the Luvale in northwest Zambia, Spring suggests, "Specialists who have cured people successfully are most in demand" (1980a:62). Individuals must experience, and the general public must see evidence of, a PMP's efficacy. One manifestation of this has been the emergence of professional associations of PMPs that attest to their members' abilities, such as that among Yoruba PMPs in Ibadan (Maclean, 1979a). Among Shona PMPs in Zimbabwe, "Medical certificates and badges are now in common use. These certificates are generally hung on the wall of the healer's place of healing" (Chavunduka, 1978:83). Other professional associations of PMPs have established "ranked titles" (Osborne, 1972:83). Thus, popular differentiation among PMPs with respect to skill and ability provides further evidence of the empirical-rational premises that pervade African pluralistic medicine (Oyebola, 1981).

Health-Related Services Considered As Both a Commodity and an Obligation

A seeming contradiction tends to emerge within most representations of African pluralistic medicine with respect to the nature of the relationship between the PMP and his or her community. On the one hand, PMPs appear to provide their services as a form of communal obligation. As detailed below, PMPs develop the ability to help others, in part, through personal sacrifice and training and, in part, through supernatural intervention (for example, the aid of ancestral spirits). The reason that supernatural forces provide PMPs with the power to aid others is to protect the broader community and a PMP is, therefore, duty bound to assist individuals from his or her community whenever possible.[62] Chavunduka relates that in Zimbabwe much of the motive for faithfully protecting others follows from a basic recognition that those who have provided one with certain healing powers could just as easily retract them. "Many [PMPs], particularly those possessed by a spirit, did not abuse their power mainly because of fear of their ancestors. It was strongly believed that ancestors could withdraw the healing spirit bestowed upon the individual if offended" (Chavunduka, 1987:68).

At the same time, for those community members who seek his or her assistance, the PMP is apt to charge a rather significant fee.[63] Among the Shona in Zimbabwe, for example, work as a PMP can be a "financially rewarding oc-

[62] See Chavunduka (1987), M. Gelfand (1964a), Gessler et al. (1995), Mburu (1977), Onyioha (1977), M.-L. Swantz (1989), and Zeller (1979a).

[63] There are many such accounts. See, for example, du Toit (1985), M. Gelfand (1964a), Guenther (1979), Hours (1987), Last (1996), Mume (1977), Onyioha (1977), Sindzingre (1985), Spring (1980b), Ulin (1979), Yoder (1982), Westerlund (1989b), Whyte (1988) and Zeller (1979b).

cupation" (Chavunduka, 1978:21). Generally speaking, there is significant variation among PMPs with respect to fees. Male Nyoro PMPs in Bunyoro, Uganda, collect fees while female PMPs do not (Beattie, 1967). In some cases, PMPs only charge full fees when a person's recovery is successful (Frankenberg and Leeson, 1976; Wolff, 1979). Osborne details the often exorbitant costs incurred by members of the Egba-Egbado Yoruba communities in southwestern Nigeria when seeking the aid of specialized PMPs.

> [Community healing] projects require the expenditure of large portions of the small resources of the households of the community. The people must purchase the talents of diviners and cult chiefs who will prescribe the proper sacrifices, rituals and feasts necessary to propitiate the ancestors and eliminate the witches. These activities require the cooperation of people who have been antagonistic towards each other. They are also costly. If the witchcraft continues, even more expensive rituals and sacrifices are required. (Osborne, 1972:84–85)

Consequently, African pluralistic-medical services can take the form of both a communal obligation and a profitable commodity. Over time, successful PMPs can rise to become some of the wealthiest members of the community. Oftentimes, PMPs abandon their communities altogether and travel to distant towns or cities to market their services to those who can better afford them. Charles Good (1987) describes the Kenyan migration of Kamba PMPs from their desolate Kitui villages to Nairobi where they are able to establish more lucrative practices. A further manifestation of these competing values is the common practice of charging indigent clients less than wealthy clients—a conscious policy of commodifying one's services.[64] The sliding-scale fee structure allows a PMP to realize as large a profit as possible while still fulfilling his or her moral obligations to the community. Such cases are numerous. Nyoro PMPs in Uganda set fees based, in part, on "the resources of the client" (Beattie, 1967:212). The fees of Gala PMPs in Ethiopia "ranged from as little as eight cents charged to poor people, to $1.25 charged to the 'local rich' for the same services" (Messing, 1977:57). Zambian PMPs, likewise, establish fees "depending on the socio-economic background of the patient" (Twumasi and Warren, 1986:130). Such examples reflect a hybrid

---

[64] The logic of commodified value can extend to the efficacy of a specific treatment or medicine. A popular expression among the Luvale of Northwest Zambia captures the importance of both the botanical item itself and its formal purchase. "'Tree or herb that I paid for, not just looked at' is a Luvale proverb meaning that without payment, transfer of the knowledge is valueless" (Spring, 1980a:76). Whyte (1988) further details the commodification of botanical products within African pluralistic medicine.

understanding of one's healing powers both as a communal obligation and as a commodified source of income and wealth.

Four African Pluralistic-Medical Ethnographies

The constellation of elements within African pluralistic medicine discussed above, while common enough, is far from universal in form and content across the continent. This follows both from the highly heterogeneous nature of African societies and from the ongoing internal and external pressures and forces that are constantly transforming and remaking these societies. To capture this dynamic and complex social reality in greater detail, four ethnographic studies of African pluralistic-medical systems, representing diverse societies, settings, and periods of change, have been selected for further consideration. Each study examines a particular ethnic group's pluralistic-medical beliefs and practices within the broader context of an integrated sociocultural reality that is subject to sustained, large-scale social change in the wake of colonial and post-colonial transformations. At the same time, these ethnographic community profiles have been selected to emphasize differences based on era, setting, ethnic group, and colonial heritage. The four studies include fieldwork from as early as the 1920s and as late as the 1970s, both urban and rural communities, and four distinct ethnic/language groups in four different national territories. In addition, the authors themselves represent a range of perspectives from a variety of academic fields—two anthropologists, a sociologist, and a medical geographer.

First published in 1937, E. E. Evans-Pritchard's widely acclaimed *Witchcraft, Oracles, and Magic Among the Azande* remains a pioneering work in the study of supernatural beliefs and practices within African societies. An anthropologist who conducted fieldwork among the Azande in southern Sudan in the 1920s at the behest of the British colonial authorities, Evans-Pritchard adhered to a conventional functionalist analysis. Few Western ethnographies of Africa written since its publication fail to cite this classic work.

The Quest for Therapy in Lower Zaire, by anthropologist John Janzen, is a seminal work in the field of African pluralistic-medical traditions. Published in 1978, this study is based on field research in collaboration with William Arkinstall (a practicing surgeon) that began among the BaKongo people in rural Lower Zaire in the mid-1960s and concluded in 1969—nine years following independence. Janzen's insights are organized around his central thesis that the study of pluralistic-medical beliefs and practices must account for the manner by which individuals, families, and clans seek medical care.

The Medicine Man Among the Zaramo of Dar es Salaam provides a rare study of African pluralistic-medical beliefs and practices in an urban environment. Published in 1990, sociologist Lloyd Swantz's study is based on fieldwork conducted in the early 1970s, a short decade following Tanzanian independence. Swantz's analysis offers some comparisons of rural and urban Zaramo society and the evolving role of PMPS in the context of an increasingly mobile population whose members are losing contact with home villages and extended kinship networks. The study concludes that for the Zaramo, mired in a period of rapid social change, PMPS in Dar es Salaam provide bridges between urban Zaramo and their rural traditions (language, rituals, taboos, and so forth), facilitating their adjustment to the new urban environment.

Ethnomedical Systems in Africa was published in 1987 and is based on fieldwork conducted from 1977 to 1979 in Mathare Valley, a massive urban shantytown in Nairobi, and in the Kilungu Hills, a region in southeast Ukambani that is the rural homeland of the Kamba people.[65] The purpose of this study by Charles Good, a medical geographer, is to examine the evolving nature of Kamba pluralistic medicine in both urban and rural settings through a series of case studies. While formally organizing his work around the distinction between urban and rural communities, Good concludes that, in fact, the notion of urban and rural spaces as separate and distinct spheres is mistaken.

The Azande in Southern Sudan

The larger Azande homeland covered a massive region that spread across separate territories controlled by three colonial powers (British, Belgian, and French) in parts of what today are Sudan, Central African Republic, and Democratic Republic of the Congo. Evans-Pritchard arrived in Sudan after accepting an assignment from the British colonial authorities to develop an ethnographic profile of the Sudanese Azande. The community he entered was, predictably, in the midst of significant social upheaval and transformation. This was attributable both to the ordinary vicissitudes of life under colonial domination and to a recent, large-scale resettlement campaign that had begun in the early 1920s to combat sleeping sickness. As a consequence, much of Evans-Pritchard's fieldwork was conducted among newly settled concentrations of Azande whose former pattern of scattered homesteads had been upset. By the time of Evans-Pritchard's study direct rule was increasing

[65] In 1979, the 1.7 million Kamba people were the fourth largest ethnic group in Kenya, after the Kikuyu (3.2 million), Luhya (2.1 million), and Luo (2 million).

after a popular king had been replaced by a district commissioner. Caught up in the throes of sudden and dramatic social disruption, the traditions and practices of neighboring, non-Azande Africans were playing an increasing role in Azande society. This was especially evident with the proliferation of secret associations led by magicians and PMPs from surrounding African communities. Indeed, Evans-Pritchard documents the significant influence of other Africans on Azande society across many sociocultural realms.[66] The Azande of the 1920s thus exemplify African society as an amalgam of cultural beliefs and practices borrowed and adapted from others in an ongoing and active exchange of ideas and experiences.

Evans-Pritchard's work is not a treatise on pluralistic medicine, per se. Rather, it is an examination of the basic precepts of the Azande cultural world which, in turn, make Azande pluralistic medicine possible. Issues of health and illness are framed within the broader category of misfortune, which is itself linked to witchcraft beliefs. Evans-Pritchard seeks to describe the roles of witchcraft and magic as organizing principles of Azande society—serving as a rudimentary cosmology as well as a stabilizing influence. For Evans-Pritchard, beliefs and practices associated with witchcraft provide a window into Azande explanations of an individual's experiences and fate. While supernatural explanations did not necessarily preclude or even take precedence over natural explanations, the role of witchcraft as a factor in personal misfortune emerged from this and later ethnographies as a central theme in descriptions of African societies. Evans-Pritchard thus begins his analysis with an extended discussion of witchcraft, by way of preparing his reader for a more nuanced understanding of Azande society.

Witchcraft resides within specific individuals and to be a witch implies that a person literally carries witchcraft, as a physical substance, in his or her body.[67] This substance is described as "an oval, blackish swelling or bag in which various small objects are sometimes found" (Evans-Pritchard, 1976:1). Witchcraft is considered an inherited trait, though, in practice, it is not necessarily the case that simply because a parent is a witch that his or her child will also be a witch. Additionally, some persons who possess the witchcraft

[66] This reinforces the difficulty of treating individual African societies as discrete case studies, in isolation from other African peoples and cultures. See Janzen (1992) in this regard. "In the era of structural-functionalism and colonial domination, the local 'tribe' was the unit of study. Rarely were comparisons, or concerns for historical directions, articulated. However, useful work was accumulating which would make the task of historical comparison possible later on" (p. 2).

[67] Note that to avoid awkward and strained circumlocutions, for the purpose of describing Evans-Pritchard's study, events and conditions related to the Azande are discussed in the present tense, notwithstanding that most of them occurred over 75 years ago and little or nothing from Evans-Pritchard's description may today apply to Azande society. The same holds for discussions of BaKongo, Zaramo, and Kamba societies.

substance in their body may not actually use it or even be aware that they possess it. In such cases, the witchcraft substance is said to be cool. This contrasts with sorcerers who are conscious agents that learn magic solely for the purpose of harming others. Thus, the role of witchcraft as a guardian of the moral order is a major point of emphasis for Evans-Pritchard. From the Azande perspective, this clearly complicates efforts to locate witchcraft narrowly within the supernatural realm, given its active role within the social realm and its effect on actual events in the natural world. It is only by adopting a holistic framework that one can make sense of this.

When someone is confronted and accused of using witchcraft against another person, the situation contains a high degree of ambiguity. On the one hand, witchcraft is thought to result from a conscious act of volition. On the other hand, all commoners are considered potential witches. Therefore, it is possible that upon first being accused of harming another with witchcraft, a person is actually made aware for the first time that he or she is a witch—a circumstance almost anyone could potentially face. For example, it may be that someone harbors enmity toward another without consciously beckoning the powers of witchcraft. The person has probably held ill feelings for others at other times throughout his or her life with no ominous result. However, the witchcraft substance grows as one ages and it may be that the witchcraft substance has only recently matured to the point of bringing harm. As a consequence, the Azande find it completely plausible for a witch to be clueless about his or her own powers (Evans-Pritchard, 1976:58).[68] Thus, to be a witch, in and of itself does not indicate that someone is dangerous or evil.[69] It is only the condition of being a witch in combination with a concrete set of social relations that leads to the nefarious use of witchcraft. The supernatural world merely potentializes witchcraft—as a material substance. The social world unleashes it, while the natural world confirms witchcraft activity via the results of autopsies.

Importantly, the mechanism by which witchcraft harms someone places the locus of control among humans and not in the spirit world. The use of witchcraft involves the "soul of the witch" physically leaving the witch's body and crossing a short distance to attack the victim's internal organs.[70] Human beings control the spirit world, the spirit world does not control human

---

[68] When someone stands accused of witchcraft the response of the accused follows a familiar ritualized pattern. He or she blows out water and states, "If I possess witchcraft in my belly I am unaware of it; may it cool. It is thus that I blow out water" (Evans-Pritchard, 1976:59).

[69] This is consistent with Austen's (1993) analysis of the moral economy of witchcraft.

[70] The concept of "souls" among the Azande remains somewhat vague. People are described as possessing two souls—a body-soul and a spirit-soul. At times, the spirit-soul can separate from the body-soul, and this is the mechanism by which witchcraft is able to afflict its victims. See

beings.[71] Thus, given that physical distance provides a degree of safety, the colonial authority's re-settlement plan with populations concentrated in villages to combat sleeping sickness took on particular significance. Yet not all misfortune is considered the result of witchcraft. There are a plurality of causes behind misfortune other than witchcraft, including basic incompetence or ignorance, broken taboos, and transgressed moral codes. It follows that the Azande rely on a variety of logical categories, including natural explanations, when interpreting misfortune. If witchcraft is involved in misfortune this does not negate the role of natural causes, as illustrated by the oft-cited collapsing granary example. Two forces are at work when a granary collapses on someone. On the one hand, natural forces are behind termites weakening the granary and the sun's heat persuading people to seek shelter. On the other hand, the forces of witchcraft are what brings these two natural events together in a manner that leads to misfortune. Azande beliefs do not deny basic empirical-rational notions of cause and effect. Rather, witchcraft is said to work as a "second spear." When hunting, the first spear causes the animal to fall. The second spear kills the animal. Both spears are necessary for a successful hunt. When witchcraft is involved in misfortune it is said to act as the second spear.[72] Hence, there is no contradiction when misfortune is simultaneously attributed to both natural and supernatural causes.

When a person suspects witchcraft the first step is to identify the witch. This requires the intervention of diviners. After a set of suspects has been identified, the poison oracle[73] ceremony is organized to discover who among them is responsible for an act of witchcraft. After the poison oracle is presented with specific names, a fowl is forced to swallow a small portion of poison. The verdict is delivered when the bird either lives or dies.[74] It is necessary, therefore, prior to the poison oracle, to have a method for identifying potential suspects. When a person falls ill, he or she does not simply draw up a list of local witches who may have afflicted him or her. Rather, the ill person

---

Evans-Pritchard (1976:151) for a description of the difficulty in translating the Azande notion of *mbisimo* or "soul."

[71] This is a point emphasized by Mary Douglas who has noted that, based on Evans-Pritchard's depiction, witchcraft does not require any mysterious spiritual beings, only the powers of humans (cited in Gillies, 1976b:xxi).

[72] Kramer and Thomas (1982) describe the need for Kamba PMPS southeast of Nairobi to address illness at "the level of eradicating the causal agent and the level of neutralizing the power of the ultimate cause" (p. 172). See also Mburu (1977) for further discussion of the second spear concept.

[73] The other Azande oracles, not detailed here, include the termite oracle, the rubbing-board oracle, and *mapingo.*

[74] Winter (1963) describes a similar practice among the Amba in western Uganda.

asks, among everyone in the area, with whom has he or she quarreled. These are the names presented to the poison oracle. "Oracle consultations express histories of personal relationships, for, as a rule, a man only places before an oracle names of those who might have injured him on account of some definite events which he believes to have occasioned their enmity" (Evans-Pritchard, 1976:46). The social world and the state of interpersonal relationships, therefore, remains at the core of Azande witchcraft beliefs and divination.

Cleansing one's body and soul is a prerequisite for those diviners who will oversee the poison oracle.[75] An unclean person would contaminate or pollute the proceedings and disrupt the proper workings of the supernatural divining forces. This suggests a degree of ambiguity within Azande society with respect to the notion of pollution as a natural versus a supernatural phenomenon. Park suggests that for the Azande (as well as the Yoruba) such attention to purity and variable degrees of accuracy and reliability among divining instruments speaks to an underlying commitment to objectivity and empirical-rational measures of truth. "If we would correctly understand Yoruba precautions against contamination of the 'objectivity' of their oracles, or Zande down-grading of devices which they believe may sometimes be rigged, we should think of such precautions as protective of the essential credibility possessed by their more solemn procedures of divination" (Park, 1967:243–244). Thus, notwithstanding the precision of their measures, Azande pluralistic-medical beliefs and practices suggest an affinity for the basic principles of experimental science.

It is the role of the PMP that allows the Azande to avoid lives filled with a perpetual fear of witchcraft. As a diviner, the PMP relies on the oracles to identify witches. As a magician, the PMP uses magic to counteract the witch's power. The sources of magic are a range of medicinal plants, trees, and roots that are taught to apprentices after they are accepted into secret associations of PMPs. Notably, it is consumption of the proper medicine that is the source of a PMP's power and not the benevolence of a Supreme Being or one's ancestral spirits. As in the case of witchcraft substance, it is a natural explanation in combination with supernatural forces that accounts for a PMP's powers. Both good and bad magic play critical roles in Azande society. Good magic is used to counteract the forces of witchcraft and sorcery. Bad magic is a harmful weapon of the sorcerer. Given the high social value placed on magic, PMPs

[75] The conditions for administering of the poison oracle reflect a basic patriarchal ethic. With rare exception, women are excluded from participating in the ritual—though certainly they can be among the accused. Given the central role of the poison oracle as a guardian of justice and the moral order, men are thus able to leverage women's exclusion to strengthen their position of control. Evans-Pritchard details the extent to which this was a source of power for men, who were thereby able to maintain women in servile social roles (Evans-Pritchard, 1976:131).

are often able to profit handsomely from its mastery, while a deep public skepticism simultaneously tends to feed the common image of the PMP as a cunning trickster.[76]

Because magic is rare and expensive, when a novice PMP is in training, substantial gifts are required of the protégé throughout the training. Indeed, the potency of the magic is thought to depend upon both the generosity of the student and the goodwill of the PMP. Paying a fee performs two functions. First, the formal exchange itself is considered an essential aspect of ritual magic. Second, the effectiveness of the magical powers that are transferred is thought to depend upon the seller's satisfaction with the transaction (Evans-Pritchard, 1976:94). This reflects both the importance of maintaining positive interpersonal relations within the social world and the manner by which a PMP's services conflate the notions of commodity and obligation. In the course of a training recorded by Evans-Pritchard, it became evident that the student was aware of certain deceptions taking place. The attitude of the student was that if a degree of trickery is necessary to enhance a PMP's mystique, this does not negate the essential role of the PMP in assisting those attacked by witchcraft. At the same time, Evans-Pritchard observes that a significant level of empirically based skepticism pervades across the Azande community (Evans-Pritchard, 1976:107).[77]

These doubts further promote a pragmatic Azande attitude toward medical beliefs and practices. Adding to this general state of uncertainty has been the introduction of medicines from neighboring African communities, beginning in the 1890s. As more and more "foreign" medicines were adopted, it was not always clear which were associated with good magic versus bad magic.[78]

Lastly, the use of magic and medicine, along with a sophisticated nosology, illustrate significant fidelity to basic principles of Western science, including a link between illness and natural causes. The Azande have utilized

---

[76] Iliffe (2002) cites a popular proverb among the Shambaa of northern Tanzania to this end. "Deception, deception, that's medicine" (p. 11).

[77] Zeller (1979a) details the role of deception as a routine feature of PMP treatment among the Baganda in Uganda. "[A] common clinical treatment was cupping. The [PMP] made an incision over the part of the patient's body where the pain was localized. He then placed the end of a cattle horn, which had a small hole cut near the end to help create a vacuum over the incision. After a sufficient amount of blood had been sucked from the wound, the [PMP] removed the horn and showed the patient the blood that had been withdrawn. Inevitably there was some foreign substance, such as the head of a lizard, a snail, a snake, or a frog in the blood which the [PMP] indicated as the source of pain. The effect was easily achieved because the [PMP] had put this substance in his mouth before starting the procedure" (p. 140).

[78] Evans-Pritchard observes nonetheless that the Azande express much confidence in the effectiveness of medicines introduced by other African communities, often assuming that others possess magic superior to their own (1976:203).

systematic, empirical observations to identify a range of natural causes of illness and develop sophisticated systems for classifying illnesses by symptom clusters, while also tracing the normal course of most illnesses. The therapeutic efficacy of various plants and roots, meanwhile, has been established via a protracted process of trial and error. For this reason, an enormous pharmacopoeia has been developed. However, when a simple illness grows more serious this suggests that both natural forces (the first spear) and witchcraft (the second spear) are at work. Accordingly, ordinary illnesses are routinely treated with an assortment of plants or roots whose effectiveness has been proven through past use. More serious illnesses are treated with a combination of botanicals and magic. It is, therefore, clear that Azande witchcraft beliefs (within the supernatural world) do not undermine simultaneous exploration of empirical-rational explanations (within the natural world) when diagnosing and treating illnesses. "Almost every disease is not only diagnosed, its probable course foretold, and its relation to a cause defined, but also each disease has its own individual treatment, which in some cases has evidently been built up on experience and in other cases, though it is probably quite ineffectual, shows a logico-experimental element" (Evans-Pritchard, 1976:196).[79] Herein lies the basis for a prevalent pragmatic attitude toward non-Azande medical systems, such as biomedicine.

Thus, in the more serious cases, a person's recovery is ultimately based on his or her natural treatment in combination with the PMP's magic. In this way, magic serves as a complement to treatment based on natural explanations of an illness. For the Azande, good magic works as a preventive measure against nefarious mystical forces (witchcraft or bad magic) sent by others. Its primary purpose is not to produce a favorable change in the world (such as to cure a person who is ill). This is the role of the person's natural treatment. Its primary purpose is to prevent mystical forces from interfering with a person's normal course of recovery. This explains the receptive, pragmatic attitude among the Azande toward the introduction of biomedicine—in combination with the PMP's contributions.[80]

---

[79] As Janzen observes in a commentary on Evans-Pritchard, "To attribute misfortune to witchcraft does not exclude the 'real' cause. The two—witchcraft and natural causes—are not mutually exclusive" (1981:188).

[80] There is one notable exception with respect to Azande openness to non-Azande medicine. It developed, however, not because of challenges to beliefs within the natural and supernatural worlds. In this case, the difficulties arose within the Azande social world—in particular, challenges to patriarchal norms. Between 1900 and 1920, following European conquest, a large number of secret, closed associations emerged among the Azande to practice magic. These were initiated by neighboring African communities. Because they were not integrated into Azande cultural norms and values, they were considered subversive and dangerous. For example, in a significant break from Azande custom, both men and women were invited to join these associations in equal numbers. Colonial

The BaKongo in Lower Zaire

John Janzen conducted his fieldwork in Manianga, a region of Lower Zaire that lies halfway between Kinshasa and the port city of Matadi. Historically, the BaKongo in this area have been primarily involved in village-based, small-scale agriculture and hunting. The disruption to BaKongo village structure and social organization throughout the period of colonial rule was massive in this regard. From the early days of Belgian colonial rule, there were efforts by medical officials and others to concentrate populations in small towns and hamlets. As a result, a variety of settlement patterns developed in Manianga. By the late 1960s, less than half the population of Manianga lived in the typical precolonial village settlement. Most had moved to the growing towns that surrounded mission stations, colonial administrative posts, commercial centers, and mines. Consequently, Janzen argues that by the 1960s, "traditional" life in Manianga had largely disappeared (1978:18). Importantly, however, and somewhat in contrast to the situation described below by Swantz (1990) among the urban Zaramo, kinship ties remained strong for BaKongo, most of whom kept contact with their home village. This explains the continuing cultural influence of clan traditions, as reflected in the role of the therapy managing group.

Janzen's analysis of BaKongo pluralistic-medical beliefs and practices is premised on a basic division between illnesses attributed to natural causes and those attributed to human causes. The rationale for this distinction follows from etiological frames of reference that presume a holistic and integrated understanding of the natural, supernatural, and social worlds. Afflictions associated with natural causes are referred to as "illnesses of God" insofar as God is the creator of the basic order within the natural world. This does not imply that God plays a direct role in causing any particular person's illness. "Illnesses of God" are generally mild conditions that respond well to treatment with medicinal plants and herbs. The identification and classification of certain illnesses as mild or more severe, as well as the development of different types of medicinal botanical treatments, requires ongoing observation, experimentation, and retesting. In this manner, the category of "illnesses of God" within BaKongo pluralistic medicine suggests acceptance of the basic empirical-rational principles of Western science.

Afflictions associated with human causes are referred to as "illnesses of Man." These illnesses are attributed to disruptions of the social world, such

---

authorities soon outlawed the movement, but the associations and their lodges continued to flourish. In this fashion, one can see how the introduction of certain medical beliefs and practices may contain the seeds for broader social disruption and dislocation. Fortunately for colonial officials, biomedicine has proven itself remarkably compatible with entrenched patriarchal practices.

as communal conflict or emotional distress—especially anger and anxiety. Generally speaking, illness is first viewed as an "illness of God" (due to natural causes) unless proven otherwise. When an illness is diagnosed as an "illness of Man" and the social conflict or emotional distress is easily identified and addressed, the treatment remains a function of resolving interpersonal relationships within the social world. When social conflict manifests itself as illness, a purification of community-wide relations is required. As a consequence, purification rituals often signal simmering conflict among factions within the community (Janzen, 1978:189). One unique manifestation of "illness of Man" among the BaKongo is the possibility of illness striking an entire clan, as in one of Janzen's case studies. In that case, "(T)he structural dimension of illness and therapy engulfed the entire clan, the local church organization within that clan, a non-kin prophet community and connections with local government" (Janzen, 1978:114). Resolution required treatment and purification of the entire community, combining natural and supernatural explanations of pollution.

When social conflict or emotional distress is complicated by the role of supernatural forces, such as witchcraft or magic, then both the supernatural world and social world are implicated in a person's illness. In such cases, both the underlying illness (its physical manifestations) and the offending supernatural forces must be addressed. Appropriate treatment requires that a clear distinction be drawn between symptoms and causes (Janzen, 1978:88). Of the possible supernatural forces, witchcraft is the most common suspect. As in the case of the Azande, witchcraft represents either a willful or an unconscious desire to harm someone through supernatural forces. Therefore, there is a fundamental distinction between an "illness of Man" that is attributed to social conflict and one that is attributed to witchcraft. All uses of witchcraft result from underlying social conflict, but not all social conflict results in the use of witchcraft. When a person is confronted with the accusation of witchcraft, his or her response is similar to that of the Azande and an accusation is met by a mix of denial and contrition (Janzen, 1978:95).

Similar to the Azande (and Zaramo), the BaKongo describe witchcraft as a physical substance residing in a person. The witchcraft substance is believed to exist within every clan. When the chief is the holder of this substance, order is maintained. Trouble can develop, however, when someone in the clan other than the chief is the holder of the witchcraft substance. One of the primary functions of the chief, in combination with diviners and magicians, is to combat witchcraft and protect the collective interest. Part of the chief's role in this regard is to counter the influences of envy and anger among clan members. This overlap of witchcraft and the social world is readily acknowledged by the BaKongo. "Since the sufferer himself or his enemies or kinsmen may be to blame, or the illness may be due to a situation for which a group takes collective responsibility, the mystical cause of witchcraft is often subordinated in diagnosis to an intense analysis of social relations" (Janzen, 1978:50). For this reason, when the colonial powers first curtailed the role of chiefs, it was feared that the dangers of witchcraft would increase.[81] Thus, as in the case of the Azande, BaKongo pluralistic-medical beliefs and practices reveal a fundamental holistic framework that combines natural, supernatural, and social worlds as well as ongoing political intrigues.

Given this intermingling of etiological explanations across the natural, supernatural, and social worlds, the BaKongo enlist a range of therapeutic interventions associated with different types of healers. The four therapeutic options identified by Janzen include PMPs, kinship medicine, purification and ritual, and biomedicine. While some therapies are more commonly associated with certain types of illnesses, the pattern of BaKongo therapeutic practices reveals a fundamental pragmatism that guides the decision making of the therapy managing group. Over the course of an individual's illness, for example, there may be frequent movement between biomedical care in a hospital or clinic and the care of PMPs, as the various therapeutic options fulfill complementary roles (Janzen, 1978:1). This reflects a holistic approach that attempts to address an individual's needs on many levels. It is, therefore, an analytical fallacy to draw up lists of illnesses with natural, supernatural, or social causes. Invariably, there are multiple and overlapping causes that explain any given illness. All four therapeutic options require fees (money or gifts) and entail additional costs such as transportation and medicine. Janzen concludes, however, that expenses are not a significant factor in selecting among the therapeutic options. In fact, the cost of BaKongo pluralistic medicine and of biomedicine are comparable when all of the costs are considered (Janzen, 1978:155). The commodified form of care is thus generalized across all four therapeutic options.

Within the broad scope of BaKongo pluralistic-medical beliefs and practices, PMPs play a central role, combining empirical-rational methods (for example, experimentation and basic physiology) with magic and an analysis of social relations. Some PMPs specialize as herbalists with no claims to combat supernatural forces while others combine the use of medicinal plants with magic to neutralize witchcraft. Given the location of the PMPs' homes and practices within the local community, as well as their intimate knowledge of community members and interpersonal relationships, a PMP is often

[81] Indeed, colonial bans on the use of the poison oracle across Africa were often seen as evidence of collusion between witches and the colonial authorities. See Marwick (1967), Middleton and Winter (1963), and Winter (1963) in this regard. "Many viewed the prohibition of both ordeals and the killing of witches as indications that the state apparatuses had aligned themselves on the side of evil, protecting evil-doers against retaliation by their innocent victims" (Westerlund, 1989b:204).

the first person consulted for an illness. The work of the PMP thus blends easily with a community's daily routine. Notwithstanding their range of specializations, a common principle uniting all PMPs is the notion of the patient as a complex social being whose therapeutic needs may just as easily require a referral to a PMP specialist as to a biomedical practitioner (Janzen, 1978:203). Kinship medicine, a second therapeutic option, refers to the role of relatives in developing a diagnosis and selecting among therapy options. Via the therapy managing group, matrilineal kinship members are situated at the fulcrum of care-seeking. This can be a chaotic and uncertain process, as the group attempts to understand the situation. "A lack of definition and agreement as to what is wrong, or what should be done, along with dissatisfaction over the solutions attempted, propel the quest for therapy from episode to episode" (Janzen, 1978:64).[82] Along with PMP or biomedical care, the therapy managing group facilitates the ill person's successful recovery and further illustrates the basic link between disruptions to the social world and illness.

Echoing kinship medicine, the primary purpose of purification and ritual, the third therapeutic option within BaKongo pluralistic medicine, is to renew and revitalize the patient as a social being and community member at the conclusion of his or her illness. Purification rites mark the end of illness and closure for the person. Without undergoing such purification, the patient remains polluted and unclean after his or her initial recovery. In some circumstances, a person's entire clan requires purification. During this process, because social conflicts will have already been resolved, there is little or no emphasis on social relationships. Rather, a prophet or priest oversees a set of ritual techniques that include purification baths, anointments, isolation, laying on hands, prayers, and songs. The sufferer is given a new social role and sometimes a new residence. Purification rituals combine the notions of pollution and contagion that derive from the natural world with the notion of spiritual cleansing derived from the supernatural world. This notion of purification as a form of closure for an ill person is, of course, all but absent in biomedicine. Consequently, Janzen observes that often after someone is treated at a biomedical clinic for his or her basic symptoms, it is still necessary to solicit a PMP's assistance for purification to address the true source of his or her illness (Janzen, 1978:215).

No area of BaKongo pluralistic medicine better reveals both a fundamental belief in the empirical-rational principles of Western science and a deep-seated respect and pragmatic attitude toward Western medicine than the routine use of biomedicine, the fourth therapeutic option. Beginning with the Swedish Covenant Mission in 1891, the introduction of biomedicine

[82] Citing McGuire (1988) and Eisenberg et al. (1998), Kleinman observes that there is, likewise, a wealth of therapeutic options in contemporary U.S. suburbia (1995:24).

has made a real and tangible impact on people's lives.[83] As a consequence, there is broad social acceptance of biomedicine among the BaKongo in general and among PMPS, who routinely refer their patients to biomedical facilities (Janzen, 1978:227).[84]

BaKongo PMPS often draw comparisons between biomedicine and the work of herbalists.[85] Indeed, for all their ridicule of African pluralistic medicine, here is a point of significant agreement between Westerners and Africans: the value of medicinal botanicals. "Medicinal plants were the only element of indigenous healing that was not denigrated by colonialists or missionaries" (Janzen, 1978:62). Thus, the BaKongo comparison of its own herbalist practices with those of biomedicine found validation among biomedical practitioners themselves. "Medicines are an area where Western and African conceptions of healing seem to meet. Just as Western drugs are easily incorporated within the African conception of therapeutic powers, African herbalism can be made acceptable to the biomedical model" (Whyte, 1988:230). From the perspective of biomedical practitioners, this follows from a reductionist ideology that is able to isolate certain biochemical agents initially identified by the systematic investigations of BaKongo PMPS. From the perspective of BaKongo pluralistic medicine, this follows from an underlying empirical-rationalist sensibility in combination with a holistic and pragmatic attitude that welcomes proven "foreign" medical traditions.

The Zaramo in Dar es Salaam

The population for Lloyd Swantz's study were the Zaramo living in the greater Dar es Salaam metropolitan area in the early 1970s. While most of the population had migrated from neighboring regions, a significant portion of the Zaramo in Dar es Salaam live in the remains of former villages that were swallowed up by the expanding city limits.[86] The urban Zaramo profiled in Swantz's study are, therefore, subject to a great many forces of sociocultural change in

---

[83] Between 1933 and 1961, for instance, despite ongoing outmigration to larger cities, advances in medical care allowed the population of Manianga to grow from 70,000 to 90,000 (Janzen, 1978:26).

[84] By contrast, biomedical practitioners have demonstrated little tolerance for BaKongo PMPS. This, however, contrasts with the attitude of Western-trained, African biomedical doctors who are known to permit PMPS inside the hospital (Janzen, 1978:227).

[85] Iliffe (2002) argues that familiarity with the work of herbalists provided many young African students of biomedicine with a basic orientation with respect to biomedical norms (p. 10).

[86] The larger Zaramo community beyond Dar es Salaam occupies parts of central and eastern Tanzania. Nearly 98% of all Zaramo are Muslim and the overlapping influences of Islamic traditions, Pazi folk religion, and the practices of neighboring ethnic groups are evident across Zaramo pluralistic-medical beliefs and practices.

the context of an ongoing pattern of urbanization that entails disruption due to both migration and forced incorporation. As the largest single ethnic group in Dar es Salaam, the Zaramo represent an influential community whose size provides a reliable source of mutual assistance and cultural orientation. The various adaptations of Zaramo pluralistic medicine throughout an uncertain and disruptive period of urban resettlement frames the analysis of Swantz.

Urban life has had a profound impact on Zaramo pluralistic-medical beliefs and practices, marginalizing certain practices (such as spirit possession) and hastening the further commodification of PMP activities. Zaramo bring an assortment of troubles to the PMPs, including physical ailments (an illness or infection), interpersonal matters (marital problems or difficulties with coworkers), and personal misfortune (unemployment or a failed business). The PMPs attribute such problems to a combination of natural, supernatural, and social causes, which are reflected in their holistic approach to patient care. "For many [Zaramo] the [PMP's] view of illness, encompassing the organic, psychic, spiritual, and social aspects of life as a whole, is thought to be closer to the truth than that of a medical practitioner who sees only organic disorder as the cause of illness" (L. Swantz, 1990:148). Underlying Zamora pluralistic-medical beliefs and practices is a strong faith in the role of witches, sorcerers, and spirits as active agents in the everyday lives of people and this strong faith highlights the central role of the intermingled supernatural and social worlds within medical diagnoses.

The distinction between witches and sorcerers mirrors that described by Evans-Pritchard among the Azande insofar as a witch is someone who possesses witchcraft as an inherent, corporeal property (L. Swantz, 1990:32). The sorcerer carries greater culpability because he or she is thought to set out consciously to learn the craft of magic and spells with evil intent.[87] In addition, witches act on their own accord, while sorcerers are usually employed by others. Thus, as in the case of witchcraft, sorcery requires an understanding of the larger social world and those with whom the patient may be in conflict.[88] Whereas tight kinship networks dominate life in the village, new networks of urban social relationships have created patterns of social conflict and competition between neighbors and coworkers (Swantz, 1990:136). Under these shifting conditions, the role of the PMP in providing magical medicine does not diminish. However, it requires a deft sociological eye on the

---

[87] For this reason, reminiscent of Evans-Pritchard, L. Swantz expresses severe doubts with respect to the existence of many persons who actually consider themselves sorcerers (1990:145).

[88] In the instances of sorcery catalogued by Swantz, the possible causes included jealousy, hatred, false suspicion, quarreling, revenge, adultery, and "inadvertent witchcraft." In the latter case, it is believed that when a witch sets out to harm someone, his or her witchcraft may occasionally reach an unintended victim by accident—an innocent bypasser.

part of the PMP to recognize the sources of conflict in the emerging urban social networks, as the influence of kinship networks ebbs. The harmful mischief of spirits is generally attributed to neglecting one's ritual obligations or to spirit possession. Ritual obligations require Zaramo to pay their respects regularly at the family spirit shrine.[89] Dereliction of these responsibilities can result in personal misfortune. In Dar es Salaam, however, spirit possession—which requires a formal exorcism in one's home village—is much less common than witchcraft, sorcery, or misfortune due to the neglect of ritual obligations. Swantz argues that given the cost and inconvenience for PMPs in Dar es Salaam to perform village-based exorcisms, the diagnosis of spirit possession is now relatively rare. This contrasts with rural Zaramo communities, where spirit possession remains common.[90]

Swantz highlights a further consequence of this shift to urban-based witchcraft and sorcery—one that reflects a more ominous change across the Zaramo social world. Parallel to the penetration of large-scale commercial markets has been a transition from community-wide rituals to individual-level rituals. Community-wide ritual healing practices are ubiquitous across rural Zaramo society and Swantz argues that their collective impact reaffirms and strengthens social cohesion within the community. "Through ritual action the social relationships are restored" (1990:138). By contrast, there is almost no community-wide ritual healing among the Zaramo in Dar es Salaam. Instead, befitting the ideology of a market society where buyer and seller are abstracted from their broader social context, the accused and accuser are treated as autonomous individuals severed from the festering urban milieu and "[the PMP] treats the individual patient psychologically in relation to other people but leaves the social group untouched" (Swantz, 1990:139). Thus, PMPs facilitate Zaramo adjustment to urban life, in part by manipulating familiar cultural elements that in another setting (and era) were community-affirming. In the new setting, however, these same practices feed a nascent individualism that is leading to a radical transformation of the social world that Swantz believes, over time, will also transform (and perhaps eliminate) the role of PMPs. This sense of Zaramo pluralistic medicine as a system in flux points both to its evolving and dynamic nature and to the open and pragmatic attitude that Zaramo adopt towards their own and other medical systems.

---

[89] In this regard, Swantz distinguishes between Zaramo ritual offerings to ancestors and ancestor worship. Typically, Zaramo clan members gather at ancestral graves or spirit huts for their annual ritual offering, or *tambiko*. Swantz argues that this is not a form of ancestor worship but merely a form of respect for prior generations through ritual offerings (1990:46).

[90] This decline in the diagnosis of spirit possession and the performance of exorcisms in contemporary African societies has also been discussed by Yoder (1982) and Westerlund (1989b).

The actual behavior of Zaramo when ill reveals this overriding pragmatic reliance on both PMPs and biomedicine and, as in the case of the BaKongo, it is quite common for Zaramo to move back and forth between the hospital and their PMP for treatment. Though government hospitals and clinics are free, PMPs are generally easier to reach and their consulting rooms are far less crowded. The primary form of medical treatment offered by PMPs—an assortment of botanical sources that represent a broad indigenous pharmacopoeia for a number of ills—points to the role of natural treatments and empirical-rational techniques for assessing cures.[91] Many of the botanical items are associated with specific spirits to facilitate healing. To heal a patient, PMPs combine the proper plants and herbs with their own ability to thwart the witchcraft, sorcery, or spirits afflicting him or her. As in the case of the Azande and BaKongo, the Zaramo contend that medication alone is often insufficient to induce recovery. It is the power of the medicines in combination with the talents of the PMP that can overcome the supernatural forces that bring illness (L. Swantz, 1990:30). The plants and herbs (the first spear), therefore, treat causes within the natural world, and the magic and spells (the second spear) treat causes located in the supernatural and social worlds. This emphasis on the natural world as a core factor in illness explains the open attitude of PMPs (and of the Zaramo more generally) toward alternative medical beliefs and practices, such as biomedicine, that treat patients based on more narrow explanations of illness. Swantz observes that the PMPs are fully prepared to send a patient to a biomedical clinic if their treatment proves ineffective (1990:29). In fact, this practice is at times reciprocated.

> It is apparent that some medical personnel in Dar es Salaam hospitals at times recommend treatment by traditional medicine men. If a problem cannot be diagnosed by the medical staff in the hospital and if patients insist that they have been bewitched or are possessed by a spirit, there may be no alternative but to discharge them. In such circumstances it is unlikely that a patient will respond to modern cures. (L. Swantz, 1990:114)

In this context, the role of PMPs in an urban setting has undergone considerable evolution. However, the primary activities of PMPs continue to center around divination,[92] treatment, and protection. These three elements operate

---

[91] The treatments prescribed in over half of the case records examined by Swantz were for physical symptoms and less than half for nonphysical symptoms (1990:36).

[92] With respect to divination techniques, Swantz distinguishes between the "traditional" PMP, the *shehe,* and the *mwalimu.* Islamic traditions rely on the *kitabu* book method in which sacred Muslim texts are consulted. Traditional Zaramo practices include throwing objects onto a *boa*

within a single logic and Zaramo PMPs consider it nonsensical to consider one in isolation from the others (L. Swantz, 1990:43). A basic treatment plan follows from this holistic framework. First, the offending witch, sorcerer, or spirit is identified through divination, which, in part, involves an inventory of interpersonal relationships. Second, the patient is treated for his or her resulting physical ailment. Third, the PMP provides the patient with protective magic to guard against further harm from supernatural forces. Protection from witchcraft, sorcery, or spirits is fundamentally a matter of addressing conflicts within the social world. The PMPs view the relationship between the accused and the accuser as essential to interpreting the underlying cause. The activity of itinerant PMPs in Dar es Salaam is a case in point. These roving PMPs travel from town to town and offer their services of witch-finding and witch-eradication. For those who suspect that they have been harmed by a witch, the PMP offers antiwitchcraft medicine to swallow. This protects him or her from future harm. Others stand accused by community members of being a witch and hope to clear their name. The PMP offers this person another form of antiwitchcraft medicine. If the person lives, clearly he or she is not a witch. If he or she dies, this confirms suspicions. Paralleling Evans-Pritchard's functionalist analysis, Swantz argues that these services allow community conflicts and quarrels within the social world to dissipate and reach resolution.

One significant difference between Zaramo and Azande beliefs concerns the use of protective magic, and this has implications for future-oriented temporal notions associated with a holistic framework and, tied to this, Zaramo acceptance of prophylactic forms of biomedicine. Unlike Azande PMPs, Zaramo PMPs claim that through their magic they can achieve specific future outcomes. This is especially popular among sports teams and students who purchase protective magic for upcoming matches or exams. Swantz cites several examples of students, sports teams, and legal defendants soliciting the aid of PMPs to secure a promising outcome (1990:146). This suggests the ability not merely to neutralize witchcraft or sorcery that may be impeding someone, but also the ability to influence positively the course of real world events. Swantz draws an analogy between this reliance on protective magic as a prophylactic agent and the Western use of vaccinations within biomedicine.[93] "This thinking is as logical to the Zaramo as that which leads to vaccination against the dangers of smallpox and polio" (Swantz, 1990:111).

---

board and Rungu spirit possession. Rungu involves a form of divination with ball rattles. There are also significant variations within each of these.

[93] This, of course, is hardly restricted to the Zaramo. The Nyoro of western Uganda were practicing forms of inoculation for smallpox prior to the arrival of biomedicine (Herbert, 1975; Iliffe, 2002). See Ajose (1957) for further prophylactic practices among the Yoruba regarding smallpox and Maier (1979) for a discussion of 19th-century public hygiene practices among the Ashanti.

Hence, biomedical beliefs and practices regarding the use of treatments in the present to thwart future threats fits well with the Zaramo holistic worldview and overlapping present and future temporalities.

The lack of a standardized process for becoming a PMP creates certain difficulties unique to urban areas.[94] In rural settings, given the high degree of familiarity among community members, monitoring who has followed the prescribed prerequisites to become a PMP is more easily policed. In urban settings, lacking formal processes (such as official certification) and with very weak informal mechanisms of enforcement, practically anyone can claim to be a PMP. The reputation of a PMP, therefore, is what distinguishes a qualified and respected practitioner from others. A PMP's fee is a reflection of this. The common attitude is that the higher a person's fee, the more powerful must be his or her medicine. At the same time, Swantz observes that urban Zaramo are increasingly treating pluralistic medicine as an impersonal, commodified, professional service. Whereas in rural areas Zaramo are able to identify a specific PMP from whom they regularly receive care, 70% of Zaramo in Dar es Salaam reported that they sought assistance from various PMPs, as the need arose (Swantz, 1990:25). The strong, personal relationship at the heart of the rural patient-PMP relationship seems to have been replaced by a more utilitarian and business-like attitude in the city. For Swantz, the commodification of PMPs' services suggests the absorption of Zaramo pluralistic medicine into routinized, commercial trade relations. At the same time, the community's discrimination between effective and ineffective PMPs based on expertise and experience suggests a semblance of empirical-rational criteria for evaluating Zaramo pluralistic medicine—beyond the vagaries of ill-defined, supernatural outcomes.

Finally, Zaramo PMPs were given a significant boost in the early 1970s when Tanzanian public law explicitly recognized and sanctioned the practice of pluralistic medicine. At the time, there was a significant shortage of biomedical physicians, and it was feared that to restrict PMPs could overwhelm government hospitals and clinics, which would be inundated by a wave of displaced patients (L. Swantz, 1990:89).[95] As a consequence, many PMPs enjoy thriving practices. Swantz estimates that the urban ratio of four PMPs for every hundred persons is comparable to that in rural areas. Often, PMPs are among the wealthiest persons in Dar es Salaam. This is due to a large clientele as well as to the fact that most PMPs maintain a low profile, hidden from tax

[94] There are several routes for young males to become PMPs. Some inherit the practice from a parent after a period of apprenticeship. Some pursue systematic Islamic training and still others become PMPs after it is said that they have inherited (or been possessed by) the *mzimu* spirit.

[95] There were 200 MDs in Dar es Salaam in the early 1970s (Swantz, 1990:14). Of these, only 25% were Tanzanians and none were Zaramo.

collectors. Care is provided by PMPs in consulting rooms inside their homes in local neighborhoods. Their homes provide no markings to indicate their practice and persons find them only by informal networks of family and friends.[96] Part of the attraction of seeking assistance from PMPs is the simple, familiar setting that contrasts with the hospital or clinic. "Apart from electric lights in some offices, no trend toward modernization can be observed in the [PMP's] office. The positive side of this is that the clients feel immediately at home with the [PMP]. There is none of the strangeness that they encounter with going to the hospital or clinic" (Swantz, 1990:23). Due to the PMPs' integration with neighborhood events and the close familiarity that this fosters, their activities are easily seen as an extension of one's everyday lived experiences.[97] The line drawn by biomedicine between episodic medical care and the continuity of one's everyday life is largely absent. Thus, on the one hand, the holistic notion of medical care as an integrated element across the many facets of one's life remains a vibrant ethic. On the other hand, the Zaramo are freely able to consult biomedical practitioners as needed without compromising their guiding holistic worldview.

The Kamba in Nairobi and in Machakos District

Charles Good's profile of Kamba pluralistic-medical beliefs and practices is based on fieldwork from the late 1970s in the rural Kilungu Hills and the squatter settlement of Mathare Valley in greater Nairobi. The traditional Kamba homeland is Ukambani, a large area east of Nairobi that is comprised of two government jurisdictions, Machakos District and Kitui District. Kilungu Hills, with an estimated population of sixty-one thousand, is located in southern Machakos. The area is characterized by dispersed homesteads and scattered villages, with a Kamba population that is primarily engaged in small-holding agricultural production—though a persistent pattern of male labor out-migration has resulted in a predominantly female workforce. Initially settled in 1939, Mathare Valley is a large, sprawling, unauthorized settlement that represents the most densely populated area of squatter residences in Nairobi.[98] It is comprised of a chain of nine villages four kilometers long, with

[96] This contrasts with many PMPs in other parts of Africa, such as those in Kinshasa in the late 1970s. "Although [PMPs] have always existed in the rural and urban areas, they have been relatively inconspicuous, especially in the urban areas. However, recently, they have made their presence felt, particularly in the cities, by advertising their services" (Bibeau et al., 1980:22).

[97] See Anyinam (1987) for a general discussion of PMP integration into Africans' daily lives and Willis (1979) in this regard with respect to the Vfipa of southwest Tanzania.

[98] It was estimated in 1979 that there were over 110,000 unauthorized housing units in Nairobi, accounting for 40% of the city's population (C. Good, 1987:197).

two-thirds of the destitute population living in the three oldest villages. These three villages are the focus of Good's study.[99] Kikuyu represent two-thirds of those living in Mathare Valley. However, the majority of PMPS in the settlement are Kamba who have migrated from Machakos and Kitui.[100] Machakos developed in the 19th century as a strategic trading post and commercial center, bringing many Arab and other African traders to the region and exposing the Kamba to a number of medical traditions. "Because of their trade and colonization activities numerous Kamba came into contact with Islamic and other African traditional medical practices. Selected elements of these foreign systems . . . were adapted and incorporated by the Kamba" (Good, 1987:75). Consequently, the influences shaping Kamba pluralistic-medical beliefs and practices are varied and have evolved in pragmatic fashion to incorporate a broad range of traditions and perspectives—including biomedicine.

As in the cases of the Azande, BaKongo, and Zaramo, a holistic orientation that integrates natural, supernatural, and social worlds represents a fundamental principle of Kamba pluralistic medicine. "(T)he Kamba traditional medical system [is] part of a unified whole, interconnected with virtually every other aspect of social life and with ideas and practices that reflected a system of cosmological and earthly order" (C. Good, 1987:90–91). The integrated and overlapping nature of the natural, supernatural, and social spheres is manifest in the two primary categories of illness, which mirror those of the BaKongo. "Illnesses of God" are attributed to natural causes. *Ngai*, the creator and preserver of all things, is depicted as a distant, impersonal God who does not directly intervene to affect events in the world. Insofar as God is the creator of everything in the natural world, however, *Ngai* is thought "responsible" for any illnesses traced to natural causes. Good observes that it is common in Mathare Valley for PMPS to treat purely natural illnesses, with no discernible links to supernatural forces (1987:221). "Illnesses of Man," by contrast, are attributed to forces that link the supernatural world (for example, witchcraft, sorcery) and the social world (for example, anger, jealousy). Akin to Evans-Pritchard, Good characterizes witchcraft as a basic organizing principle of Kamba life (1987:94). Kamba pluralistic medicine is, therefore, designed in large part to diagnose and treat illnesses caused by malevolent behavior between individuals or groups within the community. "Illnesses of Man" reflect both the status of interpersonal relationships among individuals and groups within a Kamba community and the relation-

[99] The poverty and despair of Mathare Valley is especially concentrated among women and Kikuyu. While 25% of the Nairobi population is female, over 60% of those living in Mathare Valley are female.

[100] In fact, Dawson (1987b:86–87) observes that the Kikuyu who migrated to Nairobi would often complain that they had been bewitched by neighboring Kamba migrants.

ship between members of the Kamba community and their ancestral spirits (Good, 1987:93).

Good's discussion of witchcraft and sorcery departs little from that of Evans-Pritchard, Janzen, and Swantz. At the same time, Good's profile of the Kamba places a greater emphasis on the role of *aimu* (ancestral spirits) than the other three. When Kamba die, they pass on as spirits to a land that is a precise replica of their Ukambani homeland. In spirit form, the *aimu* are directly able to impact life in the world of the living. Illness and misfortune are sometimes manifestations of this when individuals or communities break taboos or fail to adhere to recognized cultural and moral norms. "Kamba believe that *aimu* play a major, inseparable role in their physical and mental health" (Good, 1987:129).

As Good details, for all their reliance on explanations based on supernatural forces, the scientific and empirical-rational content of Kamba pluralistic medicine is significant. For example, Kamba PMPs have identified symptoms, causes, and treatments for over eighty-five diseases and syndromes based on close clinical observation and systematic, trial-and-error experimentation (Good, 1987:131). In Mathare Valley, in addition to divination, PMPs rely upon a range of empirical diagnostic techniques that include case histories, clinical measures (for example, pulse rates and temperature readings) and the examination of bodily substances, such as urine and blood. Kamba pluralistic medicine, therefore, recognizes a range of empirical-rational, scientific criteria which serve as one of the bases for medical judgments.

It follows that when Kamba in either the Kilungu Hills or Mathare Valley fall ill, there are a number of therapeutic options. These alternatives reveal the holistic framework and empirical-rational principles that guide decision making and diagnoses as well as the deeply pragmatic Kamba attitude toward biomedicine. Similar to the situation among the BaKongo, Good observes, close kin and friends regularly accompany patients when seeking care, and the choice of therapy follows from the group's assessment of an illness's underlying cause (Good, 1987:246). The first recourse is generally self-treatment through home remedies and, increasingly, Western pharmaceuticals.[101] While home remedies are routinely the first option, it is important to note that Kamba health seeking does not unfold in a linear or stagist fashion. Rather, options are freely combined and mixed in a fashion that mirrors BaKongo practices. "It is appropriate to think of the collective therapaeutic options as forming an open, inclusive 'ethnomedical system' since any one person may use some or all of these resources during the course of a particular illness—and possibly in a different order for a later illness" (Good, 1987:109).

---

[101] See van der Geest, (1988) for an analysis of a similar turn to Western pharmaceuticals in Cameroon.

Should the illness persist, the next step is frequently an herbalist, though visiting a PMP or biomedical practitioner at this point is equally likely. Two-thirds of PMPs' patients interviewed in Mathare Valley had first sought biomedical care (C. Good, 1987:241). As in the case of the BaKongo and Zaramo, when Kamba turn to biomedicine this does not suggest that they have rejected African pluralistic medicine. Rather, it is generally in combination with Kamba pluralistic medicine. While the herbalist may possess a vast knowledge of local botanical remedies from Ukambani, he or she generally does not combine this knowledge with any magical powers to combat the supernatural forces. Herbalists, in fact, maintain that they are mere vehicles for *Ngai* to provide healing through botanicals (Good, 1987:140). Returning to Ukambani to retrieve plants and herbs for their remedies is a regular sojourn for Kamba herbalists living in Mathare Valley. In this fashion, the herbalists weave an overlapping urban-rural cultural sphere, while reinforcing the essential role of the natural world as a domain within Kamba pluralistic medicine.

Readily available Western pharmaceuticals in Nairobi are often considered superior to local herbal remedies. Therefore, most PMPs engage in a combination of herbalism, divination, and supernatural treatments to combat witchcraft and sorcery. Again, however, in a fashion similar to the Zaramo in Dar es Salaam, the practical difficulties of returning to home villages for the required purification and exorcism rites have resulted in a decrease in the number of spirit-based diagnoses and a rise in the number of suspected bewitchments. The influence of biomedical practices, likewise, appears to be greater among PMPs in Mathare Valley than among those in Kilungu Hills. Biomedical resources are sparse in Kilungu Hills, which is served by two small health subcenters, two dispensaries, and a Catholic mission hospital. Coincidentally, PMPs in the Mathare Valley care for a significant number of cases in which natural causes alone are diagnosed, with no mention of witchcraft or sorcery. Good argues that the greater prevalence of natural causes diagnosed in urban areas than in Kilungu is, in part, due to urban PMPs making greater use of biomedicine than their rural counterparts (1987:221).

Assuming neither home remedies nor the herbalist's treatment are successful, a PMP will be the next likely stop. The PMPs span a range of specializations. The most common are divining, herbalism, and the use of magical powers to combat witchcraft and sorcery. Some PMPs specialize in one or two of these, while others practice all three. Once the supernatural source of a person's illness is identified via divination, the PMP must call upon his or her ability to combat witchcraft and sorcery. The ability to counteract these forces is attributed to a PMP's *Ngai*-inspired supernatural powers. Because of this, individuals do not generally become PMPs by inheritance or apprenticeship. Rather, Kamba PMPs—the majority of whom Good estimates are women—are thought to be called by the ancestral spirits to become PMPs and must experience signs of supernatural powers.[102] This links each generation of PMPs with previous (deceased) generations of Kamba and strengthens the social location of PMPs as a link to Kamba cultural traditions. One consequence of this link is that PMPs view ritual protection of the community as one of their central responsibilities and, thus, the sense of pluralistic medicine as a social obligation is strong. "Kamba believe that [the PMP's] special insights and healing powers derive from a God-given ability to communicate with the ancestral spirits. They are expected to work for the welfare and harmony of the entire community" (Good, 1987:79).

Beyond these general characteristics, the broad profiles of PMPs in Kilungu Hills differ somewhat from the profiles of those in Mathare Valley. The vast majority of PMPs in Kilungu Hills are small-holding agricultural producers who receive only a marginal income from their pluralistic-medical activities. Good identifies sixty-five PMPs in the region, two-thirds of whom are women, averaging 60 years of age and 28 years of experience. While many practice in relative isolation from other PMPs,[103] for most of the Kilungu Hills population, Kamba pluralistic medicine is easily accessible. Because people within one's social circle are often implicated in matters of witchcraft or sorcery, there is a preference for assistance from PMPs who are somewhat removed from one's network of kin and friends (Good, 1987:150). For this reason, consulting with a PMP can, at times, mirror a simple business transaction, as described by Swantz among the urban Zaramo. However, the PMP's legitimacy within Kamba pluralistic medicine is inseparable from his or her social role that also entails informal communal responsibilities—even if these may not be evident in each case that is treated. As in the case of the Zaramo in Dar es Salaam, the credibility of PMPs removed from a familiar village community can be difficult to assess. It is common practice in Mathare Valley, therefore, for PMPs to join a professional association of PMPs to confer a degree of legitimacy (Good, 1987:213).

---

[102] At the same time, C. Good observes a common pattern of intergenerational PMPs within certain family lines, suggesting a strong familial influence on who becomes a PMP. About half the PMPs in Kilungu could name at least one family member who was also a practitioner (1987:146).

[103] "Despite their close physical proximity to each other . . . specific cures for [specific illnesses] illustrate quite remarkably how [PMPs] function in professional isolation from one another. Indeed, it appears that the concept of standardization of therapy is unknown, and may be consciously avoided by trading on novelty to build and maintain one's reputation" (C. Good, 1987:168). In addition, when interviewed, two PMPs in Kilungu explained that while they openly refer people to biomedical practitioners, they generally never refer them to other PMPs. By contrast, 42% of PMPs interviewed in Mathare Valley indicated that they refer patients either to biomedical care or to another PMP (Good, 1987:306).

Biomedical care at no charge is readily available to those living in Mathare Valley.[104] By contrast, Kamba pluralistic medicine can be quite expensive. In Mathare Valley, PMPs' fees are determined by the severity and type of illness (and the amount of time needed to treat it) and what a PMP believes the person is able to pay. Under these conditions, pluralistic medicine takes the form of a commodified service and PMPs thrive in Mathare Valley. Indeed, most PMPs cite economic opportunity as a prime reason for relocating to the area from Ukambani.[105] Given the significant migration to Nairobi that this poverty fosters, the value of Kamba pluralistic medicine is, in part, its basic cultural role in easing the transition to urban life, as in the case of the Zaramo in Dar es Salaam. "[S]easoned migrants and newcomers alike will often sense [biomedical clinics] as cold, impersonal places that are not organized to deal with the personal and social adjustment problems that often accompany and precipitate their somatic illnesses. [PMPs] are valued because they can meet such needs" (C. Good, 1987:193).

For the Kamba, as for the Azande, BaKongo, and Zaramo, the holistic nature of African pluralistic medicine in combination with its integral roles across social institutions and practices suggests that its replacement as a medical system with biomedicine would be at best an inadequate substitute and at worst a disruptive and destructive social influence. Good thus attributes the continued survival of African pluralistic medicine in Mathare Valley and Kilungu Hills to its perpetuation of Kamba cultural norms and expectations with respect to physical illness and the social order (1987:298).

The arrival of biomedicine in Africa, therefore, set in motion a host of dramatic events, advancing the agendas of the colonial powers, shaping the long-term sociocultural development of a peripheralized region of the capitalist world-system, and setting the stage for an epic battle between Western and non-Western worldviews. The noble champions of modernization suggested that Western science—beyond the grasp of the primitive Africans and a mortal threat to their primordial superstitions—acted as a necessary solvent for dissolving backward African civilizations and thus offered hope and progress. This familiar storyline is simple, neat, and demonstrably false. Of course, given the context of colonial and neocolonial subjugation in which

[104] Most biomedical facilities across Kenya are located in towns and urban areas. Thus, in a country that is 85% agrarian, it is estimated that no more than 15–20% of the entire population have basic access to biomedical care (C. Good, 1987:48).

[105] The home villages for 90% of Kamba PMPs in Mathare Valley are in the impoverished Kitui region, an area that routinely experiences severe drought and famine. At the same time, the region's legendary PMPs and powerful botanical medicines are widely revered (Good, 1987:201). Thus, though the majority of Kenyans in Mathare Valley are Kikuyu, the majority of PMPs are Kamba and Luo.

major social institutions and basic forms of material culture were systematically reshaped in the image of the colonizer, such fairy tales are not surprising. Moreover, when biomedicine arrived there were certainly significant, arguably intractable, differences between its worldview (as reflected in Western science) and the worldviews associated with African pluralistic medicine. Thus, many of the conflicts between Africans and Europeans clearly reflected genuine fissures with respect to these worldviews. However, a truly impartial appraisal of these events would reveal not African but European intransigence in the face of unfamiliar medical beliefs and practices.

A deep-seated pragmatic and holistic perspective informed African attitudes toward Western belief systems. As a consequence, Africans considered very few precepts of Western science to be fundamentally irreconcilable with African worldviews. The one exception to this was the narrow epistemological base of Western science that restricted valid knowledge to observable phenomena within the natural world—thus eclipsing the supernatural and social worlds.[106] Not only were the beliefs and practices of African pluralistic medicine largely compatible with those of biomedicine, it is argued here that, among the common elements of African pluralistic medicine sketched above, one finds various antecedents hastening the adoption of a great many biomedical elements. For example, etiological explanations rooted in the natural world, a respectful, pragmatic attitude toward others' medical systems, and a tradition of rigorous professional training were all basic features of African pluralistic medicine across the continent prior to European disembarkation. Ultimately, it was not a matter of biomedicine replacing African pluralistic medicine. It was a matter of African pluralistic medicine *absorbing* biomedicine. The result, in part a function of Africa's simultaneous incorporation into the capitalist world-system, has been the transformation of biomedicine as a singular historical-cultural formation. The product of this transformation, as explored in Chapter 5, is African biomedicine, the latest incarnation of global biomedicine.

[106] In fact, Kleinman (1995) argues that, in certain ways, Western biomedicine seems the most orthodox and rigid of the natural sciences. "The medical value orientation is, ironically, not nearly as open to competing paradigms or intellectual play of idea as is 'hard' natural science, whose ways of approaching problems in cosmology and theoretical physics seem more flexible and tolerant than the anxious strictness of the 'youngest science'" (p. 30).

5
African Biomedicine

The late 20th-century advent of African biomedicine signals a uniquely African contribution to biomedicine as a singular historical-cultural formation and constituent element of the capitalist world-system.[1] Remarkable in geohistorical scope and sociocultural complexity, African biomedicine reveals the acrid residue of colonial/postcolonial Western aggressions alongside the striking African resolve to challenge and remake centuries-old Western medical beliefs and practices. Indeed, the history of biomedicine in Africa chronicles, at one and the same time, the transformation of African beliefs and practices in the wake of a formidable historical-cultural formation *and* the transformation of a formidable historical-cultural formation in the wake of African beliefs and practices. In other words, to understand contemporary African biomedicine is to grasp how it was first created by and then recreated global biomedicine. These developments follow from three analytical premises that serve as the necessary predicates for an interpretation of African biomedicine as a historical-cultural formation that

[1] It will be noted that, for the purpose of contrasting Western biomedicine with biomedicine as practiced in Africa, African biomedicine has been treated throughout this study in an undifferentiated fashion. However, as in the case of African pluralistic medicine, African biomedicine is no monolith. Across the continent there is a wide variety of local manifestations of African biomedicine to be further explored and detailed.

links day-to-day events at the village level with circuits of global accumulation over the *longue durée*.

The first analytical premise, as explored in Chapter 2, holds that biomedicine itself represents a dynamic ontological whole that is subject to ongoing development and reconstitution. As an ontological whole, biomedicine is comprised of multiple ontological spheres whose dialectical interrelationships drive its development. Thus, biomedicine as a scientific enterprise is influenced and transformed by changes in biomedicine as a symbolic-cultural expression or biomedicine as an expression of social power, and vice versa. Efforts to reduce biomedicine to a narrow set of scientific principles or discrete material forms are fundamentally flawed. Rather, biomedicine is constituted by the combinations of its scientific content, its sociocultural values, beliefs, and practices, and its imbricated social power relations. As biomedicine reaches new lands and peoples, its basic beliefs and practices are culturally contextualized and its organizing principles are reshaped and realigned. Thus, biomedicine *becomes* Western biomedicine—the universal becomes the particular—once it reaches the African shore. Even if it were possible for Western biomedicine to be exported in a mythical "pure" Western form, the lasting impact of its arrival would still be determined by local conditions. As an ontological whole, subject to the vicissitudes of historical-cultural change, biomedicine undermines the West's continuing attempts to associate it with certain primordial and universal "scientific" criteria and material forms. To be sure, African biomedicine as currently constituted owes a great deal to the West. But African biomedical beliefs and practices are no less beholden to African pluralistic medicine.

The second analytical premise, as detailed in Chapter 4, suggests that the constellation of common elements that comprise African pluralistic medicine contain the antecedents for adopting many Western biomedical beliefs and practices. Most prominently, these include natural explanations of illness and misfortune, pragmatic attitudes toward other medical systems, and holistic interpretations of the natural, supernatural, and social worlds. African pluralistic-medical etiologies tend to emphasize the confluence of natural, supernatural, and social causes with respect to illness as a subcategory of misfortune. However, it is commonly the case that a specific illness will be attributed to natural causes, such as infection or environmental contagion, without appeal to supernatural or social explanations. Thus, on the one hand, the notion of natural causes is a well-established principle of African pluralistic medicine. On the other hand, illnesses that are exclusively attributable to natural causes, and solely treated with natural botanicals, are also consistent with African pluralistic-medical beliefs and practices. The governing etiological rationale of Western biomedicine, therefore, is also a basic feature of African pluralistic medicine. At the same time, a pragmatic interest in "foreign" medical systems represents a guiding principle across African pluralistic-medical systems. African pluralistic-medical practitioners (PMPs) routinely investigate and borrow medical techniques and botanicals from neighboring ethnic communities. However, Africans have been equally eager to test and adopt various techniques and medicines from non-African peoples, such as Arab and Portuguese traders. Consequently, while the circumstances of biomedicine's 19th-century arrival may have been bloody and contentious, African pluralistic medicine was nonetheless inherently predisposed to learning and borrowing from biomedicine's basic medical corpus. Judiciously drawing from select biomedical beliefs and practices, Africans have been able to enhance their own medical systems without fundamentally compromising the underlying collective worldviews that inform African pluralistic medicine.

The holistic framework of interpretation is another antecedent element of African pluralistic medicine shaping the development of African biomedicine. One of the most consistent and widespread characteristics of African pluralistic medicine is an appeal to the natural, supernatural, and social worlds as overlapping and mutually interacting spheres. Though these three spheres are useful for distinguishing certain phenomenal forms, they in no way refer to separate and distinct worlds—as in the case of science and religion in the West, for example. In light of this, a curious contradiction remains the legacy of those ethnographic studies reviewed in Chapter 4. On the one hand, endless notepads have been filled with observations of holistic collective worldviews wherein the notion of the natural, supernatural, and social worlds as discrete categories is rejected as a Western contrivance. On the other hand, when Africans later adopt biomedicine after considerable negotiation as a therapeutic option, it is depicted as standing *outside* African pluralistic medicine—as a separate and discrete option! The myth of African/Western dualism persists in direct contradiction of the voluminous ethnographic literature. Indeed, biomedicine is no more *outside* Kamba pluralistic medicine than are those medical techniques and botanicals that the Kamba have borrowed from their Luo neighbors. The constellation of common elements within African pluralistic medicine—for instance, natural explanations of illness and misfortune, medical pragmatism, and a holistic perspective—are the clear antecedents to contemporary African biomedicine. Ultimately, Western biomedicine has been unable to supplant African pluralistic medicine because the defining features of African biomedicine first resided in African pluralistic medicine. Indeed, given the exclusive etiological premises and narrow ideological orthodoxy of Western biomedicine vis-à-vis African etiological holism and medical pragmatism, it could be argued that African pluralistic medicine was always destined to absorb biomedicine rather than vice versa.

The third analytical premise, as outlined in Chapter 3, points to the unique circumstances of biomedicine's initial journey to Africa, the incorporation of

Africa into the capitalist world-system and the resulting "globalization" of biomedicine as a singular historical-cultural formation. The importance of analyzing biomedicine in Africa as an aspect of the expanding capitalist world-system is twofold. First, biomedicine's arrival was not an isolated or accidental occurrence. The analysis of biomedicine in Africa as a complex sociocultural phenomenon is often detached from the broader colonial context and treated merely as a unique case of intercultural exchange. The geopolitical context of biomedicine's arrival, however, conditioned its reception and development. The nature of colonial rule invariably shaped African attitudes and expectations with respect to biomedicine as an instrument of invasion and subordination. As part of a concerted effort to universalize Western cultural values, beliefs, and practices more generally across a newly incorporated region of the capitalist world-system, biomedicine was purposely and strategically introduced to Africans as a direct challenge to established collective worldviews. Second, biomedicine itself is a historical-cultural formation and a constituent element within the capitalist world-system, enmeshed within a patchwork of political and economic structures and processes. As detailed in Chapter 1, because the capitalist world-system comprises a single unit of analysis, those phenomena that comprise it—such as the axial division of labor, the interstate system, or biomedicine—are "singular" or system-wide phenomena. As such, the biography of biomedicine is inseparable from its role within the capitalist world-system, and the analysis of the capitalist world-system, as a concrete whole, is incomplete absent an account of biomedicine and other historical-cultural formations. Thus, the development of biomedicine, as a singular historical-cultural formation, suggests mutually interacting global processes, wherein, as biomedicine reaches non-Western societies it transforms these societies and, in turn, these societies transform biomedicine. Confronted with biomedicine at the moment of its incorporation into the capitalist world-system, African societies both made accommodations for biomedicine (often at the end of a gun) and expanded the operating principles of biomedicine via its pragmatic integration with more inclusive African etiological perspectives. The result is African biomedicine.

The analysis of African biomedicine must, therefore, simultaneously account for several aspects of biomedicine's development as a singular historical-cultural formation. On the one hand, African biomedicine must be analyzed as an ontological whole comprised of multiple, embedded ontological spheres. Integral to this depiction are those antecedent elements of African pluralistic medicine that facilitated its absorption and transformation of Western biomedicine. On the other hand, the development of African biomedicine must be framed as a consequence of Africa's incorporation into the capitalist world-system. The emergence of African biomedicine, a contemporary moment in the *longue durée* of global biomedicine, is inseparable from the life history of the capitalist world-system and, as such, following the incorporation of Africa, African biomedicine and the capitalist world-system have become enjoined in a web of interdependent and mutually conditioning relationships.

African Biomedicine as an Ontological Whole

The sociocultural context for the discussion of biomedicine as an ontological whole in Chapter 2 was restricted to Western societies over the past two centuries and this was sufficient for the limited purposes of that analysis. When analyzing African biomedicine as both an ontological whole and a singular historical-cultural formation, however, the sociocultural context grows more complex due to the added dimensions of Africa's relation to the West and its incorporation into the capitalist world-system. The three ontological spheres—biomedicine as a scientific enterprise, as a symbolic-cultural expression, and as an expression of social power—continue to organize the presentation of African biomedicine as an ontological whole. However, the interrelationships defining African biomedicine are expanded and include: (1) the interrelationships between each ontological sphere and between the three temporal-spatial levels of abstraction within each ontological sphere; and (2) the interrelationships between African biomedicine and Western biomedicine and between African biomedicine and the capitalist world-system as a concrete whole over the *longue durée*.

From one angle of vision, the description of African biomedicine as an ontological whole, at the most basic level, appears to mirror those early European accounts of the African pluralistic medicine that they first stumbled upon. In other words, it is an attempt to capture that which is most evident at a relatively rudimentary level of observation and analysis. As such, what one first notices in Africa today are medical systems comprised of a broad collection of pluralistic beliefs and practices that represent multiple, interdependent ontological spheres. In a typical African city one can find a combination of biomedical clinics and hospitals alongside a collection of PMPS (such as diviners, herbalists, and spiritual healers).[2] In a typical African village, one will find a similar collection of PMPS along with a regional biomedical clinic and perhaps a regional public health office. Thus, one encounters a thriving pluralistic-medical system premised on an eclectic range of beliefs and practices that combine natural, supernatural, and social interpretations of illness as a subcategory of misfortune. Individuals are able then to partake of those services that best fit their needs for a given situation. Hence, one hundred

[2] See, for example, the vivid description of the Kinshasa medical system provided by Devisch et al. (2001).

years after its introduction, Western biomedicine has been effectively integrated with an expanded African pluralistic-medical system—referred to here as African biomedicine—that is comprised of multiple, embedded ontological spheres.

The outlines of African biomedicine as a scientific enterprise are made especially stark by the varied and contentious etiological explanations of illness and notions of efficacy with respect to various therapies. Within African biomedicine, there are those ongoing efforts to identify causal links between the onset of illness and phenomena or forces across the natural, supernatural, and social worlds. For this purpose, African biomedicine recognizes a variety of competing etiological premises. This, of course, contrasts with etiological explanations within Western biomedicine that pertain only to phenomena in the natural world. On the surface these etiological orientations may appear to be mutually exclusive. However, in light of the "second spear," there is nothing especially inconsistent about persons moving back and forth between therapies that appeal to different rationales. Furthermore, from the perspective of these persons, this is not a movement between discrete systems but between varying therapeutic options within a single pluralistic-medical system. This is why it can be argued that those contemporary efforts to "combine" biomedicine and African pluralistic medicine, as described below, are in fact merely efforts to create a medical delivery system that better matches how Africans approach medical care. Within African biomedicine, therefore, the scientific content is divided into those phenomena associated with causal explanations in the natural, supernatural, and social worlds.

Natural explanations within African biomedicine do not differ dramatically from those of Western biomedicine, as explored in Chapter 2. Staugård (1991), for example, concludes, "Many [African pluralistic-medical] concepts about the etiology and transmission of HIV/AIDS appear to be fully compatible with modern, scientific concepts, although expressed in different terms, within a different framework" (p. 23). The basic features of supernatural and social explanations within African biomedicine are discussed in Chapter 4 in the context of African pluralistic medicine.[3] That which is unique to African biomedicine—that which sets it apart from Western biomedicine—is the manner by which these three etiological rationales are combined and undifferentiated. Whereas Western biomedicine narrowly identifies "medicine" per se with those beliefs and practices premised upon the post-Enlightenment scientific method, African biomedicine respects the scientific method but does not worship it as the exclusive oracle of truth regarding illness. This *does not* suggest

[3] It must be recognized at the same time that all of these elements of African biomedicine, as dynamic features of an ontological whole, are also subject to continuous and ongoing development and change. See, for example, the accounts of C. Good (1987) and L. Swantz (1990).

that African biomedicine rejects or is even unduly skeptical of the explanations and treatments devised by Western biomedicine. Indeed, many PMPs enthusiastically subject their own therapies to the scrutiny of the scientific method.[4] This simply suggests that, above and beyond those health-related phenomena pertaining to natural explanations, there remains a host of factors that require supernatural or social explanations, or both, for a full understanding.

Alongside competing etiological rationales, African biomedicine as a scientific enterprise promotes ongoing efforts to establish the efficacy of various botanicals and therapies associated with forces and phenomena across the natural, supernatural, or social worlds. One might imagine that the efficacy of a specific treatment would be more easily determined than the etiology of a given illness. After all, once a treatment is administered the person either does or does not recover. This, however, is an incomplete understanding of efficacy that originates in natural explanations. For example, if the cause of an illness is attributed to supernatural forces, than it is believed that the observed cause-effect relationship between administering a natural treatment and a person's recovery (from the "first spear") will prove short-lived, and the lingering supernatural cause, left unaddressed, will strike again. The criteria for efficacy, therefore, is specific to each type of explanation. Given these difficulties with the truncated biomedical constructions of etiology and efficacy, as borrowed from the West, it seems evident that the category of "scientific enterprise" as constituted by Western biomedicine is inadequate. It has been necessary, therefore, to broaden this ontological sphere of African biomedicine to include supernatural and social explanations of illness as integral features of African biomedicine as an ontological whole. In the process, African pluralistic-medical beliefs and practices are recast in conformity with the contributions of Western biomedicine, and the original "scientific-explanatory" contents of Western biomedicine both retain their unique insights and are forced to recognize the ontological limits of those insights. The result is an ontological sphere, biomedicine as a scientific enterprise, that more accurately represents the values and beliefs of African biomedicine as it is actually practiced. It is thus, by particularizing Western biomedicine, that African biomedicine is able to "universalize" biomedicine itself as a singular historical-cultural formation.

Western biomedicine as a symbolic-cultural expression concerns those ideological constructs associated with biomedicine in the West that legitimate its values, beliefs, and practices—most especially its presumptively discrete ontological spheres. It is argued in Chapter 2 that the narrow precepts

[4] In 1985, for example, the Organization of African Unity collaborated with the Inter-African Committee on Medicinal Plants to publish a pharmacopeia of African botanicals with established efficacy (DeJong, 1991).

of biomedicine (with respect to etiology, for example) required a sophisticated ideological scaffolding for its initial popularization and eventual monopoly over the domain of medicine proper. As a result, any contradictions between biomedicine as a symbolic-cultural expression and biomedicine as a scientific enterprise were between the precepts of biomedicine and evolving collective worldviews in the West. By contrast, because the precepts of biomedicine have been pragmatically grafted onto African pluralistic medicine in a holistic fashion, African biomedicine as a symbolic-cultural expression merely reifies those inherent tensions between natural, supernatural, and social explanations within African biomedicine as a scientific enterprise. Many will object that, over time, the biomedical rationale within African pluralistic medicine is bound to crowd out other etiological explanations and, therefore, as Africa further "modernizes," its symbolic-cultural expressions will mirror those in the West. Certainly this is possible. If so, this would largely be a function of African biomedicine as an expression of social power—for example, global pharmaceutical firms seeking further markets and greater profits. For now, however, it is important to stress that the necessary conditions for the adoption and broad utilization of Western biomedicine as a scientific enterprise across the African continent *did not also require* the adoption of Western biomedicine as a symbolic-cultural expression. This follows, in part, from a deep-rooted holism and pragmatism informing collective worldviews across Africa's diverse societies, in part from the dynamic development of African biomedicine as an ontological whole, and in part from the nature of African biomedicine as a singular historical-cultural formation. This combination of factors has the potential to move the developmental pattern of African biomedicine beyond the linear, stagist modernization paradigm. As the latter dimensions are taken up below, we here emphasize the holism and pragmatism of African biomedicine as a symbolic-cultural expression.

Prior to the arrival of biomedicine, much of African pluralistic medicine blithely entertained a quiet tension between competing natural, supernatural, and social explanations of misfortune and illness. This was done through a sophisticated holistic framework of interpretation. Whereas collective worldviews in the West presumed separate and distinct ontological spheres for matters medical, spiritual, or interpersonal, collective worldviews in Africa observed their indivisibility and mutual interdependence. For the purposes of everyday communication one might refer to phenomena as pertaining to the natural, supernatural, or social sphere, however within a broader cosmology, these are differences without distinction. Overlapping etiological explanations tend to foster a persistent dynamic tension. For example, within African biomedicine it is completely consistent both, on occasion, to attribute an illness exclusively to natural causes and, at other times, to dismiss efforts to draw meaningful distinctions between the natural, supernatural, and social worlds. African biomedicine, as a symbolic-cultural expression, embodies this dynamic tension—carried over from African pluralistic medicine—between holism and discrete explanations. Consequently, the introduction of Western biomedicine heightens a pre-existing internal contradiction within African pluralistic medicine between inherently inconsistent etiological explanations and efforts to integrate and harmonize varying beliefs and practices via holistic interpretations. Importantly, the beliefs and practices of biomedicine do not introduce new or unique ideas that fundamentally oppose African pluralistic medicine. Hence, African biomedicine as a symbolic-cultural expression requires no new ideological rationales for its acceptance. At the same time, given holism as an organizing principle of African collective worldviews, biomedicine's arrival feeds and further complicates an already-existing dynamic tension between competing etiological rationales. Thus, holism explains why Africans were able to incorporate Western biomedicine while avoiding the rapid dissolution of its collective worldviews. However, it remains uncertain whether holism will be sufficient to sustain the heightened contradictions found within African biomedicine as a symbolic-cultural expression.

One of the primary sources of African pluralistic medicine's cocky self-assuredness with respect to its holistic framework vis-à-vis biomedical atomism resides primarily in its pragmatic attitude toward the medical beliefs and practices of other societies. If the African pluralistic-medical beliefs and practices encountered by the first wave of European medical officers and missionaries were truly built on "primitive superstition," as the European suggested, then surely this was a type of primitive superstition that was unique in its acceptance of competing medical cultures and belief systems. In combination with African holism, the pragmatism of African biomedicine may be what most distinguishes it from Western biomedicine as a symbolic-cultural expression. Whereas Western biomedicine is resolutely obstinate regarding its superiority over all other medical systems, African biomedicine actively engages with and shamelessly borrows from other societies' medical beliefs and practices. Because this is done within a holistic framework, "foreign" beliefs and practices are examined and occasionally replace certain long-standing beliefs and practices without disrupting or threatening underlying collective worldviews—as would *necessarily* be the case for Western biomedicine. In a radical departure from Western biomedicine, therefore, African biomedicine as a symbolic-cultural expression not only recognizes, but presumes, its continuing evolution and transformation. Western biomedicine as a scientific enterprise is, of course, open to new discoveries and ongoing development. However, it is understood that none of these new developments will challenge the essential ideological content of biomedicine, given its closed epistemological premises.[5] Western biomedicine as a symbolic-cultural expression, therefore, is not subject to further fundamental change. This would dissolve Western biomedicine. By contrast, given its pluralistic roots, African biomedicine as a symbolic-cultural expression is premised upon such change. The elements of holism and pragmatism, therefore, both explain the integration of biomedicine with African pluralistic medicine and further distinguish the dynamic nature of African biomedicine, as a symbolic-cultural expression, from the static nature of Western biomedicine.

African biomedicine as an expression of social power and Western biomedicine as an expression of social power share many common attributes. Like Western biomedicine, African biomedicine encompasses a complex social institution. Like Western biomedicine, there are ongoing attempts by competing industries and interests (for example, practitioner factions and social elites) to control this complex social institution. Like Western biomedicine, African biomedicine is inseparable from local and global processes of commodification and capital accumulation. Unlike Western biomedicine, as analyzed in Chapter 2, however, many of the key industries and interests that shape African biomedicine as an expression of social power extend well beyond its shores. Thus, while many of the same factors shape African biomedicine and Western biomedicine as expressions of social power, in the case of African biomedicine the unit of analysis must account for both local power struggles and global threats. Consequently, African biomedicine as an expression of social power is significantly shaped (and controlled) by a range of global actors, most especially those with direct commercial or professional interests—such as pharmaceutical firms, biotechnology companies, and biomedical trade and professional organizations. To highlight the hybrid nature of African biomedicine as an expression of social power, we focus on two levels. At the local level, there are ongoing struggles between PMPs and African biomedical practitioners with respect to professional recognition and the right to define and regulate medicine. At the global level, African biomedicine as an expression of social power has been subject to the predatory activi-

[5] In 1992, for example, the U.S. National Institutes of Health (NIH) established the Office of Alternative Medicine. This was upgraded to the National Center for Complementary and Alternative Medicine (NCCAM) in 1999. The declared mission of NCCAM is threefold. "To explore complementary and alternative healing practices in the context of rigorous science. To train complementary and alternative medicine researchers. To disseminate authoritative information to the public and professionals." In this fashion, NIH scientists simultaneously concede the potential medical value of complementary and alternative medicine, while restricting the criteria for assessing this value to the reductionist, etiological premises of Western scientific medicine. That which proves to be efficacious can thus be seamlessly folded into the existing repertoire of Western biomedicine.

ties of various biomedical industries abetted by a network of private and public, core-based, humanitarian donors.

For African biomedical practitioners, the decades of the 1960s and 1970s combined great hope with tremendous frustration. With the formal edifice of colonial rule lifted, African biomedical practitioners were for the first time granted the professional status and autonomy enjoyed by their Western colleagues.[6] "For most of the colonial period the medical profession as a profession scarcely existed in either Anglophone or Francophone Africa" (Last, 1986:9). However, forced to labor with antiquated equipment, inadequate supplies, and bankrupt government budgets, the dream of developing a biomedical system on par with the West remained for most far from reach. In addition, the PMPs whom colonial officials had campaigned to push to the margins of society had not only survived decades of Western repression, but they continued to enjoy broad public support. Consequently, these two factions, African biomedical practitioners and African PMPs, were poised to challenge each other's claims for a role in the postcolonial African health care system. African biomedical practitioners, with their new status and autonomy, sought to protect their privileged control over medical care. The PMPs, whose intimate connections to daily African life the African biomedical practitioners could not deny, sought recognition for their knowledge, skills, and significant contributions to African healthcare. Resulting from this competition were twin movements. As PMPs moved aggressively to professionalize their ranks, African biomedical practitioners vigorously pushed to establish and regulate the boundaries of legitimate medicine. The professionalization of African pluralistic-medical care turned on the adamant assertions of PMPs that there existed a coherent and recognizable body of knowledge and set of practices over which they had a demonstrated mastery. With no formal written guidelines on par with the ancient literature of Ayurvedic or Unani medicine to reference, PMPs relied on a system of often grueling apprenticeships to train new practitioners. The requisite knowledge and skills were passed directly from one generation to the next. Consequently, significant gaps and inconsistencies were prevalent among PMPs, and many sought a method to verify an individual's level of skill and knowledge. Establishing professional PMP associations with clear and rigorous criteria for membership was one common response.[7] The primary benefits of PMP associations included enhanced public confidence, a begrudging professional recognition, and formal control over professional criteria and standards. For African biomedicine as an expression of social power, PMP professionalization signified conformity

[6] See Iliffe's (2002) "collective biography" of African MDS in East Africa in this regard.

[7] See Bibeau (1982a), Chavunduka (1986), Fassin and Fassin (1988), Flint (2001), Green (1996), Last (1986), Oyebola (1981), Twumasi (1985), and Twumasi and Warren (1986).

with the norms of a modern consumer society and a significant loss of individual PMP autonomy, alongside closer group identification and cohesion among PMPS as an exclusive professional class. Always conceived of, at least in part, as a commodity, African biomedicine was now increasingly treated as an article of trade to be bought and sold like toothpaste or a pair of shoes. Professionalization, therefore, also prepared the path for the greater regulation of PMP therapies.

The resulting regulation of medical care in Africa required systematically categorizing various therapies as beneficial, ineffective, or harmful. The criteria for assessing this was largely controlled by African biomedical practitioners. The notion of beneficial, therefore, closely followed the biomedical logic of demonstrable efficacy discussed above. Given the PMPS' pragmatic acceptance of the basic principles of the experimental sciences, there was little debate concerning findings when a given therapy was shown to be either beneficial or harmful. There remained, however, a significant number of therapies with no demonstrable benefit or harm. Because many PMPS maintained that the benefit of these therapies, especially those pertaining to supernatural or social worlds, were not susceptible to the methods of the experimental sciences and because African biomedical practitioners could prove no harm, much of the debate turned on how to categorize and regulate these therapies within the boundaries of legitimate medicine.[8] African biomedical practitioners discounted these therapies as nonbeneficial while PMPS sought recognition for their holistic contributions to the population's health.[9] At the same time, because PMPS prefer to be free from government regulation, African biomedicine as an expression of social power has tended to push these therapies to the margins of the medical system. Thus, like Western biomedicine, African biomedicine as an expression of social power at the local and national levels is dominated by African biomedical practitioners as an organized faction of social elites[10]—in league with a retinue of national and global elites.

---

[8] See Chavunduka and Last (1986), Iliffe (2002), MacCormack (1986), and Pearce (1986).

[9] There was a further concern with respect to those therapies with little or no demonstrable medical benefit or harm. This concerned the fear of con artists. See, for example, Elling's (1981) discussion of a group of Yoruba PMPS who benefited from their role as mediators between the God of Smallpox and the population. Due to the financial rewards of this role, many PMPS actively worked to undermine smallpox eradication campaigns. See also Green's (1994) discussion of further cautions pertaining to the potential harm of African pluralistic-medical practices. While such activities can lead to serious hardship, this same criticism can be extended to the often dubious role of pharmaceutical firms in marketing their goods in peripheralized societies. See Bodenheimer (1984), A. Ferguson (1988), Gereffi (1983), Turshen (2001), and Yudkin (1980) with respect to pharmaceutical abuses.

[10] A majority of African biomedical practitioners belonging to the Nigerian Medical Association, for example, maintained that the recognition of PMPS was akin to "licensing killers" (Feierman, 1985:126).

However, unlike Western biomedicine, African biomedicine as an expression of social power at the local and national levels has been forced to reach accommodation with, and often work alongside, PMPs due to their considerable social power and continuing broad base of social support in Africa.

At the same time, an expansive and well-positioned spectrum of core-based, global actors has been able to shape African biomedicine directly as an expression of social power. These include pharmaceutical and biotechnology firms, medical equipment suppliers, and professional associations of biomedical practitioners and educators, each of whom has a stake in the growth of biomedicine globally. "Pressure from organized Western medicine helps to sideline traditional medicine, keeping it out of the policy discussions and specifically out of national health care strategic plans and official systems" (Gbodossou et al., 2005:3). A parallel sphere of global actors—a collection of influential foundations and governmental and nongovernmental organizations (NGOs)—has emerged to expedite this expansion of biomedicine via the provision of "foreign aid" in the form of humanitarian medical assistance. Not unlike officials from the World Bank and International Monetary Fund who link financial assistance to neoliberal policies (for example, structural readjustment), these avowedly humanitarian organizations largely adhere to the cultural and economic norms of Western biomedicine when designing aid and promoting market-based medicine. Laurell and López Arellano's analysis of the World Bank's *1993 World Development Report: Investing in Health* details the nature of these self-serving stipulations.

> Although the Report dedicates considerable space to the role of individuals and nonprofit organizations, its main concern is with expanding the health market. The division of clinical services into "essential" and "discretionary" is crucial to this quest, since the latter, according to the World Bank, are private goods that should be provided as commodities in the market. The Bank recognizes that this would require the creation of financial instruments to ensure consumer purchasing power . . . This acknowledgement allows the Bank to introduce the insurance companies, together with private medical providers, as prominent agents in the health field. The Report discusses at length various forms of articulating private financing and service provision to facilitate private sector involvement. (Laurell and López Arellano, 2002:198–199)

Rather transparently, and in concert with neoliberal privatization plans, much of this foreign aid is earmarked for African governments to purchase outsourced goods and services from Western biomedical firms. This model of self-aggrandizing foreign aid has been analyzed in detail elsewhere.[11] In brief, wealthy nations provide assistance to African nations with the stipulations that (1) these funds must be used to purchase goods and services from select firms from the wealthy nations and (2) these funds must be linked to neoliberal economic reforms that further open African resources and financial markets to global speculation. Frequently, these funds are provided as a loan that must be repaid as a further gesture of "good faith." In this fashion, foreign aid promotes the further development of African markets and consumers for Western biomedical products and services. O'Manique (2004:53) argues, "The World Bank's health strategy was one instrument for bringing global health policy into line with the neoliberal canon that ascribed health mainly to the private domain, through the introduction of market forces into the health sector and the allocation of public resources according to the criteria of technical efficiency and cost-effectiveness." Just as the colonial powers of the past introduced tropical medicine to reap the benefits of a healthy workforce, today Western biomedical firms continue to profit from providing health care to Africans. African biomedicine as an expression of social power, therefore, reflects a simmering cauldron of powerful forces. At the local and national levels, the professionalization and regulation of medical care drives PMPS to establish uniform standards and criteria. At the global level, a coterie of global elites, representing a collection of biomedical industrial, financial, and professional interests, devises schemes to pull Africans more tightly into the orbit of biomedical commodification.

HIV/AIDS and African Biomedicine's Embedded Ontological Spheres

As in the case of Western biomedicine, the embedded nature of the multiple ontological spheres that comprise African biomedicine is manifest across the three spatial-temporal levels of abstraction that correspond with short-term events, middle-range episodes, and the structures and processes of the capitalist world-system over the *longue durée*. In this regard, due in large part to its sociocultural complexity, the contemporary HIV/AIDS pandemic reveals in especially stark fashion the basic features of African biomedicine across these first two spatial-temporal levels. The HIV/AIDS pandemic stalks the African continent as a short-term event that has increasingly ravaged the African people throughout the second half of the postcolonial era—a middle-range episode. The period of independence began with a tremendous sense of hope and optimism, as Africa's young generation of leaders pursued ambitious

[11] Among others, see Hayter (1971), Laurell and López Arellano (2002), Perkins (2006), Richards (1977), and Stiglitz (2003).

social agendas addressing emergent African priorities and aspirations. The HIV/AIDS pandemic decisively disrupted and redirected African priorities in the postcolonial era and also made clear the limits of African independence and autonomy with respect to African biomedicine several decades after direct European rule had come to an end. Thus, we turn to the contemporary HIV/AIDS pandemic as an event shaping, and shaped by, African biomedicine in the postcolonial era.

The first large-scale global efforts to arrest the African HIV/AIDS pandemic began in the mid-1980s, two decades after nominal independence for most African nations. An analysis of the pandemic begins, therefore, with its sociohistorical and geopolitical context—the forty-year, middle-range episode of postcolonial Africa. Throughout the postcolonial era, Africa has remained among the most impoverished and underdeveloped regions of the capitalist world-system.[12] The ravages of the Atlantic slave trade over four centuries, an exploitative and extractive colonial system, Cold War proxy wars, and the contrived, colonial-era territorial states left the continent weak and battered. The social priorities of the national liberation movements of the 1950s and 1960s—education, healthcare, economic growth—have been undermined by these factors as well as by the internal strife and divisions accompanying the meager spoils of postcolonial self-rule. Consequently, throughout the postcolonial era, Africa has ranked at the bottom in the world with respect to per capita medical resources as well as to most standard measures of health and welfare.[13]

In light of extensive African poverty and growing global disparities, there have been sporadic, core-based efforts throughout the postcolonial period to address the deteriorating health of Africans. These have included campaigns to train more African biomedical practitioners, gifts of equipment, technology, and medicine, and waves of international medical volunteers, such as *Médecins Sans Frontières,* who periodically provide direct assistance. Though more could always be done, these efforts have certainly had a tangible impact on African lives (for example, the smallpox eradication campaign) and remain an important contribution to the wellbeing of Africans in the postcolonial era. Beginning in the 1970s, in addition to these efforts to expand African biomedical resources, there has been a push by African governments and some international bodies to "combine" African pluralistic medicine with biomedical care. This follows, in part, from pragmatic efforts to supplement a resource-deprived biomedical system. In 2000, the World Health Organization (WHO) estimated that for 80–85% of the African population, PMPS

---

[12] See Arrighi (2002), Baylies (2000), and Saul and Leys (1999).

[13] See UN Population Fund (2006) and WHO (2007).

were the primary source of health education and health care (Gbodossou et al., 2005:1).[14] Thus, many governments and international agencies have enlisted the assistance of PMPs both as a basic stopgap measure and as convenient cultural links for purposes of health promotion in general.[15] Echoing this sentiment, Nchinda (1976:134) observes simply that "[T]raditional medicine fulfills the four criteria of accessibility, availability, acceptability and dependability."

In the mid-1970s, WHO produced a series of influential reports investigating the potential role of PMPs as a health care resource in Africa.[16] These studies led to a joint WHO/UNICEF meeting in Alma Ata in the Kazakhstan region of the Soviet Union in 1978. It was at this meeting that the WHO adopted principles for achieving "health for all by the year 2000" through primary health care. These principles were based, in part, on the development of primary health care plans with an enhanced role for PMPs, reflecting a general sense that PMPs fulfill a strategic social role that can greatly enhance public health campaigns. In an analysis of Tanzanian PMP associations, for example, Semali (1986:95) suggests, "As the [PMPs] have indicated their willingness to collaborate and learn from modern health workers, we may then utilize their position in the society to promote health." The use of PMPs is also, however, an attempt to overcome a predictable reluctance of many Africans fully to accept biomedicine as their exclusive form of medical care. "Many a Western-trained doctor has been baffled by the lack of response and apparent stubbornness on the part of some patients to follow an otherwise scientifically sound treatment regime" (Nchinda, 1976:133).

These two strands, core-based biomedical assistance and national collaboration with PMPs, have resulted in a mixed legacy that has further complicated Western dualistic depictions of African medical systems. On the one hand, these efforts to address the dire African health needs throughout the postcolonial era have been essential and necessary interventions in a tragic humanitarian crisis. On the other hand, the form of this response typifies Western prescriptions for African ailments that, from the late 19th century forward, have been predicated on African modernization and the abdication of established collective worldviews. Consequently, descriptions of postcolo-

---

[14] This marked little or no improvement from two decades earlier when Bichmann (1979:176) estimated that 70–90% of African rural populations lacked access to public health.

[15] See Bibeau et al (1980), Dunlop (1974/1975), Green (1996), Harrison (1974), Oyebola (1986), Oyeneye (1985), and WHO (1978).

[16] These included: "Health Manpower Development: Training and Utilization of Traditional Healers and their Collaboration with Health Care Delivery Systems" in 1975; "Traditional Medicine and Its Role in the Development of Health Services in Africa" in 1976; "African Traditional Medicine" in 1976, and "The Promotion and Development of Traditional Medicine" in 1978.

nial African medical systems by Western health officials and scholars alike continue to assert a fundamental dualism between Western biomedicine and African pluralistic medicine that implicitly privileges the former.

This dualistic attitude is replete throughout the descriptions of efforts to combine biomedicine and African pluralistic medicine in the postcolonial era. For example, in their review of African efforts to combine medical systems, Kikhela et al. (1981:96) observe, "In most developing countries, particularly in Africa, two medical systems are in operation: One modeled on the modern medicine practiced in the industrial nations, and the other based on indigenous medical traditions." Bichmann (1979) distinguishes between domestic medicine, folk medicine, traditional medicine, and cosmopolitan medicine with respect to African medical care, while Devisch et al. (2001:107), citing "different understandings of the human body and the etiology of health and illness," distinguish between "the medical health care establishment," "folk healers," and "faith or spiritualist healers." Solidifying the dichotomy between biomedicine and African pluralistic medicine, Green (1988:1129) laments, "Perhaps syncretism can never develop very far due to a basic incompatibility between the two paradigms of illness and the supporting worldviews." MacCormack (1986:156) deftly attributes this dualism to Africans themselves, explaining, "From the rural patients' point of view, inadequacies in either the scientific or the traditional system can be minimized by judicious shopping in either system for therapies."

Such depictions suggest that Africans in the postcolonial era select among a range of therapeutic options depending upon the circumstances and an untenable, mythical dichotomy is reified between "modern" Western biomedicine and "primitive" African pluralistic medicine. Discrete Western analytical categories trump African holism. Notwithstanding the well documented African beliefs and practices that frame health and healing as holistic processes that intermingle the values, beliefs and practices from varying medical systems, the predominant Western image continues to treat biomedicine as a separate and distinct category within African medical systems. Bibeau et al. (1980:34) are among the few to bring a critical eye to this false dualism. "Patients should be free to move toward Western-type medicine for illnesses whose symptoms exceed the competence of traditional medicine and toward [PMPS] for treatments that modern medicine is unable or is not as competent to provide." These same authors go on to provide a remarkable description of collaborative African medicine that is not too far afield from the notion of African biomedicine developed here.

> The formula that we are proposing for integrated medicine is not a mixture of discrete elements borrowed from the two medical systems but rather a harmonizing of two medical practices, each operating

> within its own sphere and each renewing and enriching itself and the other. It is only on this basis that a new type of purely African medicine can emerge, clearly adapted to the health needs of the Zairian people. (Bibeau et al., 1980:35)

While there have thus been ongoing efforts to integrate biomedicine and African pluralistic medicine throughout the postcolonial era, it has been the HIV/AIDS pandemic in particular, beginning in the mid-1980s, that has greatly accelerated such efforts. The resulting campaigns to treat and prevent HIV/AIDS are especially intriguing given the sociocultural nature of HIV transmission and the role of poverty and social inequality as cofactors in its epidemiology. Indeed, HIV/AIDS-related health policies in Africa have often been criticized precisely for an adherence to a narrow medical model that fails to address the broader range of contributing factors, such as the nature of North-South relations.[17] Early 20th-century campaigns to combat sleeping sickness had required massive relocations to avoid tsetse flies and had presented severe challenges. The complexities of these ordeals, however, cannot compare with public health campaigns to regulate sexual behaviors and other highly stigmatized and taboo social activities. For this reason, Western and African biomedical practitioners were soon made acutely aware of their mammoth cultural inadequacies in the face of HIV/AIDS. Collaboration with PMPS was no longer merely an option. It became imperative. The resulting series of "arranged marriages" further testify to the banality of treating biomedicine and African pluralistic medicine as discrete and separate entities rather than as integral and overlapping features of a holistic medical framework. It was also to give the West its first hazy images of African biomedicine as an ontological whole.

From the perspective of biomedical practitioners, the primary role of PMPS in official HIV/AIDS public health campaigns is that of cultural ambassador and translator, though Charles Good (1988:107) also notes their important role as "an early warning system" to monitor local conditions. In general, it was not the knowledge and insights of PMPS as medical practitioners that was sought but their basic ability to overcome a paralyzing African ignorance. Indeed, further advancing the Western/African dualism Devisch et al. (2001:125) suggest that PMPS must somehow bridge two wholly distinct medical discourses. "[O]ne quickly perceives in the parallel health systems a struggle between a universalizing, positivist and modernizing knowledge and traditional, local, pluralistic attitudes and practices. In sum, different historical and socio-cultural contexts have led not only to

[17] See Farmer (2001, 2003), Mann and Kay (1991), and O'Manique (2004).

competing care systems but to competing health discourses."[18] The PMPS enjoy the trust and confidence of those Africans with whom health officials want access. Thus, one of the most perplexing challenges confronting Western biomedicine in the postcolonial era has been how to fashion a relationship with African pluralistic medicine that allows one to instrumentalize the PMPS' role in the community without appearing to legitimize the PMPS' beliefs and practices.

In the early 20th century the colonial strategy had been to marginalize and belittle PMPS and a battery of antiwitchcraft laws was designed to minimize them as a cultural influence. One hundred years later, in the face of a cataclysmic HIV/AIDS pandemic, there has been a significant sea change in Western attitudes. Today, there are open calls for collaboration and moves to incorporate rather than marginalize PMPS. This pragmatic arrangement has prompted important ruptures with standard biomedical orthodoxy, including the consideration of sociocultural factors and a halting recognition of PMP holism. These are seen as not only helpful but necessary steps to penetrate and interpret the complex sociocultural reality of HIV/AIDS effectively. The 2002 foreword to a UNAIDS Report on AIDS in East Africa reflects the guarded nature of this new cooperative relationship.

> [PMPS] make a unique contribution that is complementary to other approaches. They also tend to be the entry point for care in many African communities, and even more so for the complex HIV-related diseases that frequently jolt family dynamics and shake community stability. [PMPS] often have high credibility and deep respect among the population they serve. They are knowledgeable about local treatment options, as well as the physical, emotional and spiritual lives of the people and are able to influence behaviors. Thus, it is imperative and practical to consider [PMPS] partners in the expanded response to HIV/AIDS, and to maximize the potential contribution that can be made towards meeting the magnitude of needs for the solution to HIV/AIDS in the African context. (UNAIDS, 2002:5)

There are, therefore, two primary rationales for such collaboration. On the one hand, it is recognized that given the current distribution of global resources, it is all but unthinkable that the West will be sharing its riches to provide Africans with biomedical care except at the most minimal levels. Thus, there is a need for PMPS to "subsidize" African HIV/AIDS treatment to overcome the enormous global wealth inequalities. On the other hand, it is

[18] See also Staugård (1991) with respect to the role of PMPS as links between "the government health service and the majority of the population" (p. 22).

widely recognized that PMPs enjoy a significant degree of popularity and local trust and, at the same time, that they possess a cultural understanding and acumen that biomedical practitioners in general do not consider a feature of "real" medical training. Thus, PMPs are called upon to work with local communities in the area of HIV/AIDS prevention after biomedical practitioners provide their esteemed lackeys with the proper facts and information. "Given their counseling skills, [PMPs] have managed to persuade AIDS patients who claim to be bewitched, to take the HIV/AIDS tests and start regular treatment . . . Creating a close relationship is vital to win the patients' confidence and convince them to take the HIV test" (Nalugwa, 2003:39). Whereas the medical missionaries came to save souls, the international medical agencies have come to save bodies. In each case, however, the foreigners were challenged by a set of African pluralistic-medical beliefs and practices that interfered with their objectives. Consequently, in each case, the foreigners required an understanding of these beliefs and practices that permitted the development of a language and a manipulative, yet culturally sensitive, approach to meet their ends. Note, for example, the somewhat troubling tone of Willms et al. in their call for the development of "culturally-compelling" interventions that can go beyond previous "culturally-appropriate" interventions.

> The challenge now confronting health social scientists is to create interventions that are *culturally compelling*—that is, interventions that are not only culturally appropriate in language, idiom and expression, but persuasive in their ability to make persons feel vulnerable, alter the nature of their assumptive world, and become compelled not only to think, but also to feel and act differently. (emphasis in original, Willms et al., 2001:163)

The response of African biomedicine as a scientific enterprise to the HIV/AIDS pandemic in the postcolonial era turns on the varying interpretations of its etiology and the potential efficacy of various PMP therapies. Etiological explanations of HIV/AIDS are complicated by the common belief among PMPs that its origins lie outside Africa. In the first decades of the pandemic, it was widely believed that HIV/AIDS was introduced to Africa by Westerners and by Africans returning from the West.[19] As such, the illness is often thought to be

---

[19] It is also the case that HIV/AIDS appears to imitate many sexually transmitted diseases (STDs) that are ordinarily attributed to broken taboos. However, as Willms et al. (2001) note in their study of hiv/AIDS prevention in Zimbabwe, the differences between HIV/AIDS and the category of STDs referred to as *runyoka* seem greater than the similarities. Unlike HIV/AIDS, for example, *runyoka* only afflicts adult men, has a known cure, and is only found in Africa. Comparable illnesses elsewhere in Africa include, *boswagadi* in Botswana, *mwanza* in Gabon, *anenmi* in Ethiopia, and *chira* among the Luo in Kenya.

more susceptible to Western medicine than African pluralistic medicine and PMPs are thus generally open to Western explanations of HIV/AIDS. As noted in Chapter 4, PMPs commonly distinguish between illnesses indigenous to Africa and those introduced by Europeans, and PMPs will ordinarily defer to European medicine in the latter case. At the same time, the nature of HIV transmission, combined with two decades of medical uncertainty and elusive "cures" through Western biomedicine, has left the etiology of HIV/AIDS open to considerable PMP speculation. The manifestation of HIV/AIDS—a collection of immune-related ailments—also promotes an ad hoc, symptom-based approach to diagnosis and treatment by PMPs. Thus a number of controversies have emerged, most explosively in South Africa,[20] with regard to the actual links between HIV and AIDS and the shifting boundaries that define HIV/AIDS as a syndrome. Insofar as the etiology of HIV/AIDS occasionally has the appearance of an unsettled matter—especially in the absence of a definitive cure—the current pandemic does little to resolve the tensions between biomedical and PMP etiological rationales within African biomedicine as a scientific enterprise.

Efforts to establish the efficacy of African pluralistic-medical therapies, especially botanicals, have also helped to shape African biomedicine as a scientific enterprise in the context of the HIV/AIDS pandemic. The current pandemic has sparked great interest in the potential therapeutic value of African pluralistic medicine. A growing number of national and international organizations are actively testing the efficacy of a range of PMP botanicals.[21] In 2002, two years after the first international conference on African pluralistic medicine in Dakar, the WHO reported that twenty-one African nations had created formal institutes to investigate the efficacy of pluralistic-medical treatments. Three years earlier, Homsy et al. (1999) reported the successful development of a Ugandan botanical treatment for *herpes zoster* and chronic diarrhea for persons living with HIV. Importantly, the criteria for efficacy in these efforts are narrowly biomedical in orientation. Nalugwa, for example,

---

[20] Shortly after his 1999 election, South African President Thabo Mbeki took a number of provocative measures. He declared the toxicity of the principle HIV/AIDS drugs, AZT and other antiretroviral drugs, to outweigh their benefit, and attempted to block their use to prevent perinatal transmission, notwithstanding their well established benefits. He invited a panel of international scientists who denied the link between HIV and AIDS to help develop the South African AIDS policy and he declared Western racism and global poverty a more significant factor in the spread of AIDS than HIV.

[21] These include, the WHO's Regional Office for Africa (AFRO), The Association for the Promotion of Traditional Medicine (PROMETRA), a Dakar-based NGO established to preserve African pluralistic medicine, and the Bioresources Development and Conservation Programme (BDCP) of Nigeria. The African Union has declared the first decade of the 21st century to be the "Decade of African Traditional Medicine" and the African Advisory Committee for Health Research and Development (AACHRD) has also called for enhanced research into the efficacy of African pluralistic medicine.

describes the research initiative of the HIV/AIDS Initiative on Traditional Healthcare in Africa (HARITHAF) in the following terms. "HARITHAF is to develop and supply simplified but controlled clinical protocols to conduct rapid evaluations of the safety and efficacy of promising herbal treatments for HIV/AIDS. The herbal medicines can either be used as immuno-stimulants and antiviral agents, or to combat opportunistic infections" (Nalugwa, 2003:24). This conflicts with the more holistic orientation of most PMPS and points to a basic contradiction. On the one hand, biomedical practitioners seek the assistance of PMPS due to their close integration with local communities. On the other hand, in the process of assessing the efficacy of PMPS' treatments, they reduce them to discrete biochemical reactions, which naturally encourages PMPS to forego their more integral role in the community and focus narrowly on botanical agents. The universal criteria of biomedicine in one moment affirms the efficacy of select African pluralistic medicine and simultaneously undermines its further development.

Consequently, the HIV/AIDS pandemic as a short-term event highlights the dynamic tension within African biomedicine as a scientific enterprise between competing etiological rationales and between divergent measures of efficacy. Insofar as biomedical practitioners are able to define the terms of cooperation between themselves and PMPS, the norms and values of biomedicine largely dominate this process. Nonetheless, PMPS are not ignorant of the pivotal role they play in this exchange—such as controlling access to certain populations—and there is consequently a continuing drive to develop a more balanced working relationship. "HIV/AIDS further swelled the numbers seeking treatment and gave [PMPS] the opportunity to demand a more equal relationship with Western medicine" (Iliffe, 2006:92). As such, PMPS are able to give ground in the areas of etiology and efficacy while negotiating for greater official recognition and practitioner rights. African biomedicine as a scientific enterprise and as an expression of social power meld together. The HIV/AIDS pandemic, as a moment in the postcolonial era, therefore, reveals many of the basic strains within African biomedicine as a scientific enterprise.

Throughout the contemporary HIV/AIDS pandemic, African biomedicine as a symbolic-cultural expression has confronted two competing interpretative influences. The first juxtaposes Western biomedical atomism with African pluralistic-medical holism. The second juxtaposes Western biomedical orthodoxy with African pluralistic-medical pragmatism. Each contrast represents competing visions of medicine, corresponding with distinct beliefs and practices within African biomedicine. Concerted efforts to combat HIV/AIDS in Africa via collaborative arrangements between biomedical practitioners and PMPS have accentuated these dynamic tensions within African biomedicine as a symbolic-cultural expression. By creating formal structures of cooperative medical care that link the activities of biomedical practitioners (and their beliefs and practices) with those of PMPs, collaborative HIV/AIDS campaigns have brought to the surface a number of fundamental differences that may have otherwise remained hidden within the complex labyrinth of African biomedicine. These fundamental differences do not merely signal competing etiologies or interpretations of efficacy, but more basic cosmological differences reflected in collective worldviews. Somewhat ironically, therefore, given the practical interest in "collaboration" on the part of biomedical practitioners, the organized medical response to HIV/AIDS in Africa began by sharpening the divisions between PMPs and biomedicine as discrete elements within African biomedicine in the name of bringing practitioners together. Accordingly, it is evident that one of the basic tasks of collaboration is *not* to reconcile or resolve these disparate views but to work within a framework that somehow validates both, while tolerating the dynamic tension that inevitably results therefrom. This, in fact, is an apt characterization of African biomedical beliefs and practices.

As discussed in Chapter 2, the operating norms of Western biomedicine are premised on the fundamental interpretive assertion that the material world is separate from and not directly impacted by forces in the nonmaterial world, for example, supernatural forces. This, of course, conflicts with a fundamental interpretive assertion of African pluralistic medicine that the material world is inseparable from, and regularly impacted by, forces in the nonmaterial world. Consequently, for the biomedical practitioner, collaboration implies temporarily enduring the PMPs' "primitive" myths and superstitions, with the prospect of developing effective community links for health education and possibly testing the PMPs' botanical therapies. For the PMP, collaboration implies temporarily enduring the biomedical practitioners' limited understanding, with the prospect of assisting in a dire health crisis and possibly validating pluralistic-medical applications in other areas, such as STDs. Smiles, handshakes, and formal agreements aside, therefore, a great tension persists between African biomedical efforts to address the HIV/AIDS pandemic and these competing interpretations of material reality. Ironically, the only reason that biomedical practitioners view PMPs as useful partners is their holistic perspective that locates them at the nexus of a community's medical, spiritual, and social life and thereby positions PMPs so favorably for the purpose of health education. Collaboration is, in fact, premised on the PMPs' allegedly primitive myths and superstition. Ultimately, in the balance between biomedical and PMP interpretations of material reality, holism has arguably had a greater influence than biomedical atomism with respect to comprehensive African HIV/AIDS treatment and prevention plans.

Alongside African biomedical holism, a long-standing pragmatic attitude has been no less important in forging collaborative HIV/AIDS interventions between biomedical practitioners and PMPs. As discussed in Chapter 4, a deep-seated pragmatism within African pluralistic medicine stands in sharp contrast to a stubborn and long-standing biomedical orthodoxy. Within biomedicine, truth and understanding result from faithful adherence to specific techniques and procedures that mediate between individuals and the material world. The slightest deviation from these techniques and procedures would risk tainting one's observations with subjective bias. Consequently, there is an orthodox and unyielding commitment to "pure science" as the most accurate and objective measure of reality. It follows that medicine, as an extension of science, must apply this principle to the diagnosis and treatment of disease. African pluralistic medicine recognizes the value of this approach and often seeks to follow it. However, PMPs further contend that this is but one of the available paths to truth and understanding. While its insights are accepted with respect to a narrow range of phenomena pertaining to the natural world, PMPs believe it would be foolhardy to ignore those phenomena across the supernatural and social worlds—about which Western science offers few insights—that directly impact developments in the natural world. As is plain from the previous comments on holism in light of the HIV/AIDS pandemic, the orthodox biomedical model of medicine is clearly inadequate for addressing the full complexity of the ailment. Thus, in many ways, collaboration between biomedical practitioners and PMPs is an essential and necessary step, allowing biomedical practitioners to abandon the orthodoxy of their narrow beliefs and practices and to join the PMPs in a more nuanced and pragmatic understanding of HIV/AIDS as a multilayered reality. African biomedicine as a symbolic-cultural expression, therefore, embodies two basic tensions that further define African biomedicine as a dynamic and evolving set of beliefs and practices. In the context of African biomedicine's efforts to turn back HIV/AIDS, holism has largely subdued atomism as the primary perspective for framing the pandemic. At the same time, African pluralistic-medical pragmatism has overtaken biomedical orthodoxy in the search for paradigms to understand, and strategies to combat, HIV/AIDS in its full complexity. African biomedicine as a symbolic-cultural expression and as a scientific enterprise are thus mutually interdependent.

The contemporary HIV/AIDS pandemic has also exposed the often raw edges of African biomedicine as an expression of social power. The primary conflicts in this regard are those between biomedical practitioners and PMPs within Africa and those between the interests of Africans versus the interests of a host of global biomedical actors. Indeed, the HIV/AIDS pandemic has only further heightened a simmering competition between a cross-section of forces within African biomedicine as an expression of social power at the local, national, and global levels. At the local and national levels, HIV/AIDS has inspired calls for pragmatic collaboration across the continent. However, given the grave urgency introduced by HIV/AIDS, it has also provided the pretext for PMPS to insist upon greater social recognition and a larger role in medical care, alongside the demands of biomedical practitioners to retain the exclusive right to judge what is and is not sound medicine—and to direct state action to sanction those deemed unfit. In 2004, for example, South Africa passed the Traditional Health Practitioners Act that forbids unregistered PMPS from diagnosing or treating persons with HIV/AIDS.

At the global level, various agents on behalf of global biomedical interests, such as USAID or the World Bank's Multi-Country HIV/AIDS Project for Africa and the Caribbean (MAP), have largely usurped African autonomy with respect to establishing medical priorities and designing HIV/AIDS interventions, through conditional funding that rewards certain features of African biomedicine and deters others. For example, USAID and MAP actively promote a number of neoliberal measures, such as the privatization of health care, outsourcing HIV/AIDS programs to NGOS, and healthcare financing reform.[22] In 1995, 87% of assistance from USAID to Kenya bypassed state agencies and went directly to NGOS (Iliffe, 2006:79).[23] O'Manique (2004:63) argues that, "NGOS create new circuits of power and hierarchy in the societies within which they operate, and are not necessarily accountable to their local constituents but to those who control the purse strings." By the first decade of the 21st century, for example, the World Bank had become the largest lender for AIDS prevention in Africa, further eroding the ability of the WHO and national governments to shape the global health agenda. Consequently, in the context of the HIV/AIDS pandemic, African biomedicine as an expression of social power encompasses a highly combustible combination of self-interested factions, each vying for autonomy, control, and profits.

The HIV/AIDS pandemic has furthered two basic patterns with respect to African biomedicine as an expression of social power at the local and national levels. On the one hand, continuing a practice begun in the early period of the postcolonial era, PMPS have moved to create professional associations for greater social recognition and respect.[24] In combination with their

[22] See Hansen and Zewdie (2002) for an analysis from the perspective of two World Bank employees.

[23] Given USAID's "buy American first" rules, this assistance can also be seen as an indirect payment to U.S.-based pharmaceutical corporations and other biomedical firms.

[24] At the same time, it must be recognized that greater PMP power and influence is by no means unproblematic. PMPS often wield significant arbitrary power over women and others in society. Schoepf's (1992) cautionary description of abuses by Zairian PMPS in this regard certainly applies well beyond the borders of Zaire. "[African pluralistic medicine] rests upon etiological assumptions which many of us would not wish to bolster, particularly since women and the elderly often tend to be blamed for 'causing' illness and death. Healers and politicians sometimes seek to enhance their social power by claiming to have caused death by sorcery. Alternatively, accusations may be made against political opponents in order to reduce their effectiveness" (p. 235).

broad base of popular support across African societies, these efforts to organize have established PMPS as an often formidable faction within African biomedicine, with a clear understanding of their rights and their interests. On the other hand, biomedical practitioners have moved with equal vigor to implore the state to regulate and restrict PMPS as medical practitioners. Often relying on ties to social elites, biomedical practitioners have made significant gains in positioning themselves as the final arbiter of that which is medically appropriate and that which is not. Though still badly under-resourced, African biomedical practitioners have battled to enhance their status and influence within African biomedicine. Consequently, the formal care available for HIV/AIDS treatment through African biomedicine reveals both a greater recognition for the role of PMPS and the tightening grip of biomedical gatekeepers. The HIV/AIDS pandemic has, therefore, significantly intensified the competition between PMPS and African biomedical practitioners throughout the postcolonial era within African biomedicine.

Meanwhile, the HIV/AIDS pandemic has opened African biomedicine, as an expression of social power, to even greater pressures from a sprawling collection of global biomedical interests and their surrogates. Given the scale of the HIV/AIDS humanitarian disaster across Africa, global aid agencies have been able to leverage large-scale African suffering and dictate the terms of assistance with regard to standards of care, treatment protocols, and prevention strategies—notwithstanding the often glaring discrepancies between the values, beliefs, and practices of African biomedicine and those of global aid officers. In the mid-1980s, the United Nations and its agencies took the initial lead in devising a coordinated response to HIV/AIDS in Africa. In 1986, representatives from the WHO, the World Bank, the United States, Europe, and Japan met and established the Global Program on AIDS. (This was replaced by UNAIDS in 1994.) By the early 1990s, however, the United States, the Europeans, the World Bank, and others had each developed their own HIV/AIDS policies and programs. Consequently, USAID and the World Bank have been instrumental in establishing HIV/AIDS standards of care and treatment protocols premised on biomedical beliefs and practices that introduce sociocultural values and norms that facilitate the development of markets for biomedical goods and services both related and unrelated to HIV/AIDS. Indeed, earlier World Bank efforts to privatize medical care in Africa included the imposition of fee-for-service models. In Zambia, this resulted in an 80% drop in the use of urban health centers throughout the 1980s, further exacerbating the HIV/AIDS pandemic (Iliffe, 2006:64). By the late 1990s, in parallel fashion, a number of private/public collaborative schemes, such as the Global Public Private Partnerships, were increasingly turning the public health agenda directly over to the representatives of global biomedical interests. For instance, following the UN's Global Compact in 2000, UNAIDS moved to "partner" with five pharmaceutical companies.

The major influence of these global actors on African biomedicine as an expression of social power concerns the implicit Western biomedical values and norms embodied in the treatment and prevention protocols promoted by global aid agencies. As suggested by the foreword to the 2002 UNAIDS report cited above, the HIV/AIDS treatment and prevention strategies promoted by global aid agencies tend to emphasize cultural competence as a requisite feature of successful interventions. However, rather than developing cultural competence for the purpose of better understanding a local community's priorities, this is used to design communication strategies that allow health care workers to manipulate messages and thereby secure a community's acceptance of their pre-established priorities. The long-term implications of this approach cannot escape the long shadow of the original civilizing mission of the West and the dream of African "modernization." Indeed, rather than as an obstacle for African development, HIV/AIDS is at times portrayed as a tragically fortuitous pretext for modernity. "[T]he HIV/AIDS epidemic, so often seen as a metaphor for Africa's failure to achieve modernity, might instead be the vehicle by which medical modernity became predominant within the continent" (Iliffe, 2006:157). In this process, the beliefs and practices of African biomedicine are treated as "cultural" impediments to be understood and thereby overcome rather than as innovative African medical contributions that point to certain limitations of Western biomedical understanding. In the context of the HIV/AIDS pandemic, African biomedicine as an expression of social power, therefore, is informed by conflict at two levels. The competition between the interests of PMPS versus the interests of biomedical practitioners plays out at the local and national levels in the form of professional associations and state regulations. The competition between the interests of African biomedicine versus the interests of a global biomedical-industrial complex plays out at the global level in the form of conditional foreign aid, mediated by core-based, global aid agencies. In this fashion, the HIV/AIDS pandemic, as an event in the postcolonial era, simultaneously shapes and deepens the interrelationships between African biomedicine as a scientific enterprise, as a symbolic-cultural expression and as an expression of social power.

African Biomedicine and the Capitalist World-System over the *Longue Durée*

By readjusting the lens to turn our view away from African biomedicine at the level of the HIV/AIDS pandemic as a short-term event and the postcolonial era as a middle-run episode, we redirect our gaze to African biomedicine at the level of the capitalist world-system over the *longue durée*. From this angle of vision, African biomedicine as a singular historical-cultural formation is more clearly brought into focus and the incorporation of Africa into the capitalist world-system provides a further context for the development of African biomedicine as an ontological whole. As Western biomedicine travels the globe, it is increasingly confronted with its own ontological contradictions and with the limitations of its epistemological premises. It is thus that the centuries-old narrative of Western biomedicine is superseded by the new lineage of African biomedicine. Understood as but one of its latest incarnations, African biomedicine radically reconstitutes biomedicine as a scientific enterprise, as a symbolic-cultural expression, and as an expression of social power. Thus, as an ontological whole, African biomedicine emerges via Africa's incorporation into the capitalist world-system over the *longue durée* as the most highly developed realization of biomedicine itself.

As a scientific enterprise, African biomedicine both confronts and subverts the self-ascribed universality of Western biomedicine as it has developed over the *longue durée*. True to its imperious nature, Western biomedicine is able to reconstitute the scientific content of African pluralistic medicine largely in its own image. The 21st-century African hospital, clinic, or medical school is modeled closely after those found in the West. Furthermore, within the confines of these institutions, the rudimentary protocols of Western biomedical diagnosis and treatment are respected and adhered to. Nonetheless, these institutions are not the totality of African biomedicine. They represent but one vital and indispensable aspect of an African medical system that spans a broader range of sociocultural beliefs and practices than ordinarily found in Western medical systems. Consequently, African biomedicine as a scientific enterprise *and* as an evolving singular historical-cultural formation retains a host of competing explanatory models, combining elements of Western biomedicine with those of African pluralistic medicine. Two of the features that most distinguish Western biomedicine as a scientific enterprise are its faith in the universality of its etiological rationale and the universality of its criteria for judging the efficacy of treatments. African biomedicine as a scientific enterprise challenges each of these. Consequently, viewed over the *longue durée*, African biomedicine represents an expansion of biomedicine's etiological rationale and a challenge to its purportedly culturally neutral interpretation of efficacy.

African biomedicine is premised on overlapping and interrelated etiological explanations across the natural, supernatural, and social worlds. This neither questions nor replaces the etiological rationale of Western biomedicine. Rather, it mines the etiological explanations of Western biomedicine to maximize one's understanding of those important phenomena restricted to the natural world, while preserving those etiological explanations tied to the supernatural and social worlds. African biomedicine is able thereby to expand the etiological rationale of Western biomedicine and create a more developed and nuanced understanding of illness, as a subcategory of misfortune. African biomedicine as a scientific enterprise, framed as a moment in the life history of biomedicine as a singular historical-cultural formation, reveals the reflexive nature of historical-cultural developments across the capitalist world-system. As biomedicine travels to Africa, via the processes of incorporation and colonial subjugation, it reshapes medical systems across the continent. Similarly, those new medical systems that result, insofar as they are now constituent elements of the capitalist world-system, are creations of and represent the ongoing development of biomedicine as a singular historical-cultural formation. Those overlapping and interrelated etiological explanations that comprise African biomedicine do so as extensions of an etiological rationale that defines biomedicine as a global phenomenon across a single capitalist world-system. Developments within 21st-century African biomedicine are as much moments in the history of biomedicine as is 19th-century germ theory.

In a similar fashion, African biomedicine as a scientific enterprise undermines Western claims of culturally neutral criteria for interpreting efficacy. Given the premise of mutually interdependent natural, supernatural, and social worlds, it stands to reason that those Western measures of efficacy pertaining to phenomena in the natural world will likely prove less valid measures of phenomena in the supernatural or social worlds. From the perspective of African biomedicine, for example, to ignore the potential role of the second spear is both naive and dangerous. It is a form of malpractice that follows from a Western cultural judgment, not a fully informed medical judgment. Just as Western biomedicine debates the criteria for declaring a person clinically dead based on complex cultural considerations (see Chapter 2), African biomedicine debates the complex mix of natural, supernatural, and social factors in declaring a treatment successful or not. Again, framing these notions of African biomedical efficacy over the *longue durée,* it is evident that, as a constituent element of the capitalist world-system, African biomedicine and its scientific content are inseparable from the ongoing development of biomedicine as a singular historical-cultural formation. Thus, the extension of its etiological rationales and the exposure of the cultural limitations of its interpretations of efficacy are the inevitable results of recognizing African biomedicine as a scientific enterprise—occupying a unique moment over the life history of biomedicine more generally. In universalizing its scientific form, biomedicine particularizes its actual development.

As a symbolic-cultural expression, African biomedicine greatly weakens much of the ideological scaffolding erected by Western biomedicine over the *longue durée.* Absent the reductionist epistemological premises of Western biomedicine, African biomedicine does not internalize its cardinal dualisms—mind/body, natural/supernatural, body/soul. Consequently, African biomedicine as a symbolic-cultural expression mediates between competing modes of explanation within African biomedicine and between Western and African collective worldviews. In the context of competing explanations within African biomedicine, the result is a strong holistic orientation. In the context of competing Western and African collective worldviews, the result is a dynamic pragmatism. Thus, African biomedicine as a symbolic-cultural expression recognizes the complexity of biomedicine, as an ontological whole, far more acutely than does Western biomedicine as a symbolic-cultural expression. The holism and pragmatism of African biomedicine is, therefore, able to lead biomedicine, as a singular historical-cultural formation, beyond the dull and atavistic ideological malaise of 20th-century Western biomedicine.

Ontological atomism is a hallmark of Western biomedicine as a symbolic-cultural expression. Consequently, African biomedical holism introduces significant disruption into the life history of biomedicine. As explored in Chapter 2, Western biomedicine's most basic organizational principles presume discrete domains and separate spheres across a highly-ordered and reductionist medical field. Given the nature of the mutually-interdependent natural, supernatural, and social worlds, African biomedicine as a symbolic-cultural expression interprets the discrete ontological premises of Western biomedicine as an ideological rationalization reflecting Western cultural values and beliefs. Recognizing the limited value of this perspective, African biomedicine restricts this narrow belief system to a small but influential sect of African biomedical practitioners. Thus, it exists within, and certainly influences but does not define, African biomedicine. For biomedicine as a singular historical-cultural formation over the *longue durée*, therefore, African biomedical holism frees it of its stubborn commitment to a one-sided ontological understanding of medicine. The necessary incorporation of social conditions as integral elements of one's holistic etiological rationale—as in the case of poverty and HIV/AIDS in Africa—is thus a direct contribution of African biomedicine as a symbolic-cultural expression over the *longue durée.* African biomedical holism contextualizes without discarding the atomistic ontological premises of Western biomedicine and thereby facilitates a dialogue between PMPS and African biomedical practitioners.

In like fashion, African biomedical pragmatism tempers the obstinate orthodoxy of Western biomedicine and its insular attitude toward competing medical systems. Those medical beliefs and practices that lie beyond the narrow epistemological premises of Western biomedicine are decreed void of practical insight or logical understanding for the practice of medicine proper. Often, Western medical practitioners will study such medical systems to appropriate proprietary botanicals or for the purpose of calculated subversion—as in the case of HIV/AIDS prevention in Africa—but that is the extent of their interest. African biomedical pragmatism, therefore, is a significant departure that, in fact, initially served as the genesis for African pluralistic medicine's absorption of Western biomedicine. African biomedicine as a symbolic-cultural expression supplants the ideological orthodoxy of Western biomedicine with a pragmatic and curious attitude toward nonbiomedical beliefs and practices. Consequently, as a development over the *longue durée* of biomedicine as a symbolic-cultural expression, African biomedical pragmatism first exposes and then supersedes Western biomedical orthodoxy and its exclusionary epistemological premises. Building on the ontological innovations of African biomedicine as a scientific enterprise over the *longue durée*, African biomedicine as a symbolic-cultural expression thus provides biomedicine, as a singular historical-cultural formation, with a new set of epistemological premises that mark a holistic and pragmatic turn in its unfolding life history.

As an expression of social power, African biomedicine further entangled African medical systems within the accelerating processes of biomedical rationalization and commodification in the service of capital accumulation on a world scale over the *longue durée*. As noted, Western biomedicine's once-settled ontological content and epistemological premises were now reopened. Here was the basis for drawing a greater and greater number of African pluralistic-medical practitioners, services, and products into the maelstrom of periphery-based production across the capitalist world-system. So long as biomedicine was restricted to products and services that conformed with a narrow set of precepts, it was problematic to expand the rationalization of medical processes and the commodification of medical services beyond a narrow range of practices. As African biomedicine broke down these restrictive precepts, it became possible for biomedicine, as a global biomedical-industrial complex, to appropriate further aspects of African pluralistic medicine. In somewhat ironic fashion, therefore, the large-scale rationalization and commodification of African biomedical beliefs and practices follows, in part, from its holistic and pragmatic premises.

The rationalization of African biomedicine is directly linked to conflicts between African biomedical practitioners and PMPs and the resulting professionalization of the latter. The battle between these sets of practitioners to define medicine proper, paralleling developments in the United States in the early 20th century, has had consequences well beyond the continent. Throughout the postcolonial era there has been a concerted effort by a global consortium of biomedical interests (including pharmaceutical firms, professional organizations, the World Bank, USAID, and WHO) to expand African markets for biomedical goods and services by linking African medical systems to the logic of a commodified Western biomedicine. On the one hand, this has resulted in African medical systems that are organized in rough conformity with the principles of capitalist production. On the other hand, viewed over the *longue durée*, the incorporation of African biomedicine has significantly expanded the combination of medical beliefs and practices that comprise biomedicine and its range of commodified goods and services. Ultimately, the increasing rationalization of African biomedicine, as a singular historical-cultural formation over the *longue durée*, has unleashed two major developments. On the one hand, there has been a significant reordering of African medical systems in conformity with the logic of capitalist production on a world scale. This follows from the holistic and pragmatic premises of African biomedicine. On the other hand, the capitalist world-system, along with one of its key historical-cultural formations, has demonstrated a remarkable capacity to absorb the unique and contradictory conceptual contributions of African biomedicine, thus hastening the processes of global accumulation. This follows from the enduring epistemological agnosticism of the capitalist world-system.

The rationalization and commodification of African biomedicine as an expression of social power over the *longue durée* is directly linked to its insertion into the global circuits of accumulation. Just as the global biomedical industries were able to turn the HIV/AIDS pandemic into a profitable enterprise, medical care more generally across the capitalist world-system serves the interests of capital accumulation. Importantly, HIV/AIDS in Africa serves the interests of accumulation on a world scale not simply via the provision of profitable services—though this can itself be a lucrative activity as international donors fund NGOs who purchase goods and services from Western firms on behalf of Africans. Just as important, however, is the manner by which the World Bank, WHO, USAID, and others are able to use the provision of HIV/AIDS care to refashion African biomedicine into a market-based medical system that is increasingly dependent on Western biomedical goods and services. Hence, accumulation across the capitalist world-system over the *longue durée* is enhanced by the ability of African biomedicine and other singular historical-cultural formations to transform sociocultural beliefs and practices in conformity with global processes of rationalization and commodification. African biomedicine as an expression of social power over the *longue durée*, therefore, represents the concerted efforts of various factions to control not necessarily the underlying beliefs and practices of African biomedicine but their sociocultural applications. At the local or national level, African biomedical practitioners fight to retain the authority to define medicine and PMPs struggle for recognition and respect. The result has been the rationalization of PMPs in the guise of their professionalization and regulation. At the global level, African biomedicine as a singular historical-cultural formation has been co-opted as a unique brand of biomedicine. The result of these processes has been the ongoing domestication of African biomedicine at the behest of core-based investors from the global biomedical-industrial complex.

African Biomedicine and Transformation of the Capitalist World-System

The web of connections between African biomedicine and the capitalist world-system are by no means incidental. African biomedicine first came to be and continues to flourish as a singular historical-cultural formation across the expanding capitalist world-system. Absent its relationship to the capitalist world-system, African biomedicine remains an abstraction. Indeed, African biomedicine is no less a product of the continent's incorporation than the African railroad, telegraph, or semi-industrialized port city. The analysis of African biomedicine as a constituent element of the capitalist world-system, therefore, is inseparable from those processes of African incorporation and ongoing peripheralization. Several compelling storylines follow from this. From one angle of vision, African biomedicine appears to be a direct result of African incorporation and an instrument for its continuing peripheralization and sociocultural transformation. From a second angle of vision, as a singular historical-formation, African biomedicine suggests the capacity of African pluralistic medicine to absorb and radically reconstitute Western biomedicine. From a third angle of vision, as a constituent element of the capitalist world-system, African biomedicine seems to occupy a prime position from which to influence directly the further development of the capitalist world-system.

In the wake of Western global expansion, a variety of historical-cultural formations have played critical roles in hastening sociocultural adaptation across the African continent. From the church and the school house to the clinic and the movie house, there has been a delicate negotiation whereby the barbarian is first made aware of his or her savagery before the civilizing influence of Western cultural beliefs and practices are then generously prescribed. Acceptance of one's savagery and reverence for the West is considered the first step in a long recovery. Recognizing and moving beyond the backward and primitive superstitions of African pluralistic medicine is thus a major step in this evolution. As in the case of other historical-cultural formations, however, the transformation of African pluralistic medicine is never complete and the result is rarely an exact replica of Western biomedicine. Ultimately, it is sufficient for Africans to modify African pluralistic medicine in a fashion that roughly imitates Western biomedicine—emphasizing that which matches biomedicine, such as natural explanations and commodification, and downplaying that which conflicts with biomedicine, such as supernatural explanations. The result of this is African biomedicine, a singular historical-cultural formation that pays due deference to Western cultural beliefs and practices, while retaining a host of cardinal African pluralistic-medical features. For the capitalist world-system, the ongoing peripheralization of Africa is premised, in part, on the continuing resonance of Western cultural influences (for example, interpretations of efficacy) and the ongoing integration of African markets for biomedical goods and services (such as HIV/AIDS medical treatment). In this way, Western biomedicine transforms African societies.

Once the capitalist world-system incorporates new territory, a process of adjustment proceeds both for the new territory and for the capitalist world-system. With respect to historical-cultural formations, there are two results from incorporation. First, its influence is spread over a larger spatial territory, while certain core features are weakened or discarded. A basic premise of Western biomedicine, for example, is a narrow etiology limited to natural explanations. This conflicts with African pluralistic etiologies. The result within African biomedicine is an eclectic etiological arrangement in which natural explanations occasionally predominate but never completely subsume supernatural and social explanations. The orthodox etiological premises of Western biomedicine are weakened. Second, historical-cultural formations must reach accommodation with certain sociocultural features of the new territory and thus reconstitute its basic features. The incorporation of Africa triggered the expanded influence of Western biomedicine across the continent. In the process, biomedicine as a historical-cultural formation facilitated the process of redefining African cultural beliefs and practices in the image of the West, as Western biomedicine pushed up against African collective worldviews. In the process of integrating Western biomedicine with its own sociocultural beliefs and practices, however, African collective worldviews pushed back and Africans have been able thereby to both assimilate and refashion this uniquely Western bequest. Holism and pragmatism, for example, are integral features of African biomedicine that have now infected and reconstituted the beliefs and practices of biomedicine as a singular historical-cultural formation. In this way, African societies transform biomedicine.

One result of African incorporation, therefore, has been a modified and expanded set of values, beliefs, and practices associated with biomedicine, as a singular historical-cultural formation and constituent element of the capitalist world-system. In this manner, Africans are able to influence not merely biomedicine but an integral feature of the capitalist world-system itself. This follows from the notion within world-systems analysis that the capitalist world-system and its constituent elements are mutually conditioning. The capitalist world-system is not a discrete body to which an African appendage has merely been grafted. The capitalist world-system is comprised of interrelated and interdependent structures and processes that constitute the capitalist world-system as a concrete whole. Consequently, Africa has been drawn into this mix of structures and processes via a web of enmeshed political, economic, and historical-cultural sinews. Africa enters into a series of relationships that comprise the capitalist world-system and it is via these relationships that Africa is, on the one hand, peripheralized and, on the other hand, able to influence the character of singular historical-cultural formations. In this way, African values, beliefs and practices infiltrate the capitalist world-system, however modestly, and African collective worldviews begin to challenge certain ideological precepts of accumulation on a world scale.

The capacity to absorb the broad range of global political, economic, and historical-cultural structures and processes only speaks to the insatiable voracity and astounding flexibility of the capitalist world-system. Indeed, were the tenets of global capitalism less amenable to local sociocultural beliefs and practices, Africans may have more easily challenged the incorporation and ongoing peripheralization of the continent. The capitalist world-system has survived and expanded over the *longue durée* precisely due to its remarkable ability to integrate and transform new territories and peoples while constantly revivifying and reinventing itself. The future of African biomedicine and the future of the capitalist world-system are now inextricably linked, and it is through this relationship of mutual interdependence that both Africa and the capitalist world-system continue to transform each other in fundamental ways.

References

Abu-Lughod, Janet. 1989. *Before European Hegemony: The World-System, A.D. 1250–1350.* Oxford, UK: University Press.

Ademuwagun, Zacchaeus. 1979. "The Challenge of the Co-Existence of Orthodox and Traditional Medicine in Nigeria." In *African Therapeutic Systems*, 165–170, edited by Zacchaeus Ademuwagun, John Ayoade, Ira Harrison, and Dennis Warren. Waltham, MA: Crossroads Press.

Aidoo, Thomas. 1982. "Rural Health Under Colonialism and Neocolonialism: A Survey of the Ghanaian Experience." *International Journal of Health Services*. 12(4):637–657.

Airhihenbuwa, Collins. 1995. *Health and Culture: Beyond the Western Paradigm*. Thousand Oaks, CA: Sage Publishers.

Ajayi, J. F. Ade, 1968. "The Continuity of African Institutions Under Colonialism." In *Emerging Themes of African History*, 189–200, edited by Terence Ranger. Nairobi: East African Publishing House.

Ajose, Oladele. 1957. "Preventive Medicine and Superstitions in Nigeria." *Africa: Journal of the International African Institute*, 27:268–274.

Akerele, Olayiwola. 1987. "The Best of Both Worlds: Bringing Traditional Medicine Up to Date." *Social Science and Medicine*, 24(2):177–181.

Akisanya, A. 1977. "Traditional Medical Practices and Therapeutics in Nigeria." In *Traditional Healing: New Science or New Colonialism? (Essays in Critique of Medical Anthropology)*, 231–241, edited by Philip Singer. New York: Conch Magazine Limited.

Amin, Samir. 1974. *Accumulation on a World Scale: A Critique of the Theory of Underdevelopment*. New York: Monthly Review Press.

———. 1972. "Underdevelopment and Dependency in Black Africa: Origins and Contemporary Forms." *Journal of Modern African Studies*, 10(4):503–524.

Anyinam, Charles. 1987. "Availability, Accessibility, Acceptability and Adaptability: Four Attributes of African Ethno-Medicine." *Social Science and Medicine*, 25(7): 803–811.

Appadurai, Arjun. 1995. "The Production of Locality." In *Counterworks: Managing the Diversity of Knowledge*, 204–225, edited by Richard Fardon. New York: Routledge Press.

Apter, Andrew. 1993. "Atinga Revisited: Yoruba Witchcraft and the Cocoa Economy, 1950–1951." In *Modernity and Its Malcontents: Ritual and Power in Postcolonial Africa*, 111–128, edited by Jean Comaroff and John Comaroff. Chicago: University of Chicago Press.

Argyle, W. J. 1969. "European Nationalism and African Tribalism." In *Tradition and Transition in East Africa: Studies in the Tribal Element in the Modern Era*, 41–58, edited by P. Gulliver. Berkeley: University of California Press.

Arnold, David. 1996. "Introduction: Tropical Medicine Before Manson." In *Warm Climates and Western Medicine: The Emergence of Tropical Medicine, 1500–1900*, 1–19, edited by David Arnold. Amsterdam: Editions Rodopi B. V.

———. 1993. "Medicine and Colonialism." In *Companion Encyclopedia of the History of Medicine, Vol. II*, 1393–1416, edited by W. F. Bynum and Roy Porter. London: Routledge.

———. 1988a. "Introduction: Disease, Medicine and Empire." In *Imperial Medicine and Indigenous Societies*, 1–26, edited by David Arnold. Manchester, UK: Manchester University Press.

———. 1988b. "Smallpox and Colonial Medicine in Nineteenth-Century India." In *Imperial Medicine and Indigenous Societies*, 45–65, edited by David Arnold. Manchester, UK: Manchester University Press.

Arrighi, Giovanni. 2002. "The African Crisis: World Systemic and Regional Aspect." *New Left Review*, 15:5–36.

———. 1994. *The Long Twentieth Century: Money, Power and the Origins of Our Times*. New York: Verso Press.

Asuni, Tolani. 1979. "Modern Medicine and Traditional Medicine." In *African Therapeutic Systems*, 176–81, edited by Zacchaeus Ademuwagun, John Ayoade, Ira Harrison, and Dennis Warren. Waltham, MA: Crossroads Press.

Austen, Ralph. 1993. "The Moral Economy of Witchcraft: An Essay in Comparative History." In *Modernity and Its Malcontents: Ritual and Power in Postcolonial Africa*, 89–110, edited by Jean Comaroff and John Comaroff. Chicago: University of Chicago Press.

———. 1987. *African Economic History: Internal Development and External Dependency*. Portsmouth, NH: Heinemann Educational Books, Inc.

Bach, Robert. 1982. "On the Holism of a World-System Perspective." In *World-Systems Analysis: Theory and Methodology*, 159–180, edited by Terence Hopkins and Immanuel Wallerstein. Beverly Hills, CA: Sage.

Baer, Hans. 2001. *Biomedicine and Alternative Healing Systems in America: Issues of Class, Race, Ethnicity and Gender*. Madison, WI: University of Wisconsin Press.

———. 1989. "The American Dominative Medical System as a Reflection of Social Relations in the Larger Society." *Social Science and Medicine*, 28(11):1103–1112.

Baer, Hans A., Merrill Singer, and Ida Susser. 2003. *Medical Anthropology and the World System*, 2nd Ed. Westport, CT: Praeger.

Bakx, Keith. 1991. "The 'Eclipse' of Folk Medicine in Western Society?" *Sociology of Health and Illness*,131:20–38.

Balandier, Georges. 1966. "The Colonial Situation: A Theoretical Approach." In *Social Change: The Colonial Situation*, 34–18, edited by Immanuel Wallerstein. New York: John Wiley & Sons.

Baronov, David. 2004. "Exporting Behavior Modification Models to a U.S. Colony: Public Health Workers and HIV/AIDS Prevention in Puerto Rico." *Caribbean Studies*, 32(2):105–144.

Baylies, Carolyn. 2000. "Overview: HIV/AIDS in Africa: Global and Local Inequalities and Responsibilities." *Review of African Political Economy*,28(86):487–500.

Beasley, William. 1981. *The Modern History of Japan*. New York. St. Martin's Press.

Beattie, John. 1967. "Divination in Bunyoro, Uganda." In *Magic, Witchcraft and Curing*, 211–231, edited by John Middleton. Garden City, NY: The Natural History Press.

Beaujard, Philippe. 1988. "Plantes et médécine traditionnelle dans le su-est de Madagascar." *Journal of Ethnopharmacology*, 23:165–265.

Beck, Ann. 1985. "Old and New Approaches to Medicine in Rhodesia and Zimbabwe." In *African Healing Strategies*, 182–189, edited by Brian M. du Toit and Ismail Abdalla. New York: Trado-Medic Books.

———. 1981. *Medicine, Tradition and Development in Kenya and Tanzania, 1920–1970*. Waltham, MA: Crossroads Press.

———. 1970. *A History of the British Medical Administration of East Africa*. Cambridge, MA: Harvard University Press.

Becker, Howard, Blanche Geer, Everett C. Hughes and Anselm Strauss. 1961. *The Boys in White: Student Culture in Medical Schools*. Chicago: University of Chicago Press.

Berliner, Howard. 1985. *A System of Scientific Medicine: Philanthropic Foundations in the Flexner Era*. New York: Tavistock.

———. 1982. "Medical Modes of Production." In *The Problem of Medical Knowledge: Examining the Social Construction of Medicine*, 162–173, edited by Peter Wright and Andrew Treacher. Edinburgh: Edinburgh University Press.

———. 1975. "A Larger Perspective on the Flexner Report." *International Journal of Health Services*, 5(4):573–592.

Bibeau, Gilles. 1982a. "New Legal Rules for an Old Art of Healing: The Case of the Zairian Healer's Association." *Social Science and Medicine*, 16(21):1843–1849.

———. 1982b. "A Systems Approach to Ngbandi Medicine." In *African Health and Healing Systems: Proceedings of a Symposium*, 43–84, edited by P. Stanley Yoder. Los Angeles: Crossroads Press.

———. 1979. "The WHO in Encounter with African Traditional Medicine: Theoretical Conceptions and Practical Strategies." In *African Therapeutic Systems*, 182–186, edited by Zacchaeus Ademuwagun, John Ayoade, Ira Harrison, and Dennis Warren. Waltham, MA: Crossroads Press.

Bibeau, Gilles, Ellen Corin, Mulinda Habi Buganza, Mabiala Mandela, Matumona Mahoya, Mukana Ka Mukana, Nsiala Miaka Makengo, Rashim Ahluwalia, and Bernard Méchin. 1980. *Traditional Medicine in Zaire: Present and Potential Contribution to the Health Services*. Ottowa: International Development Research Center.

Bichmann, Wolfgang. 1979. "Primary Health Care and Traditional Medicine—Considering the Background of Changing Health Care Concepts in Africa." *Social Science and Medicine*, 13B:175–182.

Bierlich, Bernhard. 1995. "Notions and Treatment of Guinea Worm in Northern Ghana." *Social Science and Medicine,* 41(4):501–509.

Bjerke, Svein. 1989. "Witchcraft as Explanation: The Case of the Zinza." In *Culture, Experience and Pluralism: Essays on African Ideas of Illness and Healing,* 219–234, edited by Anita Jacobson-Widding and David Westerlund. Uppsala: Almqvist & Wiksell International.

Boahen, A. Abu. 1987. *African Perspectives on Colonialism.* Baltimore: Johns Hopkins University Press.

Bodenheimer, Thomas. 1984. "The Transnational Pharmaceutical Industry and the Health of the World's People." In *Issues in the Political Economy of Health Care,* 187–216, edited by John McKinlay. London: Tavistock.

Bowles, B. 1979. "The Political Economy of Colonial Tanganyika, 1939–1961." In *Tanzania Under Colonial Rule,* 164–191, edited by M. H. Y. Kaniki. London: Longman Group Limited.

Brady, Erika. 2001. "Introduction." In *Healing Logics: Culture and Medicine in Modern Health Belief Systems,* 3–12, edited by Erika Brady. Logan, Utah: Utah State University Press.

Brandt, Allan and Martha Gardner. 2000. "The Golden Age of Medicine?" In *Medicine in the Twentieth Century,* 21–39, edited by Roger Cooter and John Pickstone. Amsterdam: Harwood Academic Publishers.

Braudel, Fernand. 1972. "History and the Social Sciences." In *Economy and Society in Early Modern Europe, Essays from* Annales, 11–42, edited by Peter Burke. New York: Harper & Row Publishers.

Braverman, Harry. 1974. *Labor and Monopoly Capital: The Degradation of Work in the Twentieth Century.* New York. Monthly Review Press.

Brett, E. A. 1973. *Colonialism and Underdevelopment in East Africa: The Politics of Economic Change, 1919–1939.* Brookfield, VT: Gregg Revivals.

Brown, E. Richard. 1979. *Rockefeller Medicine Men: Medicine and Capitalism in America.* Berkeley, CA: University of California Press.

———. 1978. "Public Health in Imperialism: Early Rockefeller Programs at Home and Abroad." In *The Cultural Crisis of Modern Medicine,* 252–270, edited by John Ehrenreich. New York: Monthly Review Press.

Bruce-Chwatt, L. and Joan Bruce-Chwatt. 1980. "Malaria and Yellow Fever." In *Health in Tropical Africa During the Colonial Period,* 43–58, edited by E. E. Sabben-Clare, David Bradley, and Kenneth Kirkwood. Oxford: Clarendon Press.

Buckley, Anthony. 1985a. *Yoruba Medicine.* Oxford: Clarendon Press.

———. 1985b. "The God of Smallpox: Aspects of Yoruba Religious Knowledge." *Africa: Journal of the International African Institute,* 55(2):187–200.

Burrow, James. 1977. *Organized Medicine in the Progressive Era: The Move Toward Monopoly.* Baltimore: Johns Hopkins University Press.

Buxton, J. 1973. *Religion and Healing in Mandari.* Oxford: Clarendon Press.

Bynum, William. 1994. *Science and the Practice of Medicine in the 19th Century.* New York: Cambridge University Press.

Canary, John and John Burton. 1983. "Modern Allopathic Medicine and Public Health." In *Traditional Medicine and Health Care Coverage: A Reader for Health Administrators and Practitioners,* 90–109, edited by Robert Bannerman, John Burton, and Ch'en Wen-Chieh. Geneva: World Health Organization.

Césaire, Aimé. 1972. *Discourse on Colonialism*. New York: Monthly Review Press.

Chandler, Alfred. 1977. *The Visible Hand: The Managerial Revolution in American Business*. Cambridge, MA: Harvard University Press.

Chase-Dunn, Christopher. 1989. *Global Formations: Structures of the World-Economy*. Cambridge, MA: Basil Blackwell.

Chavunduka, G. L. 1994. *Traditional Medicine in Modern Zimbabwe*. Harare: University of Zimbabwe Publications.

———. 1987. "Development of African Traditional Medicine: The Case of Zimbabwe." In *African Medicine in the Modern World* (Seminar Proceedings No. 27), 59–72. Edinburgh: University of Edinburgh, Centre of African Studies.

———. 1986. "The Organization of Traditional Medicine in Zimbabwe." In *The Professionalization of African Medicine*, 29–50, edited by Murray Last and G. L. Chavunduka. Manchester, UK: Manchester University Press.

———. 1978. *Traditional Healers and the Shona Patient*. Gwelo: Mambo Press.

Chavunduka, G. L. and Murray Last. 1986. "Conclusions: African Medical Professions Today." In *The Professionalization of African Medicine*, 259–269, edited by Murray Last and G. L. Chavunduka. Manchester, UK: Manchester University Press.

Chhabra, S. C., R.L.A. Mahunnah and E. N. Mshiu. 1990. "Plants Used in Traditional Medicine in Eastern Tanzania. IV. Angiosperms (*Momosaceae* to *Paplionaceae*)." *Journal of Ethnopharmacology*, 29(3):295–323.

Clarke, Adele, Laura Mamo, Jennifer Fishman, Janet Shim, and Jennifer Fosket. 2003. "Biomedicalization: Technoscientific Transformation of Health, Illness and U.S. Biomedicine." *American Sociological Review*, 68:161–194.

Clyde, David. 1980. "Tanzania." In *Health in Tropical Africa During the Colonial Period*, 98–113, edited by E. E. Sabben-Clare, David Bradley, and Kenneth Kirkwood. Oxford, UK: Clarendon Press.

Comaroff, Jean. 1993. "The Diseased Heart of Africa: Medicine, Colonialism and the Black Body." In *Knowledge, Power and Practice: The Anthropology of Medicine and Everyday Life*, 305–329, edited by Shirley Lindenbaum and Margaret Lock. Berkeley: University of California Press.

———. 1982. "Medicine: Symbol and Ideology." In *The Problem of Medical Knowledge: Examining the Social Construction of Medicine*, 49–69, edited by Peter Wright and Andrew Treacher. Edinburgh: Edinburgh University Press.

———. 1978, "Medicine and Culture." *Social Science and Medicine*, 12B:247–254.

Comaroff, Jean and John Comaroff. 1993. "Introduction." In *Modernity and Its Malcontents: Ritual and Power in Postcolonial Africa*, xi–xxxvii, edited by Jean Comaroff and John Comaroff. Chicago: University of Chicago Press.

Conco, W. Z. 1979. "The African Bantu Traditional Practice of Medicine: Some Preliminary Observations." In *African Therapeutic Systems*, 58–80, edited by Zacchaeus Ademuwagun, John Ayoade, Ira Harrison, and Dennis Warren. Waltham, MA: Crossroads Press.

Corin, Ellen. 1995. "The Cultural Frame: Context and Meaning in the Construction of Health." In *Society and Health*, 272–304, edited by Benjamin Amick. Cambridge, MA: Oxford University Press.

Curtin, Philip. 1996. "Disease and Imperialism." In *Warm Climates and Western Medicine: The Emergence of Tropical Medicine, 1500–1900*, 99–107, edited by David Arnold. Amsterdam: Editions Rodopi B. V.

Davidson, A. 1968. "African Resistance and Rebellion Against the Imposition of Colonial Rule." In *Emerging Themes of African History*, 177–188, edited by Terence Ranger. Nairobi: East African Publishing House.

Davis, Matthew and Paul Darden, 2003. "Use of Complementary and Alternative Medicine by Children in the United States." *Archives of Pediatric and Adolescent Medicine*, 157:393–396.

Davis-Roberts, Christopher. 1992. "*Kutambuwa Ugonjuwa*: Concepts of Illness and Transformation Among the Tabwa of Zaire." In *The Social Basis of Health and Healing in Africa*, 376–392, edited by Steven Feierman and John Janzen. Berkeley: University of California Press.

Dawson, Marc. 1987a. "The Anti-Yaws Campaign and Colonial Medical Policy in Kenya." *International Journal of African Historical Studies*, 20:417–437.

———. 1987b. "The Social History of Africa in the Future: Medical-Related Issues." *African Studies Review*, 30(2):83–91.

———. 1979. "Smallpox Vaccine in Kenya, 1880–1920." *Social Science and Medicine*, 13B:245–251.

DeJong, Jocelyn. 1991. *Traditional Medicine in Sub-Saharan Africa: Its Importance and Potential Policy Options*. Washington DC: The World Bank, Population and Human Resources Department [Working Papers, WPS (July) 735].

Denoon, Donald. 1988. "Temperate Medicine and Settler Capitalism: On the Reception of Western Medical Ideas." In *Disease, Medicine and Empire: Perspectives on Western Medicine and the Experience of European Expansion*, 121–138, edited by Roy MacLeod and Milton Lewis. New York: Routledge.

Devisch, René, Lapika Dimomfu, Jaak Le Roy, and Peter Crossman. 2001. "A Community-Action Intervention to Improve Medical Care Services in Kinshasa, Congo: Mediating the Realms of Healers and Physicians." In *Applying Health Social Science: Best Practice in the Developing World*, 107–140, edited by Nick Higginbotham, Roberto Briceño-León, and Nancy Johnson. London: Zed Books.

Douglas, Mary. 1963. "Techniques of Sorcery Control in Central Africa." In *Magic, Witchcraft and Curing*, 123–142, edited by John Middleton. Garden City, NY: The Natural History Press.

du Toit, Brian M. 1985. "The *Isangoma*: An Adaptive Agent Among Urban Zulu." In *African Healing Strategies*, 82–95, edited by Brian M. du Toit and Ismail Abdalla. New York: Trado-Medic Books.

Dubos, René. 1959. *Mirage of Health: Utopias, Progress and Biological Change*. New York: Anchor Books.

Duggan, A. 1980. "Sleeping Sickness Epidemics." In *Health in Tropical Africa During the Colonial Period*, 19–29, edited by E. E. Sabben-Clare, David Bradley, and Kenneth Kirkwood. Oxford: Clarendon Press.

Dunlop, David. 1974–1975. "Alternatives to 'Modern' Health-Delivery Systems in Africa: Issues for Public Policy Consideration on the Role of Traditional Healers." *Rural Africana*, 26:131–140.

Eisenberg, David, Roger Davis, S. Ettner, Scott Appel, Sonja Wilkey, Maria Van Rompay, and Ronald Kessler. 1998. "Trends in Alternative Medicine Use in the United States, 1990–1997: Results of a Follow-up National Survey." *Journal of American Medical Association*, 280(18):1569–75.

Eisenberg, David, Ronald Kessler, Maria Van Rompay, Ted Kaptchuk, Sonja Wilkey, Scott Appel, and Roger Davis. 2001. "Perceptions about Complementary Therapies Relative to Conventional Therapies among Adults Who Use Both: Results from a National Survey." *Annals of Internal Medicine,* 135:344–351.

Eisenberg, Leon. 1977. "Disease and Illness: Distinctions between Professional and Popular Ideas of Sickness." *Culture, Medicine and Psychiatry,* 1:9–23.

Elder, N. C., A. Gillcrist, and R. Minz. 1997. "Use of Alternative Health Care by Family Practice Patients." *Archives of Family Medicine,* 6:181–184.

Elling, Ray. 1981. "Political Economy, Cultural Hegemony and Mixes of Traditional and Modern Medicine." *Social Science and Medicine,* 15A:89–99.

Emmanuel, Arghiri. 1972. *Unequal Exchange: A Study of the Imperialism of Trade.* New York: Monthly Review Press.

Engel, George. 1977. "The Need for a New Medical Model: A Challenge for Biomedicine." *Science,* 196:129–136.

Engelhardt, H. Tristam, Jr. 1975. "The Concepts of Health and Disease." In *Evaluation and Explanation in the Biomedical Sciences,* 125–142, edited by H. Tristam Engelhardt, Jr. and Stuart Spicker. Boston: D. Reidel Publishing Company.

Epstein, Scarlett. 1967. "A Sociological Analysis of Witch Beliefs in a Mysore Village." In *Magic, Witchcraft and Curing,* 135–154, edited by John Middleton. Garden City, NY: The Natural History Press.

Etkin, Nina. 1988. "Cultural Constructions of Efficacy." In *The Context of Medicines in Developing Countries: Studies in Pharmaceutical Anthropology,* 299–326. edited by Sjaak Van Der Geest and Susan Whyte. Dordrecht: Kluwer Academic Publishers.

———. 1981. "A Hausa Herbal Pharmacopoeia: Biomedical Evaluation of Commonly Used Plant Medicines." *Journal of Ethnopharmacology,* 4:75–98.

Evans-Pritchard, E. E. 1976 [1937]. *Witchcraft, Oracles and Magic Among the Azande.* Oxford, UK: Clarendon Press.

Ezeabasili, N. 1982. "Traditional Ibo Ideas about Disease and Its Treatments: Nigerial Perspectives on Medical Sociology." *Studies in Third World Societies,* (March):17–28.

Fábrega, Horacio. 1997. *Evolution of Sickness and Healing.* Berkeley, CA: University of California Press.

Fanon, Frantz. 1967. "Medicine and Colonialism." In *A Dying Colonialism,* 121–145. New York: Grove Press.

———. 1965. *The Wretched of the Earth.* New York: Grove Press.

Farley, John. 1992. "Parasites and the Germ Theory of Disease." In *Framing Disease: Studies in Cultural History,* 33–49, edited by Charles Rosenberg and Janet Golden. New Brunswick, NJ: Rutgers University Press.

———. 1988. "Bilharzia: A Problem of 'Native Health,' 1900–1950." In *Imperial Medicine and Indigenous Societies,* 189–207, edited by David Arnold. Manchester, UK: Manchester University Press.

Farmer, Paul. 2003. *Pathologies of Power: Health, Human Rights and the New War on the Poor.* Berkeley: University of California Press.

———. 2001. *Infections and Inequalities: The Modern Plagues.* Berkeley: University of California Press.

Fassin, Didier and Eric Fassin. 1988. "Traditional Medicine and the Stakes of Legitimation in Senegal." *Social Science and Medicine,* 27(4):353–357.

Feierman, Steven. 1985. “Struggles for Control: The Social Roots of Health and Healing in Modern Africa.” *African Studies Review*, 28(2–3):73–147.

———. 1979. “Change in African Therapeutic Systems.” *Social Science and Medicine*, 13B:277–284.

Feldman, Jamie. 1992. “The French *are* Different: French and American Medicine in the Context of AIDS.” *Western Journal of Medicine*, 157(30):5–9.

Ferguson, Anne. 1988. “Commercial Pharmaceutical Medicine and Medicalization: A Case Study from El Salvador.” In *The Context of Medicines in Developing Countries: Studies in Pharmaceutical Anthropology*, 19–46, edited by Sjaak Van Der Geest and Susan Whyte. Dordrecht: Kluwer Academic Publishers.

Ferguson, D. 1979. “The Political Economy of Health and Medicine in Colonial Tanganyika.” In *Tanzania Under Colonial Rule*, 307–343, edited by M.H.Y. Kaniki. London: Longman Group Limited.

Figlio, Karl. 1976. “The Metaphor of Organization: An Historiographical Perspective on the Bio-Medical Sciences in the Early Nineteenth Century.” *History of Science*, 14:17–35.

Finkler, Kaja. 1994. “Sacred Healing and Biomedicine Compared.” *Medical Anthropology Quarterly*, 8(2):178–197.

Fiscella, Kevin, Peter Franks, Marthe Gold, and Carolyn Clancy. 2000. “Inequality in Quality: Addressing Socioeconomic, Racial, and Ethnic Disparities in Health Care.” *Journal of the American Medical Association*, 283:2579–2584.

Flint, Karen. 2001. “Competition, Race, and Professionalization: African Healers and White Medical Practitioners in Natal, South Africa in the Early Twentieth Century.” *Social History of Medicine*, 14(2):199–221.

Foster, George. 1983. “An Introduction to Ethnomedicine.” In *Traditional Medicine and Health Care Coverage: A Reader for Health Administrators and Practitioners*, 17–24, edited by Robert Bannerman, John Burton, and Ch’en Wen-Chieh. Geneva: World Health Organization.

———. 1976. “Disease Etiologies in Non-Western Medical Systems.” *American Anthropologist*, 78(4):773–782.

Frank, Andre Gunder. 1967. *Capitalism and Underdevelopment in Latin America: Historical Studies of Chile and Brazil*, New York: Monthly Review Press.

———. 1978. *World Accumulation, 1492–1789*. New York: Monthly Review Press.

Frankenberg, Ronald and Joyce Leeson. 1976. “Disease, Illness and Sickness: Social Aspects of the Choice of Healer in a Lusaka Suburb.” In *Social Anthropology and Medicine*, 223–258, edited by Joseph Loudon. New York: Academic Press.

Gadamer, Hans-Georg. 1996. *The Enigma of Health: The Art of Healing in a Scientific Age*. Translated by Jason Gaiger and Nicholas Walker. Stanford, CA: Stanford University Press.

Gaines, Atwood. 1992. “Medical/Psychiatric Knowledge in France and the United States: Culture and Sickness in History and Biology.” In *Ethnopsychiatry: The Cultural Construction of Professional and Folk Psychiatries*, 171–201, edited by Atwood Gaines. Albany: State University of New York Press.

Gbeassor, M., Y. Kossou, K. Amegbo, C. de Souza, K. Koumaglo and A. Denke. 1989. “Antimalarial Effects of Eight African Medicinal Plants.” *Journal of Ethnopharmacology*, 25:115–118.

Gbodossou, Erick, Virginia Davis Floyd, and Charles Ibnou Katy. 2005. *AIDS in Africa: Scenarios for the Future, The Role of Traditional Medicine in Africa's Fight Against HIV/AIDS*. Dakar, Senegal: PROMETRA Document.

Gelfand, Michael. 1976. *A Service to the Sick: A History of the Health Services for Africans in Southern Rhodesia (1890–1953)*. Gwelo: Mambo Press.

———. 1964a. *Witch Doctor, Traditional Medicine Man of Rhodesia*. London: Harvill Press.

———. 1964b. "Psychiatric Disorders as Recognized by the Shona." In *Magic, Faith and Healing: Studies in Primitive Psychiatry Today*, 156–174, edited by Ari Kiev. New York: Free Press.

Gelfand, Toby. 1993. "The History of the Medical Profession." In *Companion Encyclopedia for the History of Medicine, Vol. II*, 1119–1150, edited by W. F. Bynum and Roy Porter. New York: Routledge.

Gereffi, Gary. 1983. "The Internationalization and Structure of the Global Pharmaceutical Industry." In *The Pharmaceutical Industry and Dependency in the Third World*, 167–189. Princeton, NJ: Princeton University Press.

Germani, Gino. 1975. "Stages of Modernization in Latin America." In *Latin America: The Dynamics of Social Change*, 1–43, edited by Stefan Halper and John Sterling. New York: St. Martin's Press.

Gessler, M. C., D. E. Msuya, M.H.H. Nkunya, A. Schar, M. Heinrich, and M. Tanner. 1995. "Traditional Healers in Tanzania: Sociocultural Profile and Three Short Portraits." *Journal of Ethnopharmacology*, 48(3):145–160.

Gillies, Eva. 1976a. "Causal Criteria in African Classifications of Disease." In *Social Anthropology and Medicine*, 358–395, edited by Joseph Loudon. New York: Academic Press.

———. 1976b. "Introduction." In *Witchcraft, Oracles and Magic Among the Azande*, vii–xxix, by E. E. Evans-Pritchard. Oxford: Clarendon Press.

Gillett, Grant. 2004. "Clinical Medicine and the Quest for Certainty." *Social Science and Medicine*, 58(4):727–738.

Gluckman, Max. 1968. "Social Beliefs and Individual Thinking in Tribal Society." In *Theory in Anthropology: A Sourcebook*, 453–464, edited by Robert Manners and David Kaplan Chicago: Aldine Publishing Company.

Good, Byron. 1994. "Medical Anthropology and the Problem of Belief." In *Medicine, Rationality, and Experience: An Anthropological Perspective*, 1–24, by Byron Good. Cambridge, MA: Cambridge University Press.

Good, Byron and Mary-Jo DelVecchio Good. 1993. "'Learning Medicine': The Construction of Medical Knowledge at Harvard Medical School." In *The Anthropology of Medicine and Everyday Life*, 81–107, edited by Shirley Lindenbaum and Margaret Lock. Berkeley: University of California Press.

Good, Charles. 1991. "Pioneer Medical Missions in Colonial Africa." *Social Science and Medicine*, 32:1–10.

———. 1988. "Traditional Healers and AIDS Management." In *AIDS in Africa: The Social and Policy Impact*, 97–114, edited by Norman Miller and Richard Rockwell. Lewiston, NY: The Edwin Mellen Press.

———. 1987. *Ethnomedical Systems in Africa: Patterns of Traditional Medicine in Rural and Urban Kenya*. New York: Guilford Press.

———. 1980. "A Comparison of Rural and Urban Ethnomedicine Among the Kamba of Kenya." In *Traditional Health Care Delivery in Contemporary Africa*, 3–56, edited by Priscilla Ulin and Marshall Segall. Foreign and Comparative Studies/African Series XXXV. Syracuse: Maxwell School.

Good, Mary-Jo Delvecchio. 1995. "Cultural Studies of Biomedicine: An Agenda for Research." *Social Science and Medicine,* 41(4):461–473.

Goody, Esther. 1970. "Legitimate and Illegitimate Aggression in a West African State." In *Witchcraft Confessions and Accusations*, 207–245, edited by Mary Douglas. London: Tavistock.

Gordon, Deborah. 1988. "Tenacious Assumptions in Western Medicine." In *Biomedicine Reconsidered*, 19–56, edited by Margaret Lock and Deborah Gordon. Dordrecht: Kluwer Academic Publishers.

Gottlieb, Alma. 1989. "Witches, Kings and the Sacrifice of Identity Among the Beng of Ivory Coast." In *Creativity of Power: Cosmology and Art in African Societies*, 245–272, edited by W. Aren and I. Karp. Washington DC: Smithsonian Institute.

Gray, Robert. 1963. "Some Structural Aspects of Mbugwe Witchcraft." In *Witchcraft and Sorcery in East Africa*, 143–174, edited by John Middleton and E. H. Winter. London: Routledge and Kegan Paul.

Green, Edward. 1999. *Indigenous Theories of Contagious Disease*. Walnut Creek, CA: Alta Mira Press.

———. 1996. *Indigenous Healers and the African State: Policy Issues Concerning African Indigenous Healers in Mozambique and Southern Africa*. New York: Pact Publications.

———. 1994. *AIDS and STDS in Africa: Bridging the Gap Between Traditional Healing and Modern Medicine*. Boulder, CO: Westview Press.

———. 1988. "Can Collaborative Programs Between Biomedical and African Indigenous Health Practitioners Succeed?" *Social Science and Medicine*, 27:1125–1130.

Grob, Gerald. 1994. *The Mad Among Us: A History of the Care of America's Mentally Ill*. New York: The Free Press.

Guenther, M. 1979. "Bushman Religion and the (Non)sense of Anthropological Theory of Religion." *Sociologus*, 29(2):102–132.

Guha, Ranajit. 1983. *Elementary Aspects of Peasant Insurgency in Colonial India*. Durham, NC: Duke University Press.

Gyeke, Kwame. 1997. "Tradition and Modernity." In *Tradition and Modernity: Philosophical Reflections on the African Experience*, 217–271. New York: Oxford University Press.

Hahn, Robert. 1995. *Sickness and Healing: An Anthropological Perspective.* New Haven, CT: Yale Press.

———. 1985. "Culture-Bound Syndromes Unbound." *Social Science and Medicine*, 21:165–171.

———. 1984. "Rethinking 'Illness' and 'Disease.'" *Contributions to Asian Studies*, 18:1–23.

———. 1983. "Biomedical Practice and Anthropological Theory: Frameworks and Directions." *Annual Review of Anthropology*, 12:305–333.

———. 1982. "'Treat the Patient, Not the Lab': Internal Medicine and the Concept of 'Person.'" *Culture, Medicine and Psychiatry*,6:219–236.

Hajjar, Ihab and Theodore Kotchen. 2003. "Trends in Prevalence, Awareness, Treatment, and Control of Hypertension in the United States, 1988–2000." *Journal of the American Medical Association*, 290:199–206.

Haller, John. 1997. *Kindly Medicine: Physio-Medicalism in America, 1836–1911*. Kent, OH: Kent State University Press.

Hansen, Keith and Debrework Zewdie. 2002. "International Cooperation and Mobilization." In *AIDS in Africa*, 2nd Ed., 695–709, edited by Max Essex, Souleymane Mboup, Phyllis Kanki, Richard Marlink, and Sheila Tlou. New York: Kluwer Academic/Plenum Publishers.

Harjula, Raimo. 1989. "Curse as a Manifestation of Broken Human Relationships Among the Maasai of Tanzania." In *Culture, Experience and Pluralism: Essays on African Ideas of Illness and Healing*, 125–138, edited by Anita Jacobson-Widding and David Westerlund. Uppsala: Almqvist & Wiksell International.

Harrison, Ira. 1979. "Traditional Healers as a Source of Traditional and Contemporary Powers." In *African Therapeutic Systems*, 95–97, edited by Zacchaeus Ademuwagun John Ayoade, Ira Harrison, and Dennis Warren. Waltham, MA: Crossroads Press.

———. 1974. "Traditional Healers: A Neglected Source of Health Manpower." *Rural Africana*, 26(1):5–16.

Hayter, Teresa. 1971. *Aid as Imperialism*. New York: Pelican Books.

Headrick, Daniel. 1981. "Malaria, Quinine and the Penetration of Africa." In *The Tools of Empire: Technology and European Imperialism in the Nineteenth Century*, 58–82. New York: Oxford University Press.

Helman, Cecil. 2000. *Culture, Health and Illness*. Boston: Butterworth-Heinemann.

Herbert, Eugenia. 1975. "Smallpox Inoculation in Africa." *Journal of African History*, 16(4):539–559.

Herskovits, Melville and William Bascom. 1959. "The Problem of Stability and Change in African Culture." In *Continuity and Change in African Cultures*, 1–14, edited by William Bascom and Melville Herskovits. Chicago: University of Chicago Press.

Hirschman, Albert. 1958. *The Strategy of Economic Development*. New Haven, CT: Yale University Press.

Hobsbawm, Eric. 2000. *Bandits*. New York: New Press.

———. 1989. *The Age of Empire, 1875–1914*. New York: Vintage Books.

Hofstadter, Richard. 1955. *The Age of Reform*. New York: Vintage Books.

Homsy, Jaco et al. 1999. "Evaluating Herbal Medicine for the Management of Herpes Zoster in HIV-Infected Patients in Kampala, Uganda." *Journal of Alternative and Complementary Medicine*, 5(6):553–565.

Hopkins, Terence. 1982a. "The Study of the Capitalist World-Economy: Some Introductory Considerations." In *World-Systems Analysis: Theory and Methodology*, 9–38, edited by Terence Hopkins and Immanuel Wallerstein. Beverly Hills, CA: Sage.

———. 1982b. "World-Systems Analysis: Methodological Issues." In *World-Systems Analysis: Theory and Methodology*, 145–158, edited by Terence Hopkins and Immanuel Wallerstein. Beverly Hills, CA: Sage.

Hopkins, Terence and Immanuel Wallerstein. 1987. "Capitalism and the Incorporation of New Zones into the World-Economy." *Review—Fernand Braudel Center for the Study of Economies, Historical Systems and Civilizations*, 10 (5–6):763–779.

———. 1982. "Structural Transformations of the World-Economy." In *World-Systems Analysis: Theory and Methodology*, 121–142, edited by Terence Hopkins and Immanuel Wallerstein. Beverly Hills, CA: Sage.

Hopkins, Terence and Immanuel Wallerstein et al. 1982. "Patterns of Development of the Modern World-System." In *World-Systems Analysis: Theory and Methodology*, 41–82, edited by Terence Hopkins and Immanuel Wallerstein. Beverly Hills, CA: Sage.

Hopwood, B. 1980. "Primary Health Care in Uganda, 1894–1962." In *Health in Tropical Africa During the Colonial Period*, 147–157, edited by E. E. Sabben-Clare, David Bradley, and Kenneth Kirkwood. Oxford: Clarendon Press.

Horton, Robin. 1967. "African Traditional Thought and Western Science." *Africa: Journal of the International African Institute*, 37:50–71, 155–187.

———. 1962. "The Kalabari World Views: An Outline and Interpretation." *Africa: Journal of the International African Institute*, 32(3):197–219.

Hours, Bernard. 1987. "African Medicine as an Alibi and as a Reality." In *African Medicine in the Modern World* (Seminar Proceedings No. 27), 41–58. Edinburgh: University of Edinburgh, Centre of African Studies.

Hudson, Robert. 1983. "Disease as Supernatural." In *Disease and Its Control: The Shaping of Modern Thought*, 55–74. Westport, CT: Greenwood Press.

Huntington, Samuel. 1968. *Political Order in Changing Societies*. New Haven, CT: Yale University Press.

Iliffe, John. 2006. *The African AIDS Epidemic: A History*. Athens: Ohio University Press.

———. 2002. *East African Doctors: A History of the Modern Profession*. Kampala, Uganda: Fountain Publishers.

Imperato, Pascal. 1979. "Traditional Medical Practitioners Among the Bambara of Mali and Their Role in the Modern Health Care Delivery System." In *African Therapeutic Systems*, 202–207, edited by Zacchaeus Ademuwagun, John Ayoade, Ira Harrison, and Dennis Warren. Waltham, MA: Crossroads Press.

Imperato, Pascal and D. Traoré. 1979. "Traditional Beliefs about Measles and Its Treatment among the Bambara of Mali." In *African Therapeutic Systems*, 19–21, edited by Zacchaeus Ademuwagun, John Ayoade, Ira Harrison, and Dennis Warren. Waltham, MA: Crossroads Press.

Inkeles, Alex. 1969. "Making Men Modern: On the Causes and Consequences of Individual Change in Six Developing Countries." *American Journal of Sociology*, 75:208–225.

Jansen, G. 1973. *The Doctor-Patient Relationship in an African Tribal Society*. Assen, The Netherlands: Van Orcum.

Jansen, Marius. 2000. *The Making of Modern Japan*. Cambridge, MA: Harvard University Press.

Janzen, John. 1992. *Ngoma: Discourses of Healing in Central and Southern Africa*. Berkeley: University of California Press.

———. 1989. "Health, Religion and Medicine in Central and Southern African Traditions." In *Caring and Curing: Health and Medicine in World Religious Traditions*, 225–254, edited by L. Sullivan. New York: Macmillan.

———. 1985. "Changing Concepts of African Therapeutics: An Historical Perspective." In *African Healing Strategies*, 61–81, edited by Brian M. du Toit and Ismail Abdalla. New York: Trado-Medic Books.

———. 1982. *Lemba, 1650–1930: A Drum of Affliction in Africa and the New World*. New York: Garland Publishing.

———. 1981. "The Need for a Taxonomy of Health in the Study of African Therapeutics." *Social Science and Medicine*, 15B(3):185–194.

———. 1978. *The Quest for Therapy in Lower Zaire*. Berkeley: University of California Press.

———. 1976–77. "Traditional Medicine Now Seen as National Resource in Zaire and Other African Countries." *Ethnomedizin*, 4(1–2):167–70.

Jones, R. Kenneth. 2004. "Schism and Heresy in the Development of Orthodox Medicine: The Threat to Medical Hegemony." *Social Science and Medicine*, 58(4): 703–712.

Josephson, Matthew. 1962. *Robber Barons: The Great American Capitalists, 1861–1901*. New York: Harcourt Press.

Kargbo, Thomas. 1987. "Traditional Midwifery in Sierra Leone." In *African Medicine in the Modern World* (Seminar Proceedings No. 27), 87–114. Edinburgh: University of Edinburgh, Centre of African Studies.

Katz, Richard. 1982. *Boiling Energy: Community Healing Among the Kalahari Kung*. Cambridge, MA: Harvard University Press.

Katz, Sydney and Selig Katz. 1981. "The Evolving Role of Traditional Medicine in Kenya." *African Urban Studies*, 9:1–12.

Keharo, J. 1972. "La pharmacopée africaine traditionelle et récherche scientifique." *Présence Africaine*, 475–499.

Kikhela, Nguete, Gilles Bibeau, and Ellen Corin. 1981. "Africa's Two Medical Systems: Options for Planners." *World Health Forum*, 2(1):96–99.

King, Lester. 1954. "What Is Disease?" *Philosophy of Science*, 21:193–203.

Kirmayer, Laurence. 1988. "Mind and Body as Metaphors: Hidden Values in Biomedicine." In *Biomedicine Examined*, 57–94, edited by Margaret Lock and Deborah Gordon. Dordrecht: Kluwer Academic Publishers.

Kleinman, Arthur. 1995. "What is Specific to Biomedicine?" In *Writing at the Margin: Discourse Between Anthropology and Medicine*, 21–40, Berkeley: University of California Press. NOTE: Kleinman (1995) is a significantly revised and expanded version of Kleinman (1993).

———. 1993. "What is Specific to Western Medicine?" In *Companion Encyclopedia for the History of Medicine, Vol. I*, 15–23, edited by W. F. Bynum and Roy Porter. New York: Routledge.

———. 1986. "Concepts and Model for the Comparison of Medical Systems as Cultural Systems." In *Concepts of Health, Illness and Disease: A Comparative Perspective*, 29–47, edited by Caroline Currer and Margaret Stacey. Oxford: Berg Publishers.

———. 1981. "On Illness Meanings and Clinical Interpretation: Not 'Rational Man,' but a Rational Approach to Man the Sufferer/Man the Healer." *Culture, Medicine and Psychiatry*, 5–4:373–377.

———. 1980. *Patients and Healers in the Context of Culture: An Exploration of the Borderland Between Anthropology, Medicine and Psychiatry*. Berkeley: University of California Press.

Kosik, Karel. 1976. *Dialectics of the Concrete: A Study of Problems of Man and World*. Dordrecht: D. Reidel Publishing Company.

Kramer, Joyce and Anthony Thomas. 1982. "The Modes of Maintaining Health in Ukambani, Kenya." In *African Health and Healing Systems: Proceedings of a Symposium*, 159–198, edited by P. Stanley Yoder. Los Angeles: Crossroads Press.

Kunitz, Stephan. 1994. *Disease and Social Diversity: The European Impact on the Health of Non-Europeans*. New York Oxford University Press.

Lasker, Judith. 1977. "The Role of Health Service in Colonial Rule: The Case of the Ivory Coast." *Culture, Medicine and Psychiatry*, 1:277–297.

Last, Murray. 1996. "The Professionalization of Indigenous Healers." In *Medical Anthropology: Contemporary Theory and Method*, 2nd Ed., 374–395, edited by Carolyn Sargent and Thomas Johnson. Westport, CT: Praeger.

———. 1993. "Non-Western Concepts of Disease." In *Companion Encyclopedia for the History of Medicine, Vol. I*, 634–660, edited by W. F. Bynum and Roy Porter. New York: Routledge.

———. 1986. "The Professionalization of African Medicine: Ambiguities and Definitions." In *The Professionalization of African Medicine*, 1–28, edited by Murray Last and G. L. Chavunduka. Manchester, UK: Manchester University Press.

———. 1981. "The Importance of Knowing about Not-Knowing." *Social Science and Medicine*, 15B:387–392.

Laurell, Asa Cristina and Oliva López Arellano. 2002. "Market Commodities and Poor Relief: The World Bank Proposal for Health." In *The Political Economy of Social Inequalities: Consequences for Health and Quality of Life*, 191–208, edited by Vicente Navarro. Amityville, NY: Baywood Publishing Company, Inc.

Lefebvre, Henri. 1968 [1940]. *Dialectical Materialism*. Translated by John Sturrock. London: Jonathon Cape Ltd.

Lerner, Daniel. 1958. *The Passing of Traditional Society*. Glencoe, IL: Free Press.

Leslie, Charles. 1978. "Foreword." In *The Quest for Therapy in Lower Zaire*, vi–xvi, by John Janzen. Berkeley: University of California Press.

———. 1974. "The Modernization of Asian Medical Systems." In *Rethinking Modernization*, 69–107, edited by John Poggie, Jr. and Robert Lynch. Westport, CT: Greenwood Press.

Levy, Howard. 1978. "The Military Medicinemen." In *The Cultural Crisis of Modern Medicine*, 287–300, edited by John Ehrenreich. New York: Monthly Review Press.

Leys, Colin. 1975. *Underdevelopment in Kenya: The Political Economy of Neo-Colonialism*. London: Heinemann.

Lock, Margaret. "Introduction." 1988. In *Biomedicine Reconsidered*, 3–10, edited by Margaret Lock and Deborah Gordon. Dordrecht: Kluwer Academic Publishers.

Lock, Margaret and Deborah Gordon. 1988. "Relationships Between Society, Culture and Biomedicine." In *Biomedicine Reconsidered*, 11–18, edited by Margaret Lock and Deborah Gordon. Dordrecht: Kluwer Academic Publishers.

Lonsdale, John and Bruce Berman. 1979. "Coping with the Contradictions: The Development of the Colonial State in Kenya." *Journal of African History*, 20:487–506.

Loustaunau, Martha and Elisa Sobo. 1997. *The Cultural Context of Health, Illness and Medicine*. Westport, CT: Bergin & Garvey.

Lukacs, Georg. 1971 [1923]. *History and Class Consciousness*. Cambridge, MA: MIT Press.

Lyons, Maryinez. 1994. "The Power to Heal: African Auxiliaries in Colonial Belgian Congo and Uganda." In *Contesting Colonial Hegemony: State and Society in Africa and India*, 202–226, edited by Dagmar Engels and Shula Marks. London: British Academic Press.

———. 1988a. "Sleeping Sickness, Colonial Medicine and Imperialism: Some Connections in the Belgian Congo." In *Disease, Medicine and Empire: Perspectives on Western Medicine and the Experience of European Expansion*, 242–256, edited by Roy MacLeod and Milton Lewis. New York: Routledge.

———. 1988b. "Sleeping Sickness Epidemics and Public Health in the BelgianCongo." In *Imperial Medicine and Indigenous Societies*, 105–124, edited by David Arnold. Manchester, UK: Manchester University Press.

MacCormack, Carol. 1986. "The Articulation of Western and Traditional Systems of Health Care." In *The Professionalization of African Medicine*, 151–164, edited by Murray Last and G. L. Chavunduka. Manchester, UK: Manchester University Press.

MacGaffey, Wyatt. 1983. *Modern Kongo Prophets: Religion in a Plural Society*. Bloomington: Indiana University Press.

MacLean, Una. 1987. "The WHO Programme for the Integration of Traditional Medicine." In *African Medicine in the Modern World* (Seminar Proceedings No. 27), 5–40. Edinburgh: University of Edinburgh, Centre of African Studies.

———. 1979a. "Choices of Treatment Among the Yoruba." In *Culture and Caring: Anthropological Perspectives on Traditional Medical Beliefs and Practices*, 152–167, edited by Peter Morley and Roy Wallis. Pittsburgh: University of Pittsburgh.

———. 1979b. "Traditional Healers and their Female Clients: An Aspect of Nigerian Sickness Behavior." In *African Therapeutic Systems*, 225–234, edited by Zacchaeus Ademuwagun, John Ayoade, Ira Harrison, and Dennis Warren. Waltham, MA: Crossroads Press.

———. 1976. "Some Aspects of Sickness Behavior Among the Yoruba." In *Social Anthropology and Medicine*, 285–317, edited by Joseph Loudon. New York: Academic Press.

———. 1971. *Magical Medicine, A Nigerian Case Study*. London: Allen Lane, The Penguin Press, Harmondsworth.

MacLeod, Roy. 1988. "Introduction." In *Disease, Medicine and Empire: Perspectives on Western Medicine and the Experience of European Expansion*, 1–18, edited by Roy MacLeod and Milton Lewis. New York: Routledge.

Magdoff, Harry. 1978. *Imperialism: From the Colonial Age to the Present*. New York: Monthly Review Press.

Magner, Lois. 1992. *A History of Medicine*. New York: Marcel Dekker.

Maier, Donna. 1979. "Nineteenth-Century Asante Medical Practices." *Comparative Studies in Society and History*, 21:63–81.

Maina-Ahlberg, Beth. 1979. "Beliefs and Practices Concerning Treatment of Measles and Acute Diarrhea Among the Akamba." *Tropical and Geographical Medicine*, 31:139–48.

Mamdani, Mahmood. 1996. *Citizen and Subject: Contemporary Africa and the Legacy of Late Colonialism*. Princeton, NJ: Princeton University Press.

Mann, Jonathan and Kathleen Kay. 1991. "Confronting the Pandemic: The WHO's Global Programme on AIDS, 1986–1989." *AIDS*, 5:s221–s229.

Manning, Peter and Horacio Fábrega. 1973. "The Experience of Self and Body: Health and Illness in the Chiapas Highlands." In *Phenomenological Sociology*, 251–304, edited by George Psathas. New York: John Wiley.

Maretzki, T. and E. Seidler. 1985. "Biomedicine and Naturopathic Healing in West Germany. A Historical and Ethnomedical View of a Stormy Relationship." *Culture, Medicine and Psychiatry*, 9(4):383–421.

Marks, Shula. 1996. "What is Colonial about Colonial Medicine?" *Social History of Medicine*, 10(2):205–219.

Marks, Shula and Neil Andersson. 1988. "Typhus and Social Control: South Africa, 1917–1950." In *Disease, Medicine and Empire: Perspectives on Western Medicine and the Experience of European Expansion*, 257–283, edited by Roy MacLeod and Milton Lewis. New York: Routledge.

Marshall, Lorna. 1969. "The Medicine Dance of the !Kung Bushmen." *Africa: Journal of the International African Institute*, 39(4):347–381.

Marwick, Max. 1967. "The Sociology of Sorcery in a Central African Tribe." In *Magic, Witchcraft and Curing*, 101–126, edited by John Middleton. Garden City, NY: The Natural History Press.

Matthe, David. 1989. "Ethnomedical Science and African Medical Practice." *Medicine and Law*, 7:517–521.

Maulitz, Russell. 1979. "'Physician Versus Bacteriologist': The Ideology of Science in Clinical Medicine." In *The Therapeutic Revolution: Essays in the Social History of American Medicine*, 91–108, edited by Morris Vogel and Charles Rosenberg. Philadelphia: University of Pennsylvania Press.

Mbiti, John. 1970. *African Religions and Philosophy*. New York: Doubleday, Anchor Books.

Mburu, F. 1977. "The Duality of Traditional and Western Medicine in Africa: Mystics, Myths and Reality." In *Traditional Healing: New Science or New Colonialism? (Essays in Critique of Medical Anthropology)*, 158–185, edited by Philip Singer. New York: Conch Magazine Limited.

McGuire, Meredith. 1988. *Ritual Healing in Suburban America*. New Brunswick, NJ: Rutgers University Press.

McMichael, Philip. 1990. "Incorporating Comparison Within a World-Historical Perspective: An Alternative Comparative Method." *American Sociological Review*, 55(3):385–397.

McNeill, William. 1976. *Plagues and Peoples*. New York: Anchor Books.

Memmi, Albert. 1965. *The Colonizer and the Colonized*. Boston: Beacon Press.

Merton, Robert, George Reader, and Patricia Kendall. 1957. *Introductory Studies in the Sociology of Medical Education*. Cambridge, MA: Harvard University Press.

Messing, Simon. 1977. "Traditional Healing and the New Health Center in Ethiopia." In *Traditional Healing: New Science or New Colonialism? (Essays in Critique of Medical Anthropology)*, 52–64, edited by Philip Singer. New York: Conch Magazine Limited.

Middleton, John and E. H. Winter. 1963. "Introduction." In *Magic, Witchcraft and Curing*, 1–27, edited by John Middleton. Garden City, NY: The Natural History Press.

Miller, Genevieve. 1957. *The Adoption of Inoculation for Smallpox in England and France*. Philadelphia: University of Pennsylvania Press.

Mishler, Elliot. 1981. "Viewpoint: Critical Perspectives on the Biomedical Model." In *Social Contexts of Health, Illness and Patient Care*, 1–23, edited by Elliot Mishler. Cambridge, MA: Cambridge University Press.

Molassiotis, A., P. Fernandez-Ortega, D. Pud, et al. 2005. "Use of Complementary and Alternative Medicine in Cancer Patients: A European Survey." *Annals of Oncology*, 16(4):655–663.

Morely, Peter. 1979. "Culture and the Cognitive World of Traditional Medical Beliefs: Some Preliminary Considerations." In *Culture and Caring: Anthropological Perspectives on Traditional Medical Beliefs and Practices*, 1–18, edited by Peter Morely and Roy Wallis. Pittsburgh: University of Pittsburgh Press.

Mume, J. O. 1977. "How I Acquired the Knowledge of Traditional Medicine." In *Traditional Healing: New Science or New Colonialism? (Essays in Critique of Medical Anthropology)*, 136–157, edited by Philip Singer. New York: Conch Magazine Limited.

Murdock, George. 1980. *Theories of Illness*. Pittsburgh: University of Pittsburgh Press.

Nadel, S. F. 1952. "Witchcraft in Four African Societies: An Essay in Comparison." *American Anthropologist*, 54:18–29.

Nalugwa, Sara. 2003. *Indigenous Approaches to the HIV/AIDS Scourge in Uganda*. Social Science Research Report Series, No. 30. Addis Ababa, Ethiopia: Organization for Social Science Research in Eastern and Southern Africa.

Navarro, Vicente. 1976. *Medicine Under Capitalism*. New York: Prodist.

Nchinda, T. C. 1976. "Traditional and Western Medicine in Africa: Collaboration or Confrontation?" *Tropical Doctor*, (July):133–35.

Ndamba, J., N. Nyazema, N. Makaza, C. Anderson and K. Kaondera. 1994. "Traditional Herbal Remedies Used for the Treatment Urinary Schistosomiasis in Zimbabwe." *Ethnopharmacology*, 42(2):125–32.

Ngubane, Harriet. 1977. *Body and Mind in Zulu Medicine: An Ethnography of Health and Disease in Nyuswa-Zulu Thought and Practice*. London: Academic Press.

———. 1976. "Some Aspects of Treatment Among the Zulu." In *Social Anthropology and Medicine*, 318–357, edited by Joseph Loudon. New York: Academic Press.

Nutton, Vivian. 1983. "The Seeds of Disease: An Explanation of Contagion and Infection from the Greeks to the Renaissance." *Medicine in History*, 27:1–34.

Odebiyi, A. I. and Togonu-Bickersteth Funmi. 1987. "Concepts and Management of Deafness in the Yoruba Medical System: A Case Study of Traditional Healers in Ife-Ife, Nigeria." *Social Science and Medicine*, 24(8):645–649.

Oguah, Benjamin Eruku. 1984. "African and Western Philosophy: A Comparative Study." In *African Philosophy: An Introduction*, 3rd Ed., 213–226, edited by Richard Wright. Lanham, MD: University Press of America.

Ohnuki-Tierney, Emiko. 1994. "Brain Death and Organ Transplantation: Cultural Bases for Medical Technology." *Current Anthropology*, 35(3):233–242.

Olsson, Tord. 1989. "Philosophy of Medicine Among the Massai." In *Culture, Experience and Pluralism: Essays on African Ideas of Illness and Healing*, 235–246, edited by Anita Jacobson-Widding and David Westerlund. Uppsala: Almqvist & Wiksell International.

Olumwullah, Osaak. 2002. *Dis-Ease in the Colonial State*. Westport, CT: Greenwood Press.

O'Manique, Colleen. 2004. *Neoliberalism and AIDS Crisis in Sub-Saharan Africa: Globalization's Pandemic*. New York: Palgrave Macmillan.

Onoge, Omafume. 1975. "Capitalism and Public Health: A Neglected Theme in the Medical Anthropology of Africa." In *Topias and Utopias in Health: Policy Studies*,

219–232, edited by Stanley Ingman and Anthony Thomas. The Hague: Mouton Publishers.

Onyioha, Chief K.O.K. 1977. "The Metaphysical Background to Traditional Healing in Nigeria." In *Traditional Healing: New Science or New Colonialism? (Essays in Critique of Medical Anthropology)*, 203–230, edited by Philip Singer. New York: Conch Magazine Limited.

Orley, John. 1980. "Indigenous Concepts of Disease and Their Interaction with Scientific Medicine." In *Health in Tropical Africa During the Colonial Period*, 127–134, edited by E. E. Sabben-Clare, David Bradley, and Kenneth Kirkwood. Oxford: Clarendon Press.

Osborne, Oliver. 1972. "Social Structure and Health Care Systems: A Yoruba Example." *Rural Africana*, 17:80–86.

Osherson, Samuel and Lorna Amarasingham. 1981. "The Machine Metaphor in Medicine." In *Social Contexts of Health, Illness and Patient Care*, 218–249, edited by Elliot Mishler. Cambridge, MA: Cambridge University Press.

Oyebola, D.D.O. 1986. "National Medical Politics in Nigeria." In *The Professionalization of African Medicine*, 221–236, edited by Murray Last and G. L. Chavunduka. Manchester, UK: Manchester University Press.

———. 1981. "Professional Associations, Ethics and Discipline Among Yoruba Traditional Healers in Nigeria." *Social Science and Medicine*, 15B:87–92.

Oyeneye, O. Y. 1985. "Mobilizing Indigenous Resources for Primary Health Care in Nigeria: A Note on the Place of Traditional Medicine." *Social Science and Medicine*, 20:67–69.

Paarup-Laursen, Bjarke. 1989. "The Meaning of Illness Among the Koma of Northern Nigeria." In *Culture, Experience and Pluralism: Essays on African Ideas of Illness and Healing*, 59–74, edited by Anita Jacobson-Widding and David Westerlund. Uppsala: Almqvist & Wiksell International.

Palmer, Robert. 1963. *A History of the Modern World*, 2nd Ed. New York: Alfred A. Knopf.

Park, George. 1967. "Divination and Its Social Contexts." In *Magic, Witchcraft and Curing*, 233–254, edited by John Middleton. Garden City, NY: The Natural History Press.

Patterson, David. 1981. *Health in Colonial Ghana: Disease, Medicine and Socio-Economic Change, 1900–1955*. Waltham, MA: Crossroads Press.

Paul, James. 1978. "Medicine and Imperialism." In *The Cultural Crisis of Modern Medicine*, 271–286, edited by John Ehrenreich. New York: Monthly Review Press.

Payer, Lynn. 1988. *Medicine and Culture: Varieties of Treatment in the United States, England, West Germany and France*. New York: Henry Holt & Co.

Pearce, Tola. 1986. "Professional Interests and the Creation of Medical Knowledge in Nigeria." In *The Professionalization of African Medicine*, 237–258, edited by Murray Last and G. L. Chavunduka. Manchester, UK: Manchester University Press.

———. 1980. "Political and Economic Changes in Nigeria and the Organization of Medical Care." *Social Science and Medicine*, 14B:91–98.

Perkins, John. 2006. *Confessions of an Economic Hit Man*. New York: Plume Books.

Pool, Robert. 1994. "On the Creation of Dissolution of Ethnomedical Systems in the Medical Ethnography of Africa." *Africa: Journal of the International African Institute*, 64(1):1–20.

Porter, Roy. 1997. *The Greatest Benefit to Mankind: A Medical History of Mankind*. New York: W. W. Norton.

Powles, John. 1973. "On the Limitations of Modern Medicine." *Science, Medicine and Man*, 1:1–30.

Price-Williams, D. 1979. "A Case Study of Ideas Concerning Disease among the Tiv." In *African Therapeutic Systems*, 26–30, edited by Zacchaeus Ademuwagun, John Ayoade, Ira Harrison, and Dennis Warren. Waltham, MA: Crossroads Press.

Prince, Raymond and François Tcheng-Laroche. 1987. "Culture-Bound Syndromes and International Disease Classification." *Culture, Medicine and Psychiatry*, 11:3–19.

Prins, Gwyn. 1992. "A Modern History of Lozi Therapeutics." In *The Social Basis of Health and Healing in Africa*, 339–365, edited by Steven Feierman and John Janzen. Berkeley: University of California Press.

———. 1989. "But What was the Disease? The Present State of Health and Healing in African Studies." *Past and Present*, 124:159–70.

Quah, Stella. 2003. "Traditional Healing Systems and the Ethos of Science." *Social Science and Medicine*, 57(10):1997–2012.

Ranger, Terence. 1988. "The Influenza Pandemic in Southern Rhodesia: A Crisis of Comprehension." In *Imperial Medicine and Indigenous Societies*, 172–188, edited by David Arnold. Manchester, UK: Manchester University Press.

———. 1983. "The Invention of Tradition in Colonial Africa." In *The Invention of Tradition*, 211–262, edited by Eric Hobsbawm and Terence Ranger. Cambridge, UK: Cambridge University Press.

———. 1981. "Godly Medicine: The Ambiguities of Medical Mission in Southeast Tanzania." *Social Science and Medicine*, 15B:261–77.

Reid, Marlene. 1982. "Patient/Healer Interactions in Sukama Medicine." In *African Health and Healing Systems: Proceedings of a Symposium*, 121–158, edited by P. Stanley Yoder. Los Angeles: Crossroads Press.

Reiser, Stanley. 1978. *Medicine and the Reign of Technology*. Cambridge, MA: Cambridge University Press.

Rhodes, Lorna Amarasingham. 1996. "Studying Biomedicine as a Cultural System." In *Medical Anthropology: Contemporary Theory and Method* (2nd Ed.), 165–180, edited by Carolyn Sargent and Thomas Johnson. Westport, CT: Praeger.

Richards, Lynn. 1977. "The Context of Foreign Aid: Modern Imperialism." *Review of Radical Political Economics*, 9(4):43–77.

Rodney, Walter. 1981. *How Europe Underdeveloped Africa*. Washington DC: Howard University Press.

———. 1979. "The Political Economy of Colonial Tanganyika, 1890–1930." In *Tanzania Under Colonial Rule*, 128–163, edited by M.H.Y. Kaniki. London: Longman Group Limited.

Rosen, George. 1974a. "The Fate of the Concept of Medical Police." In *From Medical Police to Social Medicine: Essays on the History of Health Care*, 142–158, New York: Science History Publications.

———. 1974b. "Hospitals, Medical Care and Social Policy in the French Revolution." In *From Medical Police to Social Medicine: Essays on the History of Health Care*, 220–245. New York: Science History Publications.

Rosenberg, Charles. 1979. "The Therapeutic Revolution: Medicine, Meaning and Social Change in Nineteenth-Century America." In *The Therapeutic Revolution: Essays in the Social History of American Medicine*, 3–26, edited by Morris Vogel and Charles Rosenberg. Philadelphia: University of Pennsylvania Press.

Rostow, W.W. 1971. *The Stages of Economic Growth: A Non-Communist Manifesto,* 2nd Ed. New York: Cambridge University Press.

Rotberg, Robert. 1966. "The Rise of African Nationalism: The Case of East and Central Africa." In *Social Change: The Colonial Situation*, 505–519, edited by Immanuel Wallerstein. New York: John Wiley & Sons.

Rowson, J. 1965. "Recherches sur quelques plantes medicinals du Nigeria." *Annales pharmaceutiques francaises*, 23:125–135.

Saul, John and Colin Leys. 1999. "Sub-Saharan Africa in Global Capitalism." *Monthly Review,* 51(3):13–30.

Schepers, Rita and Hubert Hermans. 1999. "The Medical Profession and Alternative Medicine in the Netherlands: Its History and Recent Developments." *Social Science and Medicine*, 48(3):343–351.

Schmoll, Pamela. 1993. "Black Stomachs, Beautiful Stones: Soul-Eating Among Hausa in Niger." In *Modernity and Its Malcontents*, 193–220, edited by Jean Comaroff and John Comaroff. Chicago: University of Chicago Press.

Schoepf, Brooke. 1992. "AIDS, Sex and Condoms: African Healers and the Reinvention of Tradition in Zaire." *Medical Anthropology*, 14:225–242.

Scott, James. 1985. *Weapons of the Weak: Everyday Forms of Peasant Resistance*. New Haven, CT: Yale University Press.

Semali, I. 1986. "Associations and Healers: Attitudes Towards Collaboration in Tanzania." In *The Professionalization of African Medicine*, 87–98, edited by Murray Last and G. L. Chavunduka. Manchester, UK: Manchester University Press.

Shryock, Richard. 1969. *The Development of Modern Medicine: An Interpretation of the Social and Scientific Factors Involved*. New York: Hafner Publishing Company.

———. 1953. "The Interplay of Social and Internal Factors in the History of Modern Medicine." *Scientific Monthly*, 76: 221–230.

Simpson, George. 1980. *Yoruba Religion and Medicine in Ibadan*. Ibadan: Ibadan University Press.

Sindzingre, Nicole. 1985. "Healing is as Healing Does: Pragmatic Resolution of Misfortune Among the Senufo (Ivory Coast)." *History and Anthropology*, 2:33–57.

Sindzingre, Nicole and Andreas Zempléni. 1992. "Causality of Disease Among the Senufo." In *The Social Basis of Health and Healing in Africa*, 315–338, edited by Steven Feierman and John Janzen. Berkeley: University of California Press.

Singer, Merrill. 1992. "Biomedicine and the Political Economy of Science." *Medical Anthropology Quarterly*, 6(4):400–403.

Singer, Philip. 1977. "Introduction." In *Traditional Healing: New Science or New Colonialism? (Essays in Critique of Medical Anthropology)*, 1–25, edited by Philip Singer. New York: Conch Magazine Limited.

Sklar, Martin. 1988. *The Corporate Reconstruction of American Capitalism, 1890–1916: The Market, the Law and Politics*. Cambridge, MA: Cambridge University Press.

Sofowora, Abayomi. 1982. *Medicinal Plants and Traditional Medicine in Africa*. New York: John Wiley & Sons Limited.

Spring, Anita. 1985. "Health Care Systems in Northwest Zambia." In *African Healing Strategies*, 135–150, edited by Brian M. du Toit and Ismail Abdalla. New York: Trado-Medic Books.

———. 1980a. "Traditional and Biomedical Health Care Systems in Northwest Zambia: A Case Study of the Luvale." In *Traditional Health Care Delivery in Contemporary Africa*, 57–79, edited by Priscilla Ulin and Marshall Segall. Foreign and Comparative Studies/African Series XXXV. Syracuse: Maxwell School.

———. 1980b. "Faith and Participation in Traditional Versus Cosmopolitan Medical Systems in Northwestern Zambia." *Anthropological Quarterly*, 53(2):130–41.

Starr, Paul. 1982. *The Social Transformation of American Medicine*. New York: Basic Books.

Staugård, Frants. 1991. "Role of Traditional Health Workers in Prevention and Control of AIDS in Africa." *Tropical Doctor*, 21:22–24.

———. 1986. "Traditional Health Care in Botswana." In *The Professionalization of African Medicine*, 51–86, edited by Murray Last and G. L. Chavunduka. Manchester, UK: Manchester University Press.

Stein, Howard. 1990. *American Medicine as a Culture*. Boulder, CO: Westview Press.

Stiglitz, Joseph. 2003. *Globalization and Its Discontents*. New York: W. W. Norton & Company.

Sugiyama, Shinya. 1988. *Japan's Industrialization in the World Economy, 1859–1899: Export Trade and Overseas Competition*. Atlantic Highlands, NJ: Athlone Press.

Swanson, Maynard. 1979. "The Sanitation Syndrome: Bubonic Plague and Urban Native Policy in Cape Colony, 1900–1909." *Journal of African History*, 18(3):387–410.

Swantz, Lloyd. 1990. *The Medicine Man Among the Zaramo of Dar es Salaam*. Uddevalla, Sweden: Scandinavian Institute of African Studies.

Swantz, Marja-Liisa. 1989. "Manipulation of Multiple Health Systems in the Coastal Regions of Tanzania." In *Culture, Experience and Pluralism: Essays on African Ideas of Illness and Healing*, 277–288, edited by Anita Jacobson-Widding and David Westerlund. Uppsala: Almqvist & Wiksell International.

Tanner, R.E.S. 1956. "The Sorcerer in Northern Sukumaland, Tanganyika." *Southwestern Journal of Anthropology*, 12:437–434.

Temkin, Owsei. 1977a. "Comparative Study in the History of Medicine." In *The Double Face of Janus and Other Essays in the History of Medicine*, 126–136, by Owsei Temkin. Baltimore: Johns Hopkins University Press.

———. "Health and Disease." 1977b. In *The Double Face of Janus and Other Essays in the History of Medicine*, 419–440, by Owsei Temkin. Baltimore, MD: Johns Hopkins University Press.

———. 1977c. "An Historical Analysis the Concept of Infection." In *The Double Face of Janus and Other Essays in the History of Medicine*, 456–471, by Owsei Temkin. Baltimore: Johns Hopkins University Press.

———. 1977d. "The Scientific Approach to Disease: Specific Entity and Individual Infection." In *The Double Face of Janus and Other Essays in the History of Medicine*, 441–455, by Owsei Temkin. Baltimore, MD: Johns Hopkins University Press.

Thomas, Anthony. 1975. "Healthcare in Ukambani Kenya: A Socialist Critique." In *Topias and Utopias in Health: Policy Studies*, 267–282, edited by Stanley Ingman and Anthony Thomas. The Hague: Mouton Publishers.

Tomich, Dale. 1997. "Spaces of Slavery, Times of Freedom: Rethinking Caribbean History in World Perspective." *Comparative Studies of South Asia, Africa and the Middle East*, 27(1):67–80.

———. 1994. "Small Islands and Huge Comparisons: Caribbean Plantations, Historical Unevenness and Capitalist Modernity." *Social Science History*, 18(3):339–358.

———. 1990. *Slavery in the Circuit of Sugar: Martinique in the World Economy, 1830–1848*. Baltimore: Johns Hopkins University Press.

Turner, Victor, 1967. *The Forest of Symbols*. Ithaca, NY: Cornell University Press.

———. 1964a. "An Ndemba Doctor in Practice." In *Magic, Faith and Healing: Studies in Primitive Psychiatry Today*, 230–263, edited by Ari Kiev. New York: Free Press.

———. 1964b. "Witchcraft and Sorcery: Taxonomy Versus Dynamics." *Africa: Journal of the International African Institute*, 34(4):314–25.

Turshen, Meredeth. 2001. "Reprivatizing Pharmaceutical Supplies in Africa." *Journal of Public Health Policy* 22(2):198–225.

———. 1984. *The Political Ecology of Disease in Tanzania*. New Brunswick, NJ: Rutgers University Press.

———. 1977a. "The Political Ecology of Disease." *Review of Radical Political Economy*, 9(1):45–60.

———. 1977b. "The Impact of Colonialism on Health and Health Services in Tanzania." *International Journal of Health Services*, 7(1):7–35.

Twumasi, Patrick. 1985. *The Professionalization of Traditional Medicine in Zambia*. Urbana, IL: University of Illinois Press.

Twumasi, Patrick and Dennis Warren. 1986. "The Professionalization of Indigenous Medicine: A Comparative Study of Ghana and Zambia." In *The Professionalization of African Medicine*, 117–136, edited by Murray Last and G. L. Chavunduka. Manchester, UK: Manchester University Press.

Ulin, Priscilla. 1979. "The Traditional Healer of Botswana in a Changing Society." In *African Therapeutic Systems*, 243–246, edited by Zacchaeus Ademuwagun, John Ayoade, Ira Harrison, and Dennis Warren. Waltham, MA: Crossroads Press.

UNAIDS. 2002. *Ancient Remedies, New Disease: Involving Traditional Healers in Increasing Access to AIDS Care and Prevention in East Africa*. Geneva, Switzerland: Joint United Nations Program on HIV/AIDS.

U.N. Population Fund. 2006. *State of World Population, 2006*. New York: United Nations Publications.

van der Geest, Sjaak. 1988. "The Articulation of Formal and Informal Medicine Distribution in South Cameroon." In *The Context of Medicines in Developing Countries: Studies in Pharmaceutical Anthropology*, 131–148, edited by Sjaak van der Geest and Susan Whyte. Dordrecht: Kluwer Academic Publishers.

Vaughan, Megan. 1994. "Health and Hegemony: Representation of Disease and the Creation of the Colonial Subject in Nyasaland." In *Contesting Colonial Hegemony: State and Society in Africa and India*, 173–201, edited by Dagmar Engels and Shula Marks. London: British Academic Press.

———. 1991. *Curing Their Ills: Colonial Power and African Illness*. Stanford, CA: Stanford University Press.

Vecchiato, Norbert. 1998. "Digestive Worms: Ethnomedical Approaches to Intestinal Parasitism in Southern Ethiopia." In *The Anthropology of Infectious Disease: International Health Perspectives*, 241–266, edited by Marcia Inhorn and Peter Brown. Amsterdam: Gordon and Breach.

Waitzkin, Howard. 1978. "A Marxist View of Medical Care." *Annals of Internal Medicine*, 89:264–66.

Wall, L. Lewis. 1988. *Hausa Medicine: Illness and Well-Being in a West African Culture.* Durham, NC: Duke University Press.

Wallerstein, Immanuel. 2006. *World-Systems Analysis: An Introduction.* Durham, NC: Duke University Press.

———. 2001. *Unthinking Social Science: The Limits of 19th-Century Paradigms.* Philadelphia: Temple University Press.

———. 1999. *The End of the World as We Know It: Social Science for the 21st Century.* Minneapolis: University of Minnesota Press.

———. 1993. "The TimeSpace of World-Systems Analysis: A Philosophical Essay." *Historical Geography,* 23(1–2):5–22.

———. 1989. *The Modern World System III: The Second Era of Great Expansion of the Capitalist World-Economy, 1730–1840s.* New York: Academic Press.

———. 1982. "World-Systems Analysis: Theoretical and Interpretive Issues." In *World-Systems Analysis: Theory and Methodology,* 91–103, edited by Terence Hopkins and Immanuel Wallerstein. Beverly Hills, CA: Sage.

———. 1980. *The Modern World-System II: Mercantilism and the Consolidation of the European World-Economy, 1600–1750.* New York: Academic Press.

———. 1976. "The Three Stages of African Involvement in the World-Economy." In *The Political Economy of Contemporary Africa,* 30–57, edited by Peter Gutkind and Immanuel Wallerstein. Beverly Hills, CA: Sage Publications.

———. 1974. *The Modern World-System: Capitalist Agriculture and the Origins of the European World-Economy in the Sixteenth Century.* New York: Academic Press.

———. 1970. "The Colonial Era in Africa: Changes in the Social Structure." In *Colonialism in Africa, 1870–1960:* Vol. 2, *The History and Politics of Colonialism, 1914–1960,* 399–421, edited by L. H. Gann and Peter Duignan. Cambridge, UK: Cambridge University Press.

———. 1961. *Africa and the Politics of Independence.* NY: Vintage Books.

Wallerstein, Immanuel et al. 1996. *Open the Social Sciences: Report of the Gulbenkian Commission on the Reconstruction of the Social Sciences.* Stanford: Stanford University Press.

Warren, Dennis. 1982. "The Techiman-Bono Ethnomedical System." In *African Health and Healing Systems: Proceedings of a Symposium,* 85–106, edited by P. Stanley Yoder. Los Angeles: Crossroads Press.

———. 1979a. "The Role of Emic Analyses in Medical Anthropology: The Case of the Bono of Ghana." In *African Therapeutic Systems,* 36–42, edited by Zacchaeus Ademuwagun, John Ayoade, Ira Harrison, and Dennis Warren. Waltham, MA: Crossroads Press.

———. 1979b. "Bono Traditional Healers." In *African Therapeutic Systems,* 120–124, edited by Zacchaeus Ademuwagun, John Ayoade, Ira Harrison, and Dennis Warren. Waltham, MA: Crossroads Press.

———. 1979c. The Interpretation of Change in a Ghanaian Ethnomedical Study." In *African Therapeutic Systems,* 247–250, edited by Zacchaeus Ademuwagun, John Ayoade, Ira Harrison, and Dennis Warren. Waltham, MA: Crossroads Press.

Westerlund, David. 1989a. "Introduction: Indigenous Pluralism and Multiple Medical Systems." In *Culture, Experience and Pluralism: Essays on African Ideas of Illness and Healing,* 169–176, edited by Anita Jacobson-Widding and David Westerlund. Uppsala: Almqvist & Wiksell International.

———. 1989b. "Pluralism and Change: A Comparative and Historical Approach to African Disease Etiologies." In *Culture, Experience and Pluralism: Essays on African Ideas of Illness and Healing*, 177–219, edited by Anita Jacobson-Widding and David Westerlund. Uppsala: Almqvist & Wiksell International.

Whisson, Michael. 1964. "Some Aspects of Functional Disorders Among the Kenya Luo." In *Magic, Faith and Healing: Studies in Primitive Psychiatry Today*, 283–304, edited by Ari Kiev. New York: Free Press.

Whyte, Susan. 1997. *Questioning Misfortune: The Pragmatics of Uncertainty in Eastern Uganda*. Cambridge, UK: Cambridge University Press.

———. 1989. "Anthropological Approaches to African Misfortune: From Religion to Medicine." In *Culture, Experience and Pluralism: Essays on African Ideas of Illness and Healing*, 289–302, edited by Anita Jacobson-Widding and David Westerlund. Uppsala: Almqvist & Wiksell International.

———. 1988. "The Power of Medicines in East Africa." In *The Context of Medicines in Developing Countries: Studies in Pharmaceutical Anthropology*, 217–234, edited by Sjaak van der Geest and Susan Whyte. Dordrecht: Kluwer Academic Publishers.

Wig, Narendra. 1983. "DSM-III: A Perspective from the Third World." In *International Perspectives on DSM-III*, 79–90, edited by Robert Spitzer, Janet Williams, and Andrew Skodol. Washington, DC: American Psychiatric Press.

Wightman, W. 1971. *The Emergence of Scientific Medicine*. Edinburgh: Oliver and Boyd.

Willis, Roy. 1999. *Some Spirits Heal, Others Only Dance: A Journey Into Human Selfhood in an African Village*. Oxford: Berg.

———. 1979. "Magic and 'Medicine' in Ufipa." In *Culture and Caring: Anthropological Perspectives on Traditional Medical Beliefs and Practices*, 139–151, edited by Peter Morley and Roy Wallis. Pittsburgh: University of Pittsburgh.

———. 1970. "Instant Millennium: The Sociology of African Witch-Cleansing Cults." In *Witchcraft Confessions and Accusations*, 129–140, edited by Mary Douglas. London: Tavistock Publications.

Willms, Dennis, Nancy Johnson, Alfred Chingono and Maureen Wellington. 2001. "AIDS Prevention in the *Matare* and the Community: A Training Strategy for Traditional Healers in Zimbabwe." In *Applying Health Social Science: Best Practice in the Developing World*, 163–182, edited by Nick Higginbotham, Roberto Briceño-León, and Nancy Johnson. London: Zed Books.

Winter, E. H. 1963. "The Enemy Within: Amba Witchcraft and Sociological Theory." In *Witchcraft and Sorcery in East Africa*, 277–299, edited by John Middleton and E. H. Winter. London: Routledge and Kegan Paul.

Wiredu, Kwasi. 1984. "How Not to Compare African Thought with Western Thought." In *African Philosophy: an Introduction*, 3rd Ed., 149–162, edited by Richard Wright. Lanham, MD: University Press of America.

Wolff, N. 1979. "Concepts of Causation and Treatment in the Yoruba Medical System: The Special Case of Barrenness." In *African Therapeutic Systems*, 125–131, edited by Zacchaeus Ademuwagun, John Ayoade, Ira Harrison, and Dennis Warren. Waltham, MA: Crossroads Press.

Worboys, Michael. 2000. "Colonial Medicine." In *Medicine in the Twentieth Century*, 67–80, edited by Roger Cooter and John Pickstone. Amsterdam: Harwood Academic Publishers.

———. 1996. "Germs, Malaria and the Invention of Mansonian Tropical Medicine: From 'Diseases in the Tropics' to 'Tropical Diseases.'" In *Warm Climates and Western Medicine: The Emergence of Tropical Medicine, 1500–1900*, 181–208, edited by David Arnold. Amsterdam: Editions Rodopi B. V.

———. 1976. "The Emergence of Tropical Medicine: A Study in the Establishment of a Scientific Specialty." In *Perspectives on the Emergence of Scientific Disciplines*, 75–98, edited by Gerard Lemaine, Roy MacLeod, Michael Mulkay, and Peter Weingart. Chicago: Aldine Publishers.

World Health Organization. 2007. *World Health Statistics 2007.* Geneva, Switzerland: WHO Press.

———. 1978. *The Promotion and Development of Traditional Medicine.* Technical Report Series, No. 622.

Worsley, Peter. 1982. "Non-Western Medical Systems." *Annual Review of Anthropology*, 11:315–348.

Wright, Peter and Andrew Treacher. 1982. "Introduction." In *The Problem of Medical Knowledge: Examining the Social Construction of Medicine*, 1–22, edited by Peter Wright and Andrew Treacher. Edinburgh: Edinburgh University Press.

Yoder, P. Stanley. 1982. "Issues in the Study of Ethnomedical Systems in Africa." In *African Health and Healing Systems: Proceedings of a Symposium*, 1–20, edited by P. Stanley Yoder. Los Angeles: Crossroads Press.

Young, Allan. 1979. "The Practical Logic of Amhara Traditional Medicine." In *African Therapeutic Systems*, 132–137, edited by Zacchaeus Ademuwagun, John Ayoade, Ira Harrison, and Dennis Warren. Waltham, MA: Crossroads Press.

Young, Crawford. 1994. *The African Colonial State in Comparative Perspective*. New Haven, CT: Yale University Press.

Yudkin, John. 1980. "The Economics of Pharmaceutical Supply in Tanzania." *International Journal of Health Services*, 10:455–477.

Zeller, Diane. 1979a. "Basawo Baganda: The Traditional Doctors of Buganda." In *African Therapeutic Systems*, 138–143, edited by Zacchaeus Ademuwagun, John Ayoade, Ira Harrison, and Dennis Warren. Waltham, MA: Crossroads Press.

———. 1979b. "Traditional and Western Medicine in Buganda: Co-existence and Complement." In *African Therapeutic Systems*, 251–256, edited by Zacchaeus Ademuwagun, John Ayoade, Ira Harrison, and Dennis Warren. Waltham, MA: Crossroads Press.

Zola, Irving Kenneth. 1972. "Medicine as an Institution of Social Control." *Sociological Review*, 20:487–504.

Index

David Baronov is an Associate Professor of Sociology at St. John Fisher College and is also the author of The Abolition of Slavery in Brazil: The "Liberation" of Africans Through the Emancipation of Capital and Conceptual Foundations of Social Research Methods.